Improving Patient Care

Improving Patient Care

The Implementation of Change in Health Care

Third Edition

Edited by

Michel Wensing
Faculty of Medicine, Health Services Research and Implementation Science
University of Heidelberg, Heidelberg, Germany;
Department of General Practice and Health Services Research
Heidelberg University Hospital, Heidelberg, Germany;
Department IQ healthcare, Radboud Institute for Health Sciences
Radboud University Medical Center, Nijmegen, The Netherlands

Richard Grol
Radboud University, Nijmegen, The Netherlands;
Maastricht University, Maastricht, The Netherlands

Jeremy Grimshaw
Clinical Epidemiology Program, Ottawa Hospital Research Institute
Ottawa, Ontario, Canada;
Department of Medicine, University of Ottawa, Ottawa, Ontario, Canada;
Health Knowledge Transfer and Uptake, Ottawa, Ontario, Canada

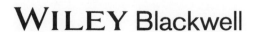

Library of Congress Cataloging-in-Publication Data

Names: Wensing, Michel, editor. | Grol, Richard, editor. | Grimshaw,
    Jeremy, editor.
Title: Improving patient care : the implementation of change in health care /
    edited by Michel Wensing, Richard Grol, Jeremy Grimshaw.
Description: Third edition. | Hoboken, NJ : Wiley-Blackwell 2020. |
    Includes bibliographical references and index.
Identifiers: LCCN 2019055404 (print) | LCCN 2019055405 (ebook) | ISBN 9781119488590 (cloth)
    | ISBN 9781119488613 (adobe pdf) | ISBN 9781119488606 (epub)
Subjects: MESH: Patient Care | Quality of Health Care | Health Care Reform |
    Organizational Innovation | Health Plan Implementation
Classification: LCC RA395.A3 (print) | LCC RA395.A3 (ebook) | NLM W 84.1 |
    DDC 362.1/0425–dc23
LC record available at https://lccn.loc.gov/2019055404
LC ebook record available at https://lccn.loc.gov/2019055405

Cover Design: Wiley
Cover Image: © mythja/Shutterstock

Set in 9.5/12.5pt STIXTwoText by SPi Global, Pondicherry, India

Contents

3   Effective Implementation of Change in Healthcare: A Systematic Approach   *45*
Richard Grol and Michel Wensing

4   Planning and Organizing the Change Process   *73*
Richard Grol and Michel Wensing

List of Contributors

Eddy Adang
Department for Health Evidence
Radboud Institute for Health Sciences
Radboud University Medical Center
Nijmegen, The Netherlands

Jozé Braspenning
Department IQ healthcare
Radboud Institute for Health Sciences
Radboud University Medical Center
Nijmegen, The Netherlands

Benjamin Brown
Centre for Primary Care and
Centre for Health Informatics
University of Manchester
Manchester
UK

Jako Burgers
Dutch College of General Practitioners (NHG)
Utrecht;
Department of Family Medicine
Care and Public Health Research Institute
(CAPHRI), Maastricht University
Maastricht, The Netherlands

Hilly Calsbeek
Department IQ healthcare
Radboud Institute for Health Sciences
Radboud University Medical Center
Nijmegen, The Netherlands

Stephen Campbell
School of Health Sciences and NIHR
Greater Manchester Patient Safety
Translational Research Centre
University of Manchester
Manchester
UK

Glyn Elwyn
Dartmouth Institute for Health
Policy and Clinical Practice
Geisel School of Medicine at
Dartmouth College
Lebanon, NH
USA

Cornelia Fluit
Department for Research in
Learning and Education
Radboudumc Health Academy
Radboud University Medical Center
Nijmegen, The Netherlands

Jeremy Grimshaw
Clinical Epidemiology Program
Ottawa Hospital Research Institute
Ottawa, Ontario;
Department of Medicine
University of Ottawa
Ottawa, Ontario
Canada

Richard Grol
Radboud University
Nijmegen;
Maastricht University
Maastricht, The Netherlands

Mirelle Hanskamp-Sebregts
Institute for Quality Assurance
Radboud Institute for Health Sciences
Radboud University Medical Center
Nijmegen;
Department IQ healthcare
Radboud Institute for Health Sciences
Radboud University Medical Center
Nijmegen, The Netherlands

Rosella Hermens
Department IQ healthcare
Radboud Institute for Health Sciences
Radboud University Medical Center
Nijmegen, The Netherlands

Ties Hoomans
Care Policy and Evaluation Centre
London School of Economics and
Political Science
London
UK

Marlies Hulscher
Department IQ healthcare
Radboud Institute for Health Sciences
Radboud University Medical Center
Nijmegen, The Netherlands

Noah Ivers
Women's College Research Institute and
Family Practice Health Centre
Women's College Hospital
Toronto, Ontario;
Department of Family and Community
Medicine, University of Toronto
Toronto, Ontario;
Dalla Lana School of Public Health
University of Toronto
Toronto, Ontario
Canada

Miranda Laurant
University of Applied Sciences
Arnhem-Nijmegen
Nijmegen;
Department IQ healthcare
Radboud Institute for Health Sciences
Radboud University Medical Center
Nijmegen, The Netherlands

Holger Pfaff
Institute of Medical Sociology
Health Services Research
and Rehabilitation Science (IMVR)
University of Cologne
Cologne, Germany

Amy Price
Stanford Medicine X
Stanford University School of Medicine
Stanford, CA
USA

Johan L. Severens
Erasmus School of Health Policy &
Management and Institute of Medical
Technology Assessment
Erasmus University Rotterdam
Rotterdam, The Netherlands

Charles Vincent
Department of Surgery and Cancer
Imperial College
London
UK

Philip van der Wees
Department IQ healthcare
Radboud Institute for Health Sciences
Radboud University Medical Center
Nijmegen, The Netherlands

Trudy van der Weijden
Department of Family Medicine
Care and Public Health Research
Institute (CAPHRI)
Maastricht University
Maastricht, The Netherlands

Michel Wensing
Faculty of Medicine
University of Heidelberg
Heidelberg;
Department of General Practice and
Health Services Research
Heidelberg University Hospital
Heidelberg, Germany;
Department IQ healthcare
Radboud Institute for Health Sciences
Radboud University Medical Center
Nijmegen, The Netherlands

Hub Wollersheim
Department IQ healthcare
Radboud Institute for Health Sciences
Radboud University Medical Center
Nijmegen, The Netherlands

Marieke Zegers
Department Intensive Care;
Department IQ healthcare
Radboud Institute for Health Sciences
Radboud University Medical Center
Nijmegen, The Netherlands

Introduction

Richard Grol[1,2] and Michel Wensing[3,4,5]

[1] Radboud University, Nijmegen, The Netherlands
[2] Maastricht University, Maastricht, The Netherlands
[3] Faculty of Medicine, University of Heidelberg, Heidelberg, Germany
[4] Department of General Practice and Health Services Research, Heidelberg University Hospital, Heidelberg, Germany
[5] Department IQ healthcare, Radboud Institute for Health Sciences, Radboud University Medical Center, Nijmegen, The Netherlands

Friesland – a province of the Netherlands – is the homeland of the famous black and white Friesian cows, and the land of milk and cheese. For centuries these cows were milked by hand, which meant the famer and his family awoke at 4 or 5 o'clock in the morning. Around 1890, reports of successful experiments with a milking machine appeared in the regional newspapers; according to the experts this machine had been shown to be both efficient and cost-effective. It milked cows with udders of different sorts very well. How quickly would this new technique spread among Friesian farmers?

The first machines were introduced in 1910, but it was not until the 1950s that they were adopted widely (Mak 1996). Why did farmers prefer to rise at the crack of dawn, even though everyone knew about the new machine? That it was the personal relationship they maintained with their cows is probably too romantic. The way to understand the reasons for this, and what a successful implementation program should have been directed toward, is to examine the farmers' motives and their living and working conditions at that time. One of the main reasons for non-adoption was that the milking machine costed money, whereas manpower provided by the family was free. At that time farmers were, for the most part, self-sufficient and their work involved little exchange of money. Perhaps equally important was their system of standards and values: the most important aim of a farming enterprise was to guarantee the continuity of the family business, not to make a profit. Taking risks was therefore at odds with their mission; following a set routine developed by their forefathers was seen as a guarantee of success. According to Mak (1996), it was not until World War II, when these standards were subjected to enormous modification, that farming practices in Friesland changed. An earlier effective introduction of milking machines would have required changes at different levels: changes in standards and values, greater skill in dealing with money, increase in farm size, and changes to milk and cheese production in factories. In short, changes in the entire process from cow to consumer, a complete change in culture at all levels.

This example demonstrates that if one wants to implement an innovation successfully, it is crucial to have a clear understanding of, and insight into, the target group's living and working conditions and standards and values, as well as of the issues involved in the implementation of an innovation itself. Simply publishing the effects or efficiency (or otherwise distributing information on the innovation's usefulness) is usually not enough to guarantee successful adoption. The real obstacles must be sought and tackled in a systematic way with a variety of appropriate methods and measures that have proven to be effective in practice. This is the message being delivered in this book.

In the field of healthcare an enormous number of valuable insights, technologies, and practices become available each year. They derive from well-planned scientific research or from careful experiments and evaluation in everyday practice. Only a small proportion of these methods and technologies are, in the short term, adopted into the daily practice of patient care. Thus patients, clients, and care users could be needlessly deprived of effective care or receive unnecessary, outdated, or, even worse, harmful care. Of course, not all innovations are improvements, but it is a general observation that in healthcare the situation is often one of "underuse, overuse and misuse of care" (Bodenheimer 1999). *Therefore, it is important that great care be taken not only to develop innovations and scientific insights, but also to take care that valuable insights and procedures are adopted into daily practice; in doing so, an important contribution can be made to the improvement of the quality of patient care and public health.*

Adopting valuable insights and procedures frequently occurs with difficulty and incompletely. Implementation of new insights or improvements in healthcare may be only partially successful and at times completely unsuccessful. Consequently, the intended results for the patients – recovery from an illness, improvement in health, better quality of life, more efficient procedures, or better collaboration between providers – are often not realized. There are many possible reasons for this, such as the nature, the effectiveness, or the applicability of the (new) proposed method of working, the professionals who need to change, or the setting in which the intended change is to take place. However, there may also be structural, financial, or organizational obstacles.

Equally, the way in which the change is implemented may be ineffective. Given that scientific knowledge on effective implementation and change in the practice of healthcare is still limited, but growing all the time, it is important to bring together this knowledge and to distill recommendations from it to aid implementation in routine patient care. That is, in sum, the purpose of this book.

The book is meant for healthcare providers, healthcare managers, staff involved in quality assessment, policy makers, and researchers in healthcare who are concerned with the question of how best to design the implementation of valuable (new and existing) insights and procedures so that they contribute to optimal patient care. This book tries to answer that question by combining the now available scientific knowledge and practical experience.

I.1 Which Changes?

The book is directed at the implementation of various changes and improvements in healthcare, including:

- adoption of practices, technologies, and healthcare delivery models, which have been well researched and found to have a proven value;
- adoption of well-developed practice guidelines in practice, both those developed centrally and those developed within a local area or institution;
- preventing, stopping, or reducing unnecessary, expensive, unsafe, or harmful practices;
- reducing undesirable variations in the care provided.

In this book, we will use words such as innovations, new procedures, new insights, and changes in care provision. What we mean by this is the introduction of improvements in healthcare. Therefore, we make no distinction between quality improvements and the implementation of new insights.

I.2 Evidence-Based Practice and Evidence-Based Implementation

It is certainly not true to say that all new technologies, procedures, guidelines, or recommendations from scientific research signify real improvements in patient care. Nor is it the case that the improvement of care provision can arise only from scientific information being made available. *In this book we concentrate on practices, technologies, and healthcare delivery models based on scientific evidence, on careful evaluation, and thus on innovations that are firmly established as being able to contribute to better, more effective, safer, more efficient, and patient-friendly care or better healthcare outcomes for patients and populations.*

That does not mean that these innovations would be able to find their way into practice on their own, without further adaptation. In many cases active contributions from the target groups will be necessary to adapt an innovation to their own setting and experiences. The importance of such "two-way traffic between practice and science" (Health Council of the Netherlands 2000), involving users and other stakeholders in the implementation of innovations, will be often emphasized in this book.

I.3 The Book's Messages

The messages delivered in this book can be summarized as follows:

- Take into account when developing a new working method, procedure, clinical guideline, or care protocol, from the outset, how it is to be implemented.
- Know and understand as completely as possible the target group and the setting in which implementation is to take place. Put yourself in the target group's position, try to see their perspective, and involve them in both the development and the implementation of the innovation.

- Employ a well-planned change intervention with a diversity of cost-effective and well-tested strategies and measures. A well-organized implementation process will contribute to successful implementation, overcoming many barriers to change.
- Careful, continuous evaluation of the actual care process and monitoring of the changes are also crucial in the ensuing success of the implementation activities.

I.4 The Book's Basic Principles

It is important for readers to keep in mind a number of principles that underpin this book:

- The book is about *optimizing patient care and prevention*; thus, it is about the quality and safety of care and about quality improvement. However, it is not a "manual for quality improvement."
- The emphasis lies on the improvement of the *primary processes in care provision* by physicians, nurses, and allied health professionals and the teams they work in. The patient is at center stage. Changes in the organization of institutions or practices can be very important, but are discussed here predominantly in terms of what they contribute to the improvement of direct patient care. Prevention of disease that is independent of patient care (e.g. control of air pollution or poverty in the population) is not covered.
- The immediate reasons for implementation may be the availability of new scientific insights and/or the availability of valuable procedures, as well as experiences from daily practice that a specific care process is not effective, efficient, or patient friendly.
- Changes may be initiated and realized in a guided process, with the emphasis on practical support for targeted individuals (*top-down*), or adaptive, with the emphasis on stakeholder involvement and needs

(*bottom-up*). We advocate a mix of these approaches.

- The book largely takes the *perspective of the implementer*, meaning the *agent of change*, the person or team who is, or who feels, responsible for the implementation of improvements in care provision. Through the book, however, processes and implementation are often also looked at through the eyes of the target group (professionals, teams, patients).

- Our *target group* for this book comprises healthcare providers, executive staff, staff involved in quality assessment, healthcare managers, and policy makers. The book also offers an introduction to and overview of the field to researchers in the field.

- Not only recommended practices, technologies, and healthcare delivery models should have "proven" value. It is equally important that the strategies for their implementation have been based as much as possible on robust research and are carefully evaluated. In this book we will show which approaches to implementation are evidence based and which have been based on experience.

I.5 The Organization of the Book

The book is organized into a number of parts, each of which contains several chapters. With this organization, the book largely follows the model that will be discussed in greater detail in Chapter 3 (see Figure I.1):

- Part I provides a general introduction, presents a set of theories on implementation and change in healthcare, describes a model for implementation (Figure I.1) that is used throughout the rest of the book, and ends with recommendations for the planning and preparation of the implementation project.

- Part II discusses the characteristics of new insights, guidelines, and procedures that can contribute to their ultimate implementation. The development of effective guidelines is then examined extensively.

- Part III is about measuring actual care provision as a basis for setting up concrete targets for improvement. It deals primarily with the development of good indicators.

- Part IV deals with the analysis of the target group and the setting, and discusses the range of factors that may play a role in implementation. Methods to carry out a "diagnostic analysis" are also presented.

- Part V describes existing dissemination and implementation strategies and current scientific knowledge of their effectiveness.

- Part VI outlines the design of an effective implementation plan, organizing its implementation in daily practice and evaluating the effects.

I.6 Changes from the Previous Edition

Compared to the previous edition of the book, which was published in 2013, the overall structure and approach have remained the same. Jeremy Grimshaw joined Michel Wensing and Richard Grol as co-editors of the book, while Martin Eccles and David Davis retired. As a substantial body of relevant new research has become available since 2013, all chapters have been updated with respect to the published literature. Several chapters (Chapters 13, 14, 16, 20, and 21) have been newly written by (largely) different author teams. In Chapters 11–18 on strategies for quality improvement and implementation of innovations, we have focused more strongly on the role of contextual factors and intervention components that are associated with effects. In Chapters 20–23 on evaluation methods, we have reduced the information on advanced methods, sample size calculation, and statistical aspects of data analysis (for which we refer to other sources).

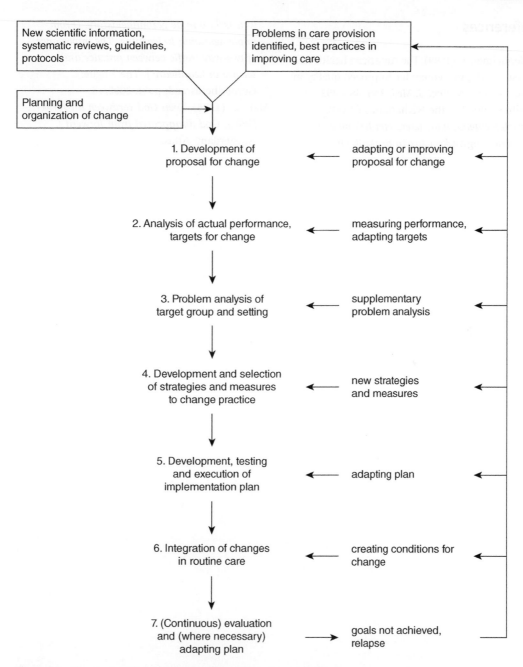

Figure I.1   The Grol and Wensing implementation of change model.

References

Bodenheimer, T. (1999). The American health care system. The movement for improved quality in health care. *N. Engl. J. Med.* 340: 488–492.

Health Council of the Netherlands (2000). *Van implementeren naar leren. Het belang van tweerichtingsverkeer tussen praktijk en wetenschap in de gezondheidszorg. [From implementation to learning. The importance of two-way traffic between practice and science in healthcare.].* The Hague: Gezondheidsraad; publ. 2000/18.

Mak, G. (1996). *Toen God verdween uit Jorwerd. [When God disappeared from Jorwerd.].* Amsterdam: Atlas.

Part I

Principles of the Implementation of Change

1

Implementation of Change in Healthcare

A Complex Problem

Richard Grol[1,2] *and Michel Wensing*[3,4,5]

[1] Radboud University, Nijmegen, The Netherlands
[2] Maastricht University, Maastricht, The Netherlands
[3] Faculty of Medicine, University of Heidelberg, Heidelberg, Germany
[4] Department of General Practice and Health Services Research, Heidelberg University Hospital, Heidelberg, Germany
[5] Department IQ healthcare, Radboud Institute for Health Sciences, Radboud University Medical Center, Nijmegen, The Netherlands

SUMMARY
• Substantial numbers of patients do not receive high-quality care: care that is accessible, safe, effective, patient centered, well-coordinated, and efficient.
• Changes in practice are often required to improve patient care and prevention. It may also demand changes in healthcare organizations and healthcare systems to facilitate practice changes.
• Different approaches to the implementation of change in patient care can be observed, each based on different assumptions and theories of human and organizational behavior.
• A combination of structured guidance ("top-down") and participation of target populations and stakeholders ("bottom-up") is often needed to achieve real and sustainable changes in practice.
• Different innovations and proposals for change demand different implementation strategies.

1.1 Introduction

The number of new insights, procedures, programs, and technologies that have become available as a result of careful development and/or scientific research is enormous. For instance, the number of clinical trials added to Medline, a large database of journals in the field of medicine, is gigantic. Subsets of this database – systematic literature analyses of clinical research studies or that portion of the literature capturing clinical guidelines – are growing at significant rates. For many problems and questions that emerge in healthcare practice and policy, a search in the research literature would identify many relevant publications.

As a consequence, knowledge about optimal patient care quickly becomes obsolete, affected by both scientific and social developments. An example of quality problems in modern times is presented in Box 1.1. A great deal of knowledge that one absorbs over the years of training to become a doctor, nurse, or paramedic is obsolete by the time training is completed. This is not a new observation (see Box 1.2). It reflects the importance of health professionals' ability to scan, absorb, and use the medical literature,

Improving Patient Care: The Implementation of Change in Health Care, Third Edition. Edited by Michel Wensing, Richard Grol, and Jeremy Grimshaw.

Box 1.1   Unsafe Cardiac Surgery: The Radboud Cardiac Surgery Case

In September 2005, details about the mortality rates at the Cardiac Surgery department of the Radboud University Nijmegen Medical Center got into the newspapers. The post-surgery mortality rate in 2004 was 6.7%, compared to 2.7% in other cardiac centers in the Netherlands. This situation initiated a process which led to major improvements in clinical practice within a few years. The Board of Directors initially denied the problem, stating that the high mortality rates were caused by the patient case mix. However, after the situation had been intensively analyzed, by both an internal committee and an external committee (appointed by the Health Care Inspectorate), the conclusion was reached that in fact these high mortality rates reflected serious problems. The high mortality and complication rates could not be attributed to more seriously ill patients (in fact, the situation was quite the opposite). Instead it was discovered that staff did not work according to prevailing clinical research evidence and protocols; there was little or no cooperation between the disciplines involved (for example, everyone used his/her own patient record); departments did not collaborate with each other; there were conflicts among cardiac surgeons; the management of the department had lost control of the situation; and little effort was invested in quality improvement. The Board of Directors of the hospital was aware of the problem, but left it to the physicians to solve it. For a long time, the national Inspectorate relied on the department's explanations.

These findings led the Inspectorate to close the department. The Board of Directors was dismissed. The management of the medical staff and the head of the department resigned. Meanwhile, many patients looked for treatment elsewhere, resulting in many empty beds. This initiated a reorganization of the Radboud University Nijmegen Medical Center in general and the cardiac surgery department in particular. The reorganization led to operations being restarted after six months. A year later, the department's mortality and complication rates were far below the national average (around 1%). The question is: What was the real cause of this change? Several hypotheses can be formulated:

- *Transparency*: publicizing the data and validating them provided both the public at large and the medical center with an insight into the fact that a real problem did exist. Good objective data on performance can contribute to the sense of urgency that something really needs to be done. This information prompted the Inspectorate as well as the patients to take measures.

- *National Inspectorate*: the decision of the Inspectorate to close the center and to demand radical changes put the organization under great pressure to implement improvements in a quick and thorough way.

- *Leadership*: the new management of the department, the medical staff, and the medical center made high quality and patient safety into an absolute priority and supervised the implementation of many changes to achieve this, including, among other actions, a revised and more intensive internal audit method.

- *Organization of care processes*: the surgical process was redesigned with the help of all disciplines involved, daily consultation on the patients as well as a joint medical file were introduced, and cooperation with the aim of a safer surgical process became a core objective.

- *Competency and motivation of professionals*: less than competent or dysfunctional surgeons were suspended, new surgeons who were prepared to work in the new system were appointed, and competencies were brought up to the required standard.

We would suggest that these changes all contributed to the improved quality and outcomes of care, probably in concert to achieve the complex change needed at Radboud. However, they represent hypotheses which need to be tested. This book presents the available scientific knowledge in this field.

Box 1.2 Development of Knowledge, a Not So Recent Example

In 1348, King Philip VI of France asked the medical faculty of the University of Paris for a scientific explanation of the plague epidemic, known as the Black Death, which killed about a third of the population of Europe. After extensive research, the Sorbonne came up with the cause – a threefold conjunction of Saturn, Jupiter, and Mars in the 14th grade of Aquarius. For a long time, this was generally accepted as being the definitive explanation in both Europe and the Arab world (Achterhuis 1998). What will we make of our explanations of the most important diseases of our time and the effectiveness of certain treatments 100 years from now?

---

described in subsequent chapters (Candy 2000). The legitimate concerns about the validity and relevance of published research and technologies (leading to "research waste") imply a need for careful selection of items for implementation into practice.

The store of new knowledge about good patient care is growing at an ever-increasing pace, but the percentage of valuable insights subsequently introduced into routine patient care and prevention is considerably lower. Taken at face value, this fact would imply that investing resources in research, guidance, and technology would seem to be a useless exercise. This was the case in the past; it may still be the case today. Although Semmelweis had demonstrated the importance of antiseptics in the nineteenth century, many surgeons operating after 1900 still used their bare hands, with adverse consequences. Even today, many institutions pay too little attention to washing and disinfecting hands before and after medical or nursing interventions, with huge consequences for patients and healthcare costs (Teare et al. 2001; Bolon 2011).

1.2 The Implementation Problem

The spread of information in the current information age, with new media and tools to transfer knowledge, is probably taking place faster than it did in the past. Nevertheless, clinicians,

researchers, and policy makers have noticed that it takes a long time before research results or insights find their way into daily practice. In many cases healthcare professionals only learn and adopt new information gradually. To some extent this is understandable, considering the high workload of most of them, and even positive given the need for a careful assessment of recommended practices. It was estimated that a healthcare professional faces 75 trials and 11 new systematic reviews a day (Bastian et al. 2010), which is substantially more than a decade earlier (Haines 1996).

Even if clinicians are informed about new insights on optimal patient care, changes do not necessarily take place within their daily routines. The same applies to decision makers in prevention programs and healthcare systems. The scientific literature is replete with examples from which it would appear that patients are not given the care that, according to recent scientific or professional insights, is desirable. For instance, a representative analysis of clinical care given to almost 7000 patients in the USA showed that on average less than 60% of the patients received the care they should receive, based on best evidence (McGlynn et al. 2003; Asch et al. 2006; Runciman et al. 2012). Even after successful implementation of improvements, professionals' adherence to clinical practice guidelines was proven to decrease after a year in about half of the cases (Ament et al. 2015; see Box 1.3).

Box 1.3 Adherence to Guidelines in Primary Care in the Netherlands

In a National Study of Primary Care, 104 primary care practices collected data to determine their adherence to prevailing clinical guidelines developed by the Dutch College of General Practitioners (Braspenning et al. 2004). In total, data were compiled for 58 indicators. Although the average overall score for the indicators was 74%, wide variations existed between clinical problems, the nature of the performance (for example, the score for medication prescription was 62% and for referral 89%), and among primary care practices.

In what follows you will find some data from studies, which will give you an idea of the nature and the extent of the implementation problem in specific fields of healthcare.

1.2.1 Effective Care

Worldwide, there are many examples of the need for improvement of healthcare practice. In the USA, for example, the overall acute myocardial infarction 30-day mortality rates remain high, having only declined from 18.8% in 1995 to 15.8% in 2006 (Krumholz et al. 2009), while Canadian rates have decreased from 13.5% in 1995 to 10.6% in 2003 (Johansen et al. 2010). While demonstrating significant reductions, a portion of these deaths remains preventable. In 2001 11% of patients in the Netherlands with an acute myocardial infarction died within 30 days following hospital admission; in 2013 this was 7.6%, similar to Switzerland and the UK, but worse than Australia (4.1%). The percentages for cerebral infarction were 16% in 2001 and 9% in 2013. The five-year survival rates for various types of cancer are better in countries such as Finland, Norway, and Switzerland than in the Netherlands. The five-year survival rate for colon cancer was on average 63% (range 51–71%) in the OECD (Organisation for Economic Co-operation and Development) countries in recent years (OECD 2017).

Improvements are also possible in the treatment of the chronically ill. For example, a study among diabetes patients at outpatient clinics of internal medicine showed that only 23% of the patients managed to have the target value of HbA1c. The average score for a set of process indicators was 64% (Dijkstra et al. 2004). In this study, care and care outcomes improved considerably when the clinic provided structured multidisciplinary care and (specialized) nurses. Similarly, in 2007, a US study found that only 34% of hypertensive patients received adequate treatment to maintain the recommended blood pressure (Ardery et al. 2007). Hospital admissions for asthma and chronic obstructive pulmonary disorder (COPD) ranged from 58/100 000 in Japan to 427/100 000 in Hungary, with an average in the OECD countries of 236/100 000 in 2015 (OECD 2017).

1.2.2 Safe Care

Patients may be unnecessarily harmed by such inadequate care, not to mention the frustrations or costs that are incurred. Figures from the USA reveal a high number of deaths (45–99 000 deaths per year) as a result of poor practice and medical (mis)management (AHRQ 2010). Studies have been performed in various countries investigating adverse events for patients in hospitals. A systematic analysis of the results of those studies showed an average of 9.2% of patients suffering from adverse events, of which more than 40% were estimated to be preventable (De Vries et al.

2008). Medical records of patients in 19 hospitals in the Netherlands were studied in 2016 (Wagner 2017). The study showed that 3.1% (1035) of the patients who died in hospital suffered a potentially avoidable death.

Medication is an important cause of unsafe care. The HARM study indicated that there are 40 000 hospital admissions every year through medication errors in ambulatory patients in the Netherlands (Van den Bemt 2002). Furthermore, 5.5% of patients contracted an infection in hospital in 2016 (RIVM 2017). The scope of this problem is global. For example, 7.5% of Canadian patients contract a nosocomial infection (Baker et al. 2004); between 3 and 20% of US patients suffer some form of hospital-related adverse event (Institute of Medicine 2000). Similar results are found in Australia and New Zealand (Wilson et al. 1995; Davis et al. 2002). A study found about 380 000 opioid-related hospital admissions in 13 states in the USA in a three-year period (2013–2015), suggesting overprescribing of these strong analgesics (Blanchard et al. 2018).

Insufficient hand hygiene in hospital is a classic example of a safety problem. Although clear evidence exists in this area, stipulating when hands need to be cleaned, compliance – most notably by physicians – is known to be poor. For instance, a study of 47 wards in three hospitals, in which nursing performance was closely observed (3500 observations), showed average rates of adherence per hospital to the infection prevention guidelines of 37, 33, and 19% (Brink-Huis et al. 2010). Erasmus et al. conducted a systematic review of 96 studies on compliance with hand hygiene guidelines in hospital care. The overall median compliance rate was 40%, with lower rates for doctors (32%) than for nurses (48%; Erasmus et al. 2010). Needless to say, there is a lot of room for improvement.

There is also room for improvement to avoid other aspects of unsafe care, for example patient falls and nutrition. A study in 10 hospitals and 10 nursing homes in the Netherlands showed that an incident or error in the area of pressure ulcers, falling, or urinary tract infections happened every week in 9% of the patients (Van Gaal et al. 2014). Similar figures can be found in almost all developed countries. In 2004, 11% of nursing home residents in the USA had pressure ulcers (Park-Lee and Caffrey 2009). The Australian Institute of Health and Welfare (2018) reported that in 2015–2016 there were 3.2 falls per 1000 hospitalizations; fall rates were higher in public hospitals than in private hospitals.

1.2.3 Efficient Care

While it is true that best evidence care is occasionally not offered to patients, it is frequently the reverse that holds true: unnecessary, expensive, and out-of-date care is also offered or provided. These inefficient clinical actions have considerable consequences in terms of personal and societal costs. Null et al. (2005) indicated that 7.5 million unnecessary surgical procedures were undertaken yearly in the USA, a country which sees approximately 53.3 million procedures annually (Cullen et al. 2009). In about 20% of their decisions, physicians in the Netherlands took unnecessary actions (Braspenning et al. 2004), including, for example, inappropriately prescribing antibiotics for acute ear infections (30%), referral to a physiotherapist for acute back pain (20%), not prescribing the first-choice medicine for stomach complaints (25%), or unnecessary prostate-specific antigen (PSA) testing for men with micturition problems (71%). Analyses of medical records in hospitals showed large numbers of "low value actions" that contribute little to health outcomes in patients (Colla et al. 2014). Examples were X-rays in case of low back pain (22%) or anti-psychotic medication as treatment for problematic behavior in case of dementia (31%). Stopping practices with unproven or low value for patients is just as important as the implementation of valuable innovations (Prasad and Ionnidis 2014).

1.2.4 Access to Care

Access to care implies the absence of financial, geographical, or time barriers to care as required. Waiting times and times for diagnosis or treatment are important indicators of timely access to care. For instance, a study by El Sharouni et al. (2003) about waiting time outcomes for radiotherapy for cancer patients showed that the average waiting time was 80 days in the Netherlands. This resulted in 41% of the patients going from having a possibly curable illness to having a possibly incurable illness. Waiting times for cataract surgery ranged from 464 days in Poland to 37 days in the Netherlands, with an average of 121 days in the OECD countries in 2015 (OECD 2017). Box 1.4 provides another example.

1.2.5 Patient-Centered Care

Patient centeredness is about the delivery of treatments and communication in a manner which involves patients in decision making and puts them at center stage when dealing with their problems. In a study in 10 European countries, 17 400 patients from primary care were asked for their experiences of care, using a validated questionnaire (EUROPEP; Grol et al. 2000). Scores were collated on two dimensions: communication and information from the physician, and organization of care. On average, patients were very positive about their primary care practices: 80% were positive or very positive about treatment, communication, information, and organization of care, with substantial variation between countries (Petek et al. 2011). The judgment of the waiting times before a consultation with the general practitioner (GP), however, was much more negative. Compared to a similar study in 1998, the evaluations were more or less the same (Petek et al. 2011).

1.2.6 Variation in the Provision of Care

Studies often point to an enormous variation in performance. In some regions or hospitals, patients are more likely to undergo surgery for back pain, removal of the uterus, or surgical reduction of the prostate than in other regions or hospitals. While variation is not necessarily problematic, it is plausible that a considerable number of patients do not receive the

---

Box 1.4 Organization of Care for Patients Suffering from Breast Cancer

Quick diagnosis and treatment of breast cancer can prevent aggravation of the situation. Schouten et al. (2010) mapped the times to treatment of 1600 breast cancer patients, who were treated by 20 different teams:

	Average	Spread (standard deviation)
Admission time for the first appointment (advice max. 5 days)	6.8 days	6.2 days
Time between first outpatient visit and diagnosis (advice max. 1 day)	5.4 days	8.6 days
Time between diagnosis and operation (advice max. 21 days)	18.5 days	16.5 days

Apart from the fact that diagnoses can be made much quicker in many places, the huge variety among institutions is remarkable. Also, much can be gained by multidisciplinary deliberation on patients (average 25%) and preoperative counseling of patients (average 55%).

recommended care, or, worse, receive unnecessary or possibly even damaging care. A survey of 276 patients suffering from lung cancer in hospitals in the east of the Netherlands measured the organizational quality of care on the basis of carefully constructed indicators (using scientific literature, guidelines, expert panels, and patient panels). Considerable variation was noted in patient throughput among the participating hospitals. For example, regarding finalizing the diagnosis within the recommended 21 days, the scores among hospitals varied between 58 and 73%. Regarding the start of the therapy as recommended (within 35 days after the first visit), scores varied between 38 and 66% (Ouwens et al. 2007).

Variation is also found between healthcare systems in different countries. In 2008, a survey among nearly 10 000 chronically ill patients in 8 countries showed that the percentage of diabetic patients that received recommended care (regular HbA1c measurement, examination of feet and fundi, and blood pressure measurement) varied between an average 35% in France and up to 60–65% in England and the Netherlands (Schoen et al. 2009). Likewise, the percentages of adults in the USA who had received an HbA1c measurement, retinal eye examination, and foot examination in the past year were 79.4, 66.7, and 64.6%, respectively (Coffey et al. 2004).

1.3 Various Approaches to the Implementation of Change in Patient Care

Partly on the basis of the figures presented so far, there is agreement between all parties involved in healthcare that care given could be improved in a number of ways: offering safer, more effective, more patient-centered, better-coordinated, and more efficient care. However, when it comes to how this can be achieved, opinions differ. Various stakeholders and disciplines have proposed a variety of approaches (Grol 1997; Grol 1999):

- *Healthcare professionals* are often inclined to take improvements into their own hands and to promote continuing professional development and achieve consensus on recommended practice for and among themselves. Professional hierarchies may support the adoption of chosen practices.
- *Biomedical researchers* more frequently classify, rate, and catalogue scientific developments within a field, making this information available to professionals through systematic reviews, rigorously developed clinical guidelines, and computerized decision support systems.
- *Healthcare researchers*, who may work for or on behalf of the government, map out health system and professional performance, indicating variations between care providers, institutions, and regions. Quality of care is measured with the help of "performance indicators"; this information is then channeled back to care providers as feedback or "mirrored information" and is increasingly made public.
- *Organizational and management experts* study how care processes can be optimized and how organizational conditions for optimal care can be created. They advise managers in healthcare organizations on organizational processes and leadership.
- *Patient representatives, ethicists, and lawyers* argue for the central role of patients, defending their right to better information provision and a more influential role in decisions about their illness. In addition, patients can be involved in the planning and design of healthcare services.
- *Health insurers and governments*, frequently assisted by *health economists*, are accountable for improving the overall quality of care, while at the same time controlling its costs. This is often done by selectively budgeting, financial incentives, or regulations, and by making rules for tariffs and volume.

Thus, in the daily practice of optimizing patient care, different parties are inclined to opt for different strategies to improve care.

These different approaches or strategies are an expression of the different assumptions that concern the effective implementation of improvements in patient care – that is, different beliefs concerning changing human behavior and the functioning of groups and organizations. The example in cardiac surgery in Box 1.1 provides an illustration of this.

The pressing question is: Which strategy is the most effective for a particular problem in a specific context? We need a better understanding of these strategies in order for us to choose the right method, for the right setting, at the right time. This book intends to provide assistance in this process. A number of approaches to the improvement of clinical practice are described below, highlighting the assumptions on which they are based (Grol 1997). Table 1.1 provides a summary.

- The *marketing approach* emphasizes the importance of developing and disseminating an attractive message. Such a message

includes an interesting and appealing proposal for change that accommodates the needs and wishes of the target group and helps them to achieve their personal goals. Proposals may be adjusted to fit a local situation and are most often disseminated through a variety of communication channels, for example by mass and professional media, and personal contacts.

- The *cognitive approach* traditionally regards professionals (and patients) as individuals who make decisions after considering and weighing rational arguments. If care providers do not adopt a particular working practice, it is because they lack sufficient or convincing information about its effectiveness. Modern cognitive theory, however, has emphasized the importance of heuristics, which may lead to bias and suboptimal decisions. Therefore, in this approach the most important strategy is to provide care providers with this information in the form of balanced summaries of scientific literature and

Table 1.1 Approaches aimed at the implementation of improved care.

Approach	Focus	Examples of strategies
Marketing	Attractive product adjusted to needs of targeted population	Segmentation of targeted population Various distribution channels
Cognitive	Rational decision making, cognitive heuristics	Systematic literature reviews Evidence-based guidelines
Motivational	Individual intrinsic motivation	Educational feedback on performance Problem-based learning
Reinforcement	Prompts, rewards, sanctions	Reminders delivered during action Economic incentives
Social interaction	Influence by important others, role models	Peer review Outreach visits Opinion leaders Patient-directed methods
Management	Structural and organizational systems and conditions	Redesigned care processes Total quality management Leadership
Control	Authority, power on the basis of sanctions	Legislation and regulations Financial sanctions Complaint procedures, disciplinary measures

Source: Data from Grol (1997).

evidence-based guidelines that can bear the scrutiny of criticism, as well as in the form of computerized decision support.

- The *motivational approach* is based on the assumption that change is mainly created by individuals' internal motivation to achieve optimal competency and performance of care providers (and patients). Strategies to improve clinical practice therefore emphasize intrinsic motivation, for instance by being based on experiences and problems that professionals are faced with in their daily work or which are experienced by patients. The use of feedback on aspects of professional performance is a crucial mechanism of learning and improving, which often depends on internal motivation. "Problem-based learning" and "portfolio learning" are learning methods that fit in well with this approach.

- The *reinforcement approach* is based on behavioral theory, which is applied in behavior change as well as economics. It emphasizes the role of reinforcement of behaviors, using prompts, rewards, and sanctions. In this approach, human behavior is seen as something that can be influenced by external forces. An important strategy in this respect is financial incentives, which may be related to performance (pay for performance). Prompts or reminders during performance of an action are another strategy that fits with the approach.

- The *social interaction approach* is based on the assumption that learning and change come about by the example, interactions, and influence of other individuals considered to be important. Like most other people, care providers are "social animals," often looking to others such as valued colleagues or opinion leaders for approval, support, and exemplary behavior that they can emulate. Moreover, patient care is increasingly provided in teams and networks of healthcare professionals. Important improvement strategies in this approach include using opinion leaders, outreach visits (especially visits by respected colleagues or experts),

peer assessment, adaptations in the patient care team, and using patients to influence professionals by asking questions or putting pressure on them.

- The *management approach* is directed toward creating the organizational conditions essential for change, such a specific organizational culture or type of leadership. Here the assumption is that poor-quality care is a systems problem; the complexity of such systems has been emphasized. Changing the system, redesigning the care processes, or changing roles and tasks, improving the internal culture, and continuously monitoring and improving care are increasingly considered as important methods required to optimize patient care. Examples of this approach are quality and safety management.

- The *control approach* describes the final set of measures, based on power to influence people's performance, using authority or sanctions. Many people do their utmost to avoid negative consequences of their actions and are sensitive to what happens to them in terms of earnings or privileges. Also, many healthcare professionals consider specific types of power as legitimate, such as power that is based on democratic procedures or on demonstrated clinical competency. Legislation and issuing rules, relicensing, recertification and compulsory accreditation, budgeting and contracts, and complaints procedures and disciplinary jurisdiction fit this type of approach to implementing improved care.

Obviously, there are other approaches, a large number of which are described in this book. Each of these is based on specific theories or beliefs about behavioral change. Some theories emphasize changing the behavior of the individual professional; others are directed at organizational systems and processes. Some assume that change must come about from inside an individual, for instance from an inner need or motivation, whereas others assume that external factors or pressures are needed for the optimal result. Likewise, some theories emphasize that patient care is the performance of teams, networks, and healthcare organizations, which should thus be the focal point of change. As a consequence, some theories put the emphasis on self-regulation and personal responsibility for those who have to change, whereas others assume that this approach rarely leads to the desired result.

In Chapter 2, we provide an overview of theories that are relevant for change in healthcare practice, which can be used for designing and evaluating implementation and improvement strategies. As far as optimizing quality and safety of patient care is concerned, there is no convincing evidence that any one of the approaches described is more effective than any other in a particular situation. For this reason, *the focus of this book is not on one specific approach, but on an integration of different approaches* within a practically applicable implementation framework (see Chapter 3).

1.4 What Is Implementation?

Implementation can be described as "a planned process and systematic introduction of innovations and/or changes of proven value; the aim being that these are given a structural place in professional practice, in the functioning of organizations or in the health care

structure" (ZON 1997). Implementation science has been defined as "scientific study of methods to promote the systematic uptake of research findings and other evidence-based practices into routine practice, and, hence, to improve the quality and effectiveness of health services and care" (Eccles and Mittmann 2006).

Many terms for realizing improvements in practice are used internationally, such as innovation, implementation, dissemination, diffusion, adoption, knowledge transfer, education, quality improvement, and care modernization. A survey in nine countries among organizations providing grants on terms which were used for "implementation of knowledge in the policy and practice of care" showed a range of different terms, each with its own definition (Box 1.5; Tetroe et al. 2008). The diversity in terms reflects the variation in thinking in scientific circles and in the policies that cover this subject.

The popularity of the terms varies across the world and, to some extent, also across decades. In Canada, for example, terms such as "knowledge translation" and "knowledge transfer" are frequently employed to indicate the adoption of knowledge into policy and practice. Further, the terms "knowledge exchange" and "integrated knowledge translation" enjoy some popularity; they represent the two-way traffic between researchers and professionals in the field of practice and policy. In Europe and

---

Box 1.5   Terms in the International Literature for Knowledge Translation

Applied health research	Knowledge communication	Research into practice
Capacity building	Knowledge cycle	Research mediation
Competing, cooperation	Knowledge exchange	Research transfer
Diffusion	Knowledge management	Research translation
Dissemination	Knowledge mobilization	Science communication
Exploitation	Knowledge transfer	Teaching
Getting knowledge into practice	Knowledge translation	The third mission
Impact	Linkage and exchange	Translation
Implementation	Popularization of research	Translational research
	Knowledge cycle	Transmission
		Utilization

Source: Data from Tetroe et al. (2008).

the USA, the terms "dissemination and implementation" are in widespread use, although other terms are also employed. The term "quality improvement" emerged in the 1980s across the world, while "safety management" emerged in the 1990s. Both have become established fields of work, particularly in hospitals. Another term, "care innovation," seems to be used mainly for information technologies and organizational changes. Individual professional workers in the field are more inclined to speak about "continuing education" or "continuing professional development," whereas biomedical and clinical researchers, when they refer to implementation, frame this concept mainly in terms of the dissemination or knowledge transfer. Davis and Tailor-Vaisey (1997) aimed to provide definitions for some terms.

In this book, we adhere to the long-standing definition of implementation by ZON, a large funder of health research in the Netherlands, given at the beginning of this section. Still relevant, it recognizes several important elements (Hulscher et al. 2000). The ZON definition of implementation from 1997 specifies the following components:

- *Planned process and systematic introduction*: introduction of the improvement in clinical practice is well planned, and the strategies to achieve change are based on an analysis of the problems, the target group, and the setting. These types of strategies may be directed at care providers, the patient/client, and/or organizational or structural aspects of care. While simple dissemination of knowledge on better care provision may result in an increase in knowledge or an attitude change on its own, it is unusual for this to lead to changes in behavior in practice. Effective implementation therefore demands a planned process, in which it is essential that effective dissemination, transfer of knowledge to practice, and attitude change take place prior to the promotion of the actual implementation of the innovation. In most cases, an iterative or incremental

approach will be preferable in which, on the basis of experience gained, the next step will be taken and the method of implementation adjusted and improved. "Systematic" does not mean that, prior to the introduction, a definitive plan is made from which there is no deviation possible.

- *Innovations and/or improvements (of proven value)*: this element concerns the introduction of innovations, procedures, or organizational processes that are new, better, or different from those accepted or employed in a specific setting. These may be new therapies or diagnostic procedures that have *proved* their worth in well-designed clinical trials. This may also be a guideline based on a systematic review of the scientific literature, a new procedure to prevent medication errors, or a "time-out" or checklist procedure in surgery. The innovation can also include a new form of management of care for patients with diabetes or heart failure that has been found to work well and that leads to the desired end. The innovation need not be fully or completely developed; in fact, the optimal time to adjust and tailor an innovation to suit the specific circumstances experienced in practice is during the implementation process.
- *Giving it a structural place*: implementation should lead to sustainable change. However, in practice there is often a relapse, particularly when support is withdrawn after a project has finished.
- *(Professional) practice, the functioning of organization(s), or the structure of healthcare*: changes can take place at different levels. This book on implementation assumes that changes in the organization or structure of the care provided are bound to have consequences for the patient and the primary care process. The changes are usually aimed at improved effectiveness or efficiency or at making the care more patient centered, with direct effects for patients. Implementation considers organizational and structural changes from this perspective.

Broadly speaking, two contrasting approaches to the implementation of knowledge or improved procedures can be distinguished (Hulscher et al. 2000; Wensing et al. 2000): the "guidance approach" and the "participation approach" (Kitson et al. 1998; Van Woerkom and Adolfse 1998). In implementation practice one usually uses elements from both. When using the term *guidance approach*, one might think of the "health technology cycle" or the "innovation cycle" (ZON 1997), which work as follows. After the primary research and synthesis of the research findings have taken place, dissemination and implementation follow. There is a clear starting point, and steering takes place externally and, for the most part, from above. The starting point is often the availability of new evidence, insights, or procedures that are considered to be worth introducing. Alternatively, the available knowledge may be summarized in response to a problem in healthcare. Dissemination and support, for example the provision of tools and practical help, aim to enhance the uptake of the recommended practices. Critics of this approach suggest that little attention is paid to the diversity of needs in the target group and that the model makes little use of the unique knowledge and experience present within that group.

In contrast, the *participation approach* (Van Woerkom and Adolfse 1998; Gagliardi et al. 2016) uses the needs and experiences from practice as its departure point for knowledge generation and implementation (Box 1.6).

The exact starting point for the change is often difficult to determine. It takes place incrementally, step by step, and in some cases there may not be a strongly felt prior need to implement a concrete innovation or working method. Communication and feedback between people in daily practice determine whether the change will or will not be achieved. The phases of development, testing, dissemination, and introduction of an innovation intertwine. A criticism leveled at this approach is that it does not always introduce an optimal or evidence-based routine. The approach actually describes how change is often brought about in practice, but the methods for participation of stakeholders and co-creation of strategies are often not well specified and not validated.

In this book we assume that elements from both approaches are crucial for effective implementation of change in healthcare. An example of a method which combines aspects of both approaches is *knowledge brokering* (Lomas 2007). Knowledge brokering encompasses all activities that put decision makers (physicians, policy makers, etc.) in contact with researchers and improve their communication with each other, leading to a better understanding of one another's targets and professional cultures, influencing each other's work, creating new forms of cooperation, and stimulating the use of research data in decision making. The basis for this construct is that researchers, policy makers, and physicians do not always understand one another very well, necessitating the need for a two-way flow in order to

---

Box 1.6   Approaches to Implementation

Guidance approach	Participation approach
Steered from external party	Steered from practice
Linear implementation	Incremental implementation
Clear start to implementation	Unclear moment of start
Driven by supply of knowledge or technology	Driven by need for knowledge or technology
Often positive about change	Neutral about change
No attention paid to diversity of needs in practice	Risk that suboptimal practice is implemented

Source: Data from Van Woerkom and Adolfse (1998).

reduce mutual distrust (Innvaer et al. 2002). Effective knowledge exchange depends on personal networks, whereby mutual communication in the network serves as the engine that gets the implementation going (Greenhalgh et al. 2004). To be more specific, this means that there is a need for well-trained *intermediaries* between researchers and policy makers and people from the practice of healthcare (Lomas 2007).

1.5 Which Recommended Practices Should Be Adopted?

A recommended practice (guideline, technology, healthcare delivery model) does not necessarily imply an improvement of current practice. In some situations, it is important to resist change to preserve valuable practices. Nevertheless, the premise of this book is that changes are often desirable or necessary improvements in patient care or prevention. These improvements may involve evidence-based insights, procedures, techniques, or guidelines for good care practice. Alternatively, they may be positive experiences using a certain care process ("best practice") or new technology. In the latter case, evaluation is recommended, as initial experiences may be biased or non-replicable in other populations and settings. The starting point for any change may be the emergence of new insights and technologies, or the need to respond to important problems in healthcare practice.

1.5.1 New Insights and Technologies

Many insights about optimal care derive from research carried out into the efficacy and efficiency of specific interventions in clinical practice and prevention. The evidence-based medicine movement is oriented toward helping care providers, patients, and policy makers make decisions on how to act when faced with health problems by basing their decisions, wherever possible, on the best

scientific evidence (Sackett et al. 1997). With this in mind, international work groups, within the framework of the Cochrane Collaboration (http://www.cochrane.org), painstakingly summarize scientific insights in a specific area. A crucial aspect of this work is a critical assessment of the methodological quality (or risk of bias) of published research, because many studies use inadequate or suboptimal methods, resulting in "research waste" (Ioannidis et al. 2014).

Once located and assessed, the studies and the systematic analyses of the literature are added to a large database, the Cochrane Database of Systematic Reviews. In terms of ambition, this worldwide activity has already been compared to the Human Genome Project, in which all human genes are being mapped (Naylor 1995). The initial idea was that clinicians would consult these databases regularly when solving problems in the healthcare setting, reflecting a critical attitude toward using the scientific literature. Research has shown, however, that while clinicians are eager to obtain support for their decisions, they find it difficult to consult databases such as these (McColl et al. 1998; Tomlin et al. 1999; Guyatt et al. 2000). Methods to make access to literature easier, for instance via the internet, on personal digital devices, or by integrating them into computerized decision support systems, have therefore been developed and applied.

Compiling scientific evidence in the form of clinical practice guidelines is one such useful method. Guidelines are a potentially important resource for introducing insights into the best forms of patient care in an easily accessible form and for these being adopted. However, before this can be achieved, they have to meet certain requirements. At the moment, guidelines for good care are being formulated all over the world by a wide range of parties, including governments, insurers, professionals, and patients' organizations. Internationally, evidence-based tables and guidelines are exchanged in and supported by the Guidelines International Network (GIN, www.g-i-n.net).

Guidelines from a variety of sources have different aims and development methods, and therefore their quality varies. In the past they were often based on the consensus view of experts; gradually guidelines' development has become more systematic, incorporating recent scientific insights into their development methods (Schünemann et al. 2014). On the one hand, guidelines form an important resource with which to implement new, valuable insights and they are thus an important intermediate step in the process of implementation of scientific knowledge. On the other hand, effective implementation strategies are needed to ensure that guidelines find their way into daily practice. Guidelines can take the format of documents of hundreds of pages, so support tools are needed to transfer the key message into practice.

1.5.2 Problems in Healthcare Practice

Many innovations in healthcare practice are not the direct results of the introduction of scientific findings or evidence-based guidelines. In many cases, the driving force behind the desired improvement in care (which may or may not be based on factual information about variations in care provision) is that existing practice does not lead to the intended result, that mistakes are being made, that patients are not satisfied, or that working methods are inefficient or unsafe. This realization then can become the point of departure for a structured approach to realize improvements, using experiences and best practices from other places. This book will also present these kinds of approaches.

It is usually possible to identify relevant studies on the topic of interest. Nevertheless, the transferability to the population and setting of interest may be problematic, or the research questions may not entirely match. No matter how carefully the search for, and analysis of, the medical literature is carried out, there is good scientific evidence for only a small minority of current clinical actions and decisions. Thus, there is a large gray area in which the experiences and preferences of those involved play an important role (Naylor 1995). Furthermore, the reality often means longer-running, complex care processes that include multiple care providers – physicians, nurses, and allied health professionals – for which the approach consists of a logical series of linked interventions or actions (Grol and van Weel 2009; Grol 2010). Seeing care provision as processes and chains of actions and the need to analyze and improve these processes and chains in their entirety take pride of place in the "total quality management" approach (Berwick 1998), as well as in models of integrated care and the like (Gabbay et al. 2011).

1.6 A Systematic Approach to "Sustainable Change"

The implementation of recommended practices in patient care and prevention could therefore be actuated both by new scientific insights and by awareness that care does not function well. The subsequent actions should lead to a change, which will in turn become part of the normal provision of care and the routines of practice. This often appears to be very difficult. Studies show that the outcomes of many implementation and improvement projects are rather small and ebb away quickly. It is crucial to invest in better knowledge on how to improve healthcare practice: "stop admiring the problems and start investing in evidence to solve them" (Dixon-Woods 2019). Implementation of innovations in resource-poor communities and countries – where the potential health gains are often highest – obviously meets with additional challenges (Yapa and Bärnighausen 2018).

Summarizing the state of the art regarding implementation, one conclusion could be that different innovations and proposals for changes in patient care demand different implementation strategies (Grol and Grimshaw 2003; Grimshaw et al. 2004). There is no such thing as one best practice for all innovations in all settings. Different target groups and situations create varying implementation problems. A good diagnostic analysis of the target group and the setting is needed, in turn directing a well-structured implementation plan. In most cases, this means using a variety of improvement strategies to be applied in a certain order. Throughout the process, continuous evaluations check whether the change is under way and the target is reached. Ideally, the complete process is well prepared and organized: most experts in the field of implementation agree on the necessity of a systematic approach to implementation of improvements in patient care. From time to time there is a breakthrough, whereby with little effort or means, important improvements are made in a short period of time. In most cases, however, the implementation strategy needs to plan for changes in a step-by-step process, thereby ensuring that all conditions for change have been realized. In Chapter 3, we present a framework for a systematic approach to implementation, based on existing models, the so-called implementation of change model (see Figure 3.1).

References

Achterhuis, H. (1998). *Prometheus en het menselijk tekort*. [Prometheus and human failing]. In: Tobben in Voorspoed (ed. H. Achterhuis). Amsterdam: Meulenhof.

Agency for Healthcare Research and Quality (2010). *National Healthcare Quality and Disparities Reports*. Rockville, MD: AHRQ.

Ament, S., de Groot, J., Maessen, J. et al. (2015). Sustainability of professionals' adherence to clinical practice guidelines in medical care: a systematic review. *BMJ Open* 5: e008073.

Ardery, G., Carter, B.L., Milchak, J.L. et al. (2007). Explicit and implicit evaluation of physician adherence to hypertension guidelines. *J. Clin. Hypertens.* 9: 113–119.

Asch, S.M., Kerr, E.A., Keesey, J. et al. (2006). Who is at greatest risk for receiving poor-quality health care? *N. Engl. J. Med.* 354: 1147–1156.

Australian Institute of Health and Welfare (2018). *Hospital Performance: Falls Resulting in Patient Harm in Hospitals*. Sydney, Australia: Australian Institute of Health and Welfare.

Baker, G.R., Norton, P.G., Flintoft, V. et al. (2004). The Canadian Adverse Events Study: the incidence of adverse events among hospital patients in Canada. *CMAJ* 170: 1678–1686.

Bastian, H., Glasziou, P., and Chalmers, I. (2010). Seventy-five trials and eleven systematic reviews a day: how will we ever keep up? *PLoS Med.* 7: e1000326.

Berwick, D. (1998). Developing and testing changes in delivery of care. *Ann. Intern. Med.* 128: 651–656.

Blanchard, J., Weiss, A.J., Barrett, M.L. et al. (2018). State variation in opioid treatment policies and opioid-related hospital admissions. *BMC Health Serv. Res.* 18: 971.

Bolon, M. (2011). Hand Hygiene. *Infect. Dis. Clin. N. Am.* 25: 21–43.

Braspenning, J.C.C., Schellevis, F.G., and Grol, R. P.T.M. (2004). *Tweede Nationale Studie naar ziekten en verrichtingen in de huisartsenpraktijk. Kwaliteit huisartsenzorg belicht. [Second national study of diseases and performances in general practice. Quality of general practice care]*. Nijmegen/Utrecht: WOK/NIVEL.

Brink-Huis, A., Schoonhoven, L., Grol, R. et al. (2010). *Helping Hands. Comparing Short-Term and Sustained Effects of Strategies to Improve Nurses' Adherence with Hand Hygiene Prescriptions*. Nice: International Forum on Quality and Safety in Health Care.

Candy, P.C. (2000). Preventing "information overdose": developing information-literate practitioners. *J. Contin. Educ. Heal. Prof.* 20: 228–237.

Coffey, R.M., Matthews, T.L., and McDermott, K. (2004). *Diabetes Care Quality Improvement: A Resources Guide for State Action*. Rockville, MD: Agency for Healthcare Research and Quality.

Colla, C., Morden, N., Sequist, T. et al. (2014). Choosing wisely: prevalence and correlates of low value healthcare services in the United States. *J. Gen. Intern. Med.* 30: 221–228.

Cullen, K.A., Hall, M.J., and Golosinskiy, A. (2009). *Ambulatory Surgery in the United States, 2006*. Washington, DC: US Department of Health and Human Services, Center for Disease Control and Prevention, National Center for Health Statistics.

Davis, D. and Tailor-Vaisey, A. (1997). Translating guidelines into practice: a systematic review of theoretic concepts, practical experience and research evidence in the adoption of clinical practice guidelines. *CMAJ* 157: 408–416.

Davis, P., Lay-Yee, R., Briant, R. et al. (2002). Adverse events in New Zealand public hospitals I: occurrence and impact. *N. Z. Med. J.* 115: U271.

Dijkstra, R.F., Braspenning, J.C., Huijsmans, Z. et al. (2004). Patients and nurses determine variation in adherence to guidelines at Dutch hospitals more than internists or settings. *Diabet. Med.* 21: 586–591.

Dixon-Woods, M. (2019). *Improving Quality and Safety in Healthcare*. Harveian Oration. London: Royal College of Physicians.

Eccles, M.P. and Mittmann, B.S. (2006). Welcome to implementation science. *Implement. Sci.* 1: 1.

El Sharouni, S.Y., Kal, H.B., and Battermann, J.J. (2003). Accelerated regrowth of non-small-cell lung tumours after induction chemotherapy. *Br. J. Cancer* 89: 2184–2189.

Erasmus, V., Daha, T., Brug, H. et al. (2010). Systematic review of studies on compliance with hand hygiene guidelines in hospitals. *Infect. Control Hosp. Epidemiol.* 31: 283–294.

Gabbay, R.A., Bailit, M.H., and Mauger, D.T. (2011). Multipayer patient-centered medical home implementation guided by the chronic care model. *Jt. Comm. J. Qual. Patient Saf.* 37: 265–273.

Gagliardi, A.R., Berta, W., Kothari, A. et al. (2016). Integrated knowledge translation (IKT) in health care: a scoping review. *Implement. Sci.* 11: 38.

Greenhalgh, T., Robert, G., Macfarlane, F. et al. (2004). Diffusion of innovations in service organizations: systematic review and recommendations. *Milbank Q.* 82: 581–629.

Grimshaw, J.M., Thomas, R.E., MacLennan, G. et al. (2004). Effectiveness and efficiency of guideline dissemination and implementation strategies. *Health Technol. Assess.* 8: 1–84.

Grol, R. (1997). Beliefs and evidence in changing clinical practice. *BMJ* 315: 418–421.

Grol, R. (1999). *Effectieve en doelmatige zorg: feit of fantasie? Inaugurale rede. [Effective and Efficient Care: Fact or Imagination? Inaugural Speech]*. Nijmegen: Radboud University Nijmegen.

Grol, R. (2010). Has guideline development gone astray? Yes. *BMJ* 340: c306.

Grol, R. and Grimshaw, J. (2003). From best evidence to best practice: effective implementation of change in patients' care. *Lancet* 362: 1225–1230.

Grol, R. and van Weel, C. (2009). Getting a grip on guidelines: how to make them more relevant for practice. *Br. J. Gen. Pract.* 59: e143–e144.

Grol, R., Wensing, M., Mainz, J. et al. (2000). J. Patients in Europe evaluate general practice care: an international comparison. *Br. J. Gen. Pract.* 50: 882–887.

Guyatt, G., Meade, M., Jaeschke, R. et al. (2000). Practitioners of evidence based care. *BMJ* 320: 954–955.

Haines, A. (1996). The science of perpetual change. *Br. J. Gen. Pract.* 46: 115–1159.

Hulscher, M., Wensing, M., and Grol, R. (2000). *Effectieve implementatie: Theorieën en strategieën. [Effective Implementation: Theories and Strategies]*. The Hague: ZONMW.

Innvaer, S., Vist, G., Trommald, M., and Oxman, A. (2002). Health policy-makers' perceptions of their use of evidence: a systematic review. *J. Health Serv. Res. Policy* 7: 239–244.

Institute of Medicine (2000). *To Err Is Human: Building a Safer Health System*. Washington, DC: Institute of Medicine.

Ioannidis, J.P.A., Greenland, S., Hlatky, M.A. et al. (2014). Increasing value and reducing waste in research design, conduct, and analysis. *Lancet* 383: 166–175.

Johansen, H., Brien, S.E., Fines, P. et al. (2010). Thirty-day in-hospital revascularization and mortality rates after acute myocardial infarction in seven Canadian provinces. *Can. J. Cardiol.* 26: e243–e248.

Kitson, A., Harvey, G., and McCormack, B. (1998). Enabling the implementation of evidence based practice: a conceptual framework. *Qual. Health Care* 7: 149–158.

Krumholz, H.M., Wang, Y., Chen, J. et al. (2009). Reduction in acute myocardial infarction mortality in the United States. *JAMA* 302: 767–773.

Lomas, J. (2007). The in-between world of knowledge brokering. *BMJ* 334: 129–132.

McColl, A., Smith, H., White, P. et al. (1998). General practitioners' perceptions of the route to evidence based medicine: a questionnaire survey. *BMJ* 316: 361–365.

McGlynn, E.A., Asch, S.M., Adams, J. et al. (2003). The quality of health care delivered to adults in the United States. *N. Engl. J. Med.* 348: 2635–2645.

Naylor, C. (1995). Grey zones of clinical practice: some limits to evidence-based medicine. *Lancet* 345: 840–842.

Null, G., Dean, C., Feldman, M., and Rasio, D. (2005). Death by medicine. *J. Orthomol. Med.* 20: 21–34.

OECD (2017). Health at a glance. http://www.oecd.org/health/health-systems/health-at-a-glance-19991312.htm (accessed November 4, 2019).

Ouwens, M., Hermens, R., Termeer, R. et al. (2007). Quality of integrated care for patients with nonsmall cell lung cancer. Variations and determinants of care. *Cancer* 110: 1782–1790.

Park-Lee, E. and Caffrey, C. (2009). *Pressure Ulcers among Nursing Home Residents: United States, 2004*. Washington, DC: US Department of Health and Human Services, Centers for Disease Control and Prevention, National Center for Health Statistics.

Petek, D., Kunzi, B., Kersnik, J. et al. (2011). Patients' evaluations of European general practice – revisited after 11 years. *Int. J. Qual. Health Care* 23: 621–628.

Prasad, V. and Ionnidis, J.P.A. (2014). Evidence-based de-implementation for contradicted, unproven, and aspiring healthcare practices. *Implement. Sci.* 9: 1.

RIVM (2017). *PREZIES landelijk surveillance netwerk ziekenhuisinfecties [PREZIES National Surveillance Network Hospital Infections]*. Bilthoven: RIVM.

Runciman, W.B., Hunt, T.D., Hannaford, N.A. et al. (2012). CareTrack: assessing the appropriateness of health care delivery in Australia. *Med. J. Aust.* 197: 100–105.

Sackett, D., Richardson, W., Rosenberg, W., and Haynes, R. (1997). *Evidence-Based Medicine: How to Practice and Teach*. London: Churchill Livingstone.

Schoen, C., Osborn, R., How, S.K.H. et al. (2009). In chronic condition: experiences of patients with complex health care needs, in eight countries. *Health Aff.* 28: w1–w16.

Schouten, L.M.T., Hulscher, M.E.J.L., and Grol, R.P.T.M. (2010). Determinants of success in quality improvement collaboratives: what factors relate to effectiveness? In: *Quality improvement collaborative. Cost-effectiveness and determinants of success* (ed. L.M.T. Schouten). Thesis. Nijmegen: Radboud University Nijmegen.

Schünemann, H.J., Wiercioch, W., Etxeandia, I. et al. (2014). Guidelines 2.0: systematic development of a comprehensive checklist for a successful guideline enterprise. *CMAJ* 186: E123–E142.

Teare, L., Cockson, B., and Stone, S. (2001). Hand hygiene. *BMJ* 323: 411–412.

Tetroe, J., Graham, I., Foy, R. et al. (2008). Health research funding agencies' support and promotion of knowledge translation: an international study. *Milbank Q.* 86: 125–155.

Tomlin, Z., Humphrey, C., and Rogers, S. (1999). General practitioners' perceptions of effective health care. *BMJ* 318: 1532–1535.

Van den Bemt, P. (2002). *Drug safety in hospitalized patients*. Thesis. Groningen: Rijksuniversiteit Groningen.

Van Gaal, B.G., Schoonhoven, L., Mintjes-de Groot, J.A. et al. (2014). Concurrent incidence of adverse events in hospitals and nursing homes. *J. Nurs. Scholarsh.* 46: 187–198.

Van Woerkom, C. and Adolfse, L. (1998). Interactieve kennisontwikkeling en -benutting. [Interactive development and use of knowledge]. *J. Syst. Integr.* 1: 10–19.

de Vries, E.N., Ramrattan, M.A., Smorenburg, S. M. et al. (2008). The incidence and nature of in-hospital adverse events: a systematic review. *Qual. Saf. Health Care* 17: 216–223.

Wagner, C. (2017). *Patientveiligheid in ziekenhuizen: 12.5 jaar onderzoek, successen en nieuwe uitdagingen [Patient safety in hospitals: 12.5 years research, successes and new challenges]*. Utrecht: Nivel.

Wensing, M., van Splunteren, P., Hulscher, M. et al. (2000). *Praktisch nieuw. Implementatie van vernieuwingen in de gezondheidszorg. [Practically New. Implementation of Innovations in Healthcare]*. Assen: Van Gorcum.

Wilson, R.M., Runciman, W.B., Gibberd, R.W. et al. (1995). The quality in Australian health care study. *Med. J. Aust.* 163: 458–476.

Yapa, H.M. and Bärnighausen, T. (2018). Implementation science in resource-poor countries and communities. *Implement. Sci.* 13: 154.

ZON (1997). *Met het oog op toepassing. Beleidsnota Implementatie Zorg Onderzoek Nederland 1997–1999. [With a View to Application. Policy Document Implementation ZON 1997–1999]*. The Hague: ZON.

2

Theories on Implementation of Change in Healthcare

Michel Wensing[1,2,3] and Richard Grol[4,5]

[1] *Faculty of Medicine, University of Heidelberg, Heidelberg, Germany*
[2] *Department of General Practice and Health Services Research, Heidelberg University Hospital, Heidelberg, Germany*
[3] *Department IQ healthcare, Radboud Institute for Health Sciences, Radboud University Medical Center, Nijmegen, The Netherlands*
[4] *Radboud University, Nijmegen, The Netherlands*
[5] *Maastricht University, Maastricht, The Netherlands*

SUMMARY

- Many theories, models, and frameworks for the implementation of innovations have been proposed, based on different scientific views on change of individual and organizational performance.
- Some theories focus on change within the individual professionals, others on change within the social setting, the organization, societal regulations, or economic structures.
- A number of theories from different disciplines are presented in this chapter, ordered in four categories: theories that focus on individual behaviors, theories about social processes, theories about organizational systems, and theories about economic and societal structures.
- The evidence for the validity of theories in healthcare settings is mixed and overall limited.

2.1 Introduction

Occasionally, the implementation of new scientific findings, new procedures, or best practices happens quickly and easily. For example, the finding from randomized controlled trials showing that myringotomy in cases of acute otitis media in children was no more effective than a conservative approach of waiting and giving medication was rapidly and widely adopted in practice. Publication of this finding was sufficient for physicians to stop performing this procedure within a short time – perhaps because most children and parents disliked it so much. However, producing change is usually much more challenging, particularly if the innovation requires complex changes in clinical practice, better collaboration between health professionals, changes in patient behavior, or changes in the organization of care.

New evidence, best practices, or new procedures rarely implement themselves. In most cases, a large number of factors determines whether or not implementation is successful. Determinants of implementation can be organized according to the following categories (Grol 1992; Damschroeder et al. 2009; Wensing et al.

Improving Patient Care: The Implementation of Change in Health Care, Third Edition. Edited by Michel Wensing, Richard Grol, and Jeremy Grimshaw.
© 2020 John Wiley & Sons Ltd. Published 2020 by John Wiley & Sons Ltd.

2010; Flottorp et al. 2013), characterized here as features of:

- *The innovation itself*: some innovations are more evidence based, better formulated, more credible, and/or better adapted to the needs of clinical practice or fit better to the norms and values of the target group than others.
- *The target group of professionals intended as users of the innovation*: their knowledge, skills, opinions, attitudes, values, routines, and/or personalities can facilitate or impede implementation.
- *The patients*: their attitudes, knowledge, behaviors, routines, needs, and preferences can also stimulate or hinder successful implementation.
- *The social and practice setting*: the attitude of colleagues, the culture in the team or social network, and the view of opinion leaders, as well as the style of leadership in the organization, can be of influence.
- *The organizational system, regulations, and economic structures*: these can exert powerful influences on practice routines and on the successful implementation of innovations.
- *The strategies for dissemination and implementation used*: these will have more or less effect depending on the choice of the intervention methods, their intensity and duration, and the source and change agents involved.

In developing effective strategies and interventions for change, a rigorous analysis and sound insight into these factors is of importance (Grol and Wensing 2004). For this understanding to be fully developed, knowledge regarding the hypotheses and theoretical assumptions underlying each factor is needed. Often, implementation of change is based on implicit beliefs or preconceptions of human behavior and of changing that behavior (Grol 1997). Making these ideas explicit and testing their validity in practice contribute to the effectiveness of implementation strategies. If systematic methods are applied, this can also contribute to the accumulation of scientific knowledge on how to improve healthcare practice, management, and policy. The latter would further support future improvement and implementation activities in healthcare; valid theories have high practical value.

Theories on implementation of change explain which conditions, factors, and interventions contribute to the implementation of an innovation. Such theories can be found in a large number of disciplines and scientific areas – for example in psychology, sociology, educational science, communication science, organizational science, economics, and political science. In addition to theories from specific disciplines, many theories, models, and frameworks for implementation practice and research have been proposed. A systematic review identified 159 theories, although the search was restricted to publications from the year 2000 onward (Striffler et al. 2018). However, most (60%) were used on only one empirical study. Restricted by the context of one chapter, we cannot present an exhaustive overview of theories. Instead, our aim is to offer a number of relevant examples of theories at different levels of healthcare related to individual healthcare professionals, the influence of the social context on change, the organization of care, and the wider political and economic context.

Rossi et al. (1999) divided theories into impact theories and process theories. *Impact theories* (also called determinant frameworks; Nilsen 2015) describe hypotheses and assumptions about how a specific intervention will facilitate a desired change, as well as the causes, effects, and factors determining success (or the lack of it) in improving healthcare. *Process theories* (also called theories of change) refer to implementation activities: how they are best planned, organized, and scheduled in order to be effective and how the target group will utilize and be influenced by the activities. Nilsen (2015) further distinguishes classic theories, implementation theories, and evaluation frameworks to the taxonomy. These further categories relate to the origins or purpose of the theories. In this chapter we focus primarily on *impact theories*; process theories are elaborated in Chapter 3. Throughout the chapter, two practical and commonplace examples will be used to illustrate the theories: hand hygiene and diabetes care (see Box 2.1).

2.2 Theories on Factors Related to Individual Professionals

Several theories describe individual factors which influence change. These concern the way professionals make decisions and associated factors, such as their attitudes and motivation with respect to realizing a particular change. Social or structural factors may be included in these theories, but they are treated as context for the decisions and behaviors of individuals. The following theories will be described:

- Cognitive theories
- Educational theories
- Motivational theories.

2.2.1 Cognitive Theories

Cognitive theories focus on the thinking and decision making of individual professionals and offer links to changing these processes. *Rational decision-making theories* assume an analytical model in which professionals consider and balance the advantages and disadvantages of different alternatives. Decision support may provide information and guidance, which play a role in this process. In this context, the provision of convincing information on risks and benefits and pros and cons is seen as crucial for performance change. In our hand hygiene example, this theory views the lack of compliance with existing guidelines primarily as a knowledge and decision-making problem. The professionals need to be well informed about and convinced by the scientific evidence on the consequences of inappropriate hand hygiene, and they need to perceive the benefits of regular washing to weigh against the disadvantages of the extra work or time involved.

Other cognitive theories show how decisions are actually made, and what factors influence these processes. A *cognitive–psychological approach* states that clinicians do not necessarily act rationally, but decide primarily on the basis of heuristics, which are derived from previous experiences and contextual information (Brehaut and Eva 2012). When they diagnose a health problem, they employ "illness scripts," cognitive structures in which they have organized their knowledge about a specific health problem and in which previous experiences with specific patients are seen as crucial for further decision making. These cognitive scripts have also been described as "mindlines" (Wieringa and Greenhalgh 2015). Experienced physicians diagnose patients more quickly because they have more cases available mentally and use the contextual information of such cases better (Hobus 1994). However, they may use obsolete knowledge as the basis of their performance.

Many cognitive mechanisms have been described, which may prevent rational decision making (Koele and van der Pligt 1993). For instance, individuals prefer consistency in thinking and acting and will make choices that may not be rational, but fit with existing opinions, needs, and behaviors (Festinger 1954). When they do not like repetitive hand washing or doubt the effect of it, they will interpret or seek information that confirms their beliefs and doubts. Individuals may also look for external explanations for specific events (such as hospital infections) instead of internal ones, in order to make them more acceptable to themselves or bring them more in line with existing perceptions (Jones et al. 1972).

Dual process theories distinguish between two information-processing routes: a central or systematic route, in which messages are carefully considered and compared to other

---

Box 2.1   The Complexity of Changing Practice: The Cases of Hand Hygiene and Diabetes

In many healthcare systems, the reduction of *hospital-acquired infections* remains high on the agenda. Such infections are estimated to affect about 1 in 11 patients, with high mortality and an increased length of stay in the hospital of a factor of 2.5. The extra cost per patient with an infection in the UK was about £3000 (Stone 2001). Between 15 and 30% of the infections are considered to be preventable. One of the main possible improvements is better hand washing and disinfecting by professionals between patient contacts. The importance of hand hygiene has been recognized since the mid-1800s, starting with Ignaz Semmelweis's discovery that hand disinfection reduced maternal morbidity in obstetric patients. Since then, we have been regularly bombarded with evidence of the importance of good hand hygiene (Pratt et al. 2001; Stone 2001). The treatment effect is so substantial that "if hand hygiene were a new drug it would be used by all." Nevertheless, compliance by health workers in general and physicians in particular is suboptimal and sometimes poor (Teare et al. 2001). Many hospitals have guidelines on the prevention of infections, but these are often not followed, and physicians largely overestimate their own routines in hand hygiene (Handwashing Liaison Group 1999). Thus, a well-established evidence base is available, summarized in disseminated clinical guidelines on the prevention of hospital infections. Most clinical professionals have been educated, at least by formal methods, on its importance. And yet, performance remains poor.

Factors influencing *diabetes care* and compliance with national clinical practice guidelines for internal medicine physicians were measured by a survey in the Netherlands (N = 96 partnerships). The survey showed considerable differences in the organization of healthcare (e.g. the presence or absence of a diabetes nurse, diabetes team meetings, and separate surgery for diabetes patients; Dijkstra 2004). Barriers to optimizing care were shown to be diverse and related to the following areas:

Perceived barrier		
Professional		
Cognitions	Lack of evidence for guideline recommendations	36%
	Guideline not read	35%
	Lack of knowledge regarding best practice	35%
Attitude	Guidelines are too rigid	58%
	Resistance against proposed way of working	52%
Social context		
	Lack of support from hospital management	46%
	Physicians disagree with respect to best practice	36%
Organizational context		
	Working according to the guidelines means additional work for internal medicine physicians	84%
	Working according to the guidelines costs extra time	56%
	Lack of supportive staff	48%
	Lack of capacity eye specialist	45%
Economic context		
	No financial compensation	59%

Problems in improving the care proved to be related not only to individual care providers, but also to the social, organizational, and economic context in which they function. Different theories on innovation and implementation can offer ideas for effective change of care for this patient group. Ideally, an effective plan for change should take all these into account.

messages and opinions; and a peripheral or heuristic route, in which the focus is predominantly on cues, such as attractive "packaging" of the message, the perceived credibility of the source, and the response of others to the message (Evans and Stanovich 2013). It may be assumed that messages which are processed through the systematic route are more likely to persist.

Thus, using various cognitive theories, a lack of hand hygiene by physicians can be explained by a lack of relevant scientific information or doubts regarding the implications of the evidence, by incorrectly balancing advantages and disadvantages, or by attributing infections to causes outside their control. In this context, it may be important to focus on the way professionals collect and process information and make decisions about their daily work. For instance, professional conferences are a crucial means for transfer of new knowledge in medical disciplines. Well-developed high-quality practice guidelines and computerized decision support can support the uptake of knowledge in routine practice.

2.2.2 Educational Theories

Many modern educational theories focus less on cognition than on the motivation to learn and improve. For instance, *adult learning theories* state that individuals learn better and are more motivated to change when they base their learning on problems experienced in practice, rather than when they are confronted with abstract information, such as guidelines (Norman and Schmidt 1992; Mann 1994; Merriam 1996; Holm 1998; Walker and Leary 2009). Professionals have a large reservoir of experiences which can be used as a source for learning and changing (Smith et al. 1998). In particular, older professionals who have acquired much experience have more individual learning needs and have frequently developed sophisticated competencies in self-directed learning.

How can we apply this set of theories to our clinical example? In order to improve hand hygiene in a hospital, the care providers involved need to experience a problem first of all, for instance that their behavior leads to infections in patients, and they need to be motivated to do something about it. The theory offers a framework to structure an appropriate approach: first to discuss experiences with this complex problem; then subsequently to explore experiences with effective solutions within the professionals' own work setting.

Principles of *problem-based* and *self-directed learning* can be used effectively in the implementation of change or innovations in healthcare, although the assumptions behind the theory remain contested (Norman 2002) and the evidence regarding their effectiveness is still limited (Smits et al. 2002). In many countries, projects are conducted in which physicians plan, perform, monitor, and evaluate their own learning and change process – so-called portfolio learning (Holm 1998). However, not all care providers possess the information, competency, and motivation to do this or to do it well. Learners who excel at self-directed learning have been described by a variety of adjectives: methodical, logical, reflective, analytical, flexible, responsible, creative, independent, open, and motivated (Mann 1994) – not a simple set of requirements for successful learning.

Another factor seen as important in educational theories is that the change process is linked to the *personal learning style* of professionals. Lewis and Bolden (1989) distinguish between four learning styles: *activists* (individuals who like new experiences and therefore accept but also abandon innovations quickly), *reflective professionals* (individuals who want to consider all options very carefully before changing), *theoretical learners* (individuals who prefer a rigorous analysis and good thinking to explain why a change would be needed), and *pragmatists* (individuals who prefer to act on the basis of practical experience with an innovation). Many care providers prefer a pragmatic learning style (Nylenna et al. 1996; Mammen et al. 2007). A program targeted at improving diabetes care or hand hygiene should ideally take into account the individual learning needs and personal motives of professionals as well as their personal learning styles.

Finally, the role of social interaction has been much emphasized in some theories of learning, and it has also found some application in the design of implementation strategies in healthcare (Thomas et al. 2014). *Social constructivist education theory* emphasizes that users (should) also influence the creation of knowledge, an idea that is known as "integrated knowledge translation" (Graham et al. 2006). In programs for the improvement of healthcare, such as hand hygiene, this implies stakeholder involvement from the earliest phase onward.

2.2.3 Motivational Theories

Motivational theories focus strongly on the role of attitudes, perceptions, and intentions toward the desired performance. These include theories such as those developed by Fishbein and Ajzen (1975), Ajzen (1988), and Kok et al. (1991). One of the most frequently used theories is that of *planned behavior*, which postulates that any given behavior of a professional (clinician, nurse, manager, allied health professional) is influenced by their individual intentions to perform that specific behavior, and, in turn, that these intentions are determined largely by attitudes concerning the behavior, by perceived social norms, and by perceived control related to the behavior (Ajzen 1991). Each of these factors can be addressed in implementation. The attitude concerning a specific behavior (such as hand washing before and/or after each contact with a patient) is determined by the expected outcomes of this behavior (i.e. it will lead to fewer infections in the hospital) and the positive or negative appraisal of these outcomes (i.e. that these outcomes are or are not worth the extra effort). Perceived social norms are influenced

by the behaviors seen in others (e.g. whether others wash or disinfect their hands regularly, particularly clinical leaders) and the importance attached to these norms. The perceived or experienced control, or self-efficacy expectations (Bandura 1986), represents the belief that one can really achieve the desired change in the specific setting (regular hand washing under time pressure, for example).

A consortium of British psychologists analyzed 131 concepts from 31 theories on behavior change and categorized these into 12 domains, using motivational theories of behavior as the foundation (Michie et al. 2005). The resulting framework (theoretical domains framework) has been widely applied in research on factors associated with implementation (Francis et al. 2012). For instance, Walker et al. (2001) used the framework in a study of physicians' intention to prescribe antibiotics for uncomplicated sore throat. Attitudes and expected impact correlated highly with intention to prescribe antibiotics. In subsequent work, a taxonomy of 93 psychological behavior change techniques has been developed (Michie et al. 2013) and a comprehensive framework for planning behavior change interventions (the "behaviour change wheel") has been proposed (Michie et al. 2011).

One has also to take into account that professionals may have different motives in relation to envisaging and preparing for change. For instance, research among nurses and physiotherapists showed that the most important reason to take part in training was the wish to improve professional competency (Tassone and Heck 1997). Fox and Bennett (1998) distinguished between 10 different factors influencing change processes of physicians, such as curiosity, personal and financial well-being, career planning, wish to improve competency, pressure from patients, and pressure from colleagues.

In conclusion, in designing programs to improve diabetes care or hand hygiene, one needs to account for and address these different motivational factors to realize successful change. For instance, one will need to help motivate the target group regarding the desired behavior, allow them to experience that colleagues and others in their social environment think the change is very important, and provide them with the confidence that change will indeed be feasible and achievable.

2.3 Theories on Social Processes

Theories which focus on the influence of social processes on change emphasize the importance of factors in the interaction between people, such as mutual influence taking place in group processes or teams, the influence of key individuals and opinion leaders, the role of social networks, and the role of leaders. Some theories, many with overlapping elements, are presented here:

- Social learning theory and other broad theories
- Theories on communication
- Social network theories
- Theories on teamwork
- Theories on professionalization
- Theories on leadership.

2.3.1 Social Learning Theory

The social cognitive or social learning theory of Bandura (1986) is a broad theory of human behavior, which is related to classic behavioral theories. It explains the behavior of individuals in terms of personal, behavioral, and contextual factors. *Contextual factors* include characteristics of the setting in which the healthcare professional operates and in which reinforcement of performance takes place. Important contextual factors are the material or nonmaterial rewards of others (e.g. positive comments by peers or opinion leaders) as well as modeling the behavior of others. Such modeling implies the observation in others that it is possible to demonstrate the behavior (such as consistently cleaning hands before and after each patient contact) and that this leads to the expected results and will be rewarded. *Personal factors* are those concerned with the skill of the individual to learn by experience, by doing, and by observation of the behavior of others. *Behavioral factors*, finally, are concerned with the ability to actually perform the desired behavior, such as hand washing. Relating this to our example of inadequate hand hygiene, the theory particularly addresses the issue of care providers observing each other and the performance of "leaders" in the setting, as well as the importance of positive reinforcement of the desired performance by peers and important others in the work setting.

A similar categorization was proposed by Michie and colleagues. They distinguished between capability, opportunity, and motivation (Michie et al. 2011). In this perspective, change is primarily perceived as an individual process; social environment, organization, and broader structures are considered "context." Coming from another scientific background, the normalization process theory of May (2013) defines a different set of factors: potential (individual psychological factors), capacity (opportunities in the context), and capability (guidance by implementation programs). Key factors in May's theory are perceived coherence (whether the innovation makes sense for participants), cognitive participation (whether they are committed and engaged), collective action (work to make the innovation function), and reflexive monitoring (reflection on and appraisal of the innovation). A key assumption in this approach is that these processes mainly occur in interactions with others, thus the results are socially constructed. Normalization process theory has been applied in a range of studies (McKevoy et al. 2014).

2.3.2 Theories on Communication

Several theories describe how effective communication can influence attitudes and behavior, which is implicitly or explicitly included in many approaches to implementation and improvement in healthcare (Manojlevic et al. 2015). For instance, the *persuasion communication model* states that, for effective communication, one needs to be exposed and attentive to the message, understand its arguments and conclusions, accept these arguments, remember the content of the messages, and, finally, change attitude. For this process to be successful, the communication should be tailored to each phase. The characteristics of the sender of the message (such as status and credibility) and those of the receiver (such as intelligence, previous knowledge, and involvement) are important in this process. For a program aiming to improve hand washing, it is important to provide the opportunity for the receiver of the message to carefully consider and accept it, and to use convincing messages, repeatedly communicated by credible sources. Characteristics of the message that are related to its ability to convince the recipient include novelty, perceived validity, personal relevance, and functionality. In examples such as hand hygiene and diabetes care, it may be possible to find new and effective ways to communicate messages to targeted health professionals.

2.3.3 Social Network Theories

Theories on the diffusion of innovations state that the adoption of new ideas and technologies is influenced by the structure of social networks (Rogers 2003). Healthcare providers exchange information, refer patients to each other, make arrangements, and have other types of interactions. The patterns in these interactions comprise a naturally emerging social network, which often becomes relatively stable over time. Theory on social networks argues that individuals in the margins of a social network are frequently the source of information on innovations, because they tend to participate in different networks simultaneously (e.g. in a healthcare organization and in a professional group; Valente 1996). As innovations are now easily disseminated through the internet, it remains to be seen whether this claim is valid nowadays.

A social network influences behaviors in several ways. First, it influences the spread of innovations. For instance, a high density of connections in a network seems favorable for the rapid dissemination (also called contagion) of innovations. Also, the social influence processes in networks often result in the selection of similar individuals in a network, which enhances social influence processes. Second, it influences the allocation of tasks and thus collaboration between health professionals and coordination of care. A number of theories, often based on social exchange and game theory, specify the determinants of collaboration (Dijkstra and Van Assen 2017), but their relevance in healthcare remains to be explored. For instance, individuals with a central position in the network (e.g. case managers for specific types of patients) may play a key role in this process. The influence of social networks is not necessarily facilitated or mediated by individual decision making, thus it is often not actively perceived or experienced by individuals despite its impact (Mittman et al. 1992; Greer 1988).

The role of *local opinion leaders* is a practically useful component of social network theories. They are considered, within their setting, as respected persons with great influence in a specific field. They are not necessarily the innovators, but can be regarded as role models for the network, and they act as facilitator, supporter, and problem solver in the change process. Through their place in the network or their informal contacts, they can easily facilitate the diffusion of information. Opinion leaders represent the social norms within the network and therefore others trust them to appraise innovations against existing social norms and the specific demands of the local situation. The presence of such important key persons within social networks in healthcare has been confirmed in a number of studies, while other studies in healthcare settings suggest that their role is limited (Doumit et al. 2011).

A program on improving hand hygiene and disinfection in hospitals or improving diabetes management in primary care using these theories would focus on the interactions in teams and networks, on the values of the opinion leaders within the networks, and on the ways members influence each other. It is crucial to enlist key persons in the network and provide them with role-modeling skills and competencies. Stability and frequent contact in a network of healthcare providers contribute to the influence of the network on behaviors. Interactions between teams who have gone through the changes and teams who have not yet done so is also important, for example by letting a person from a successful team join another team temporarily.

2.3.4 Theories on Teamwork

Increasingly, patient care is delivered by teams of health professionals. Enhancing teamwork is seen as a way to tackle the fragmentation of care and to improve care for specific patient groups. It has been embraced by many health professions, in particular nursing (RWJF 2011). Clinical teams may be mono-, multi-, or interprofessional; they typically meet regularly to coordinate patient care. Effective clinical teams define and assign tasks and roles, train individuals to perform these roles and tasks, and establish clear structures and processes for communication (Grumbach and Bodenheimer 2004). *Theories on teamwork* in social psychology have specified many factors which have an impact on the processes and outcomes of teamwork. They include, for instance, the presence of a team leader (Shortell et al. 2004), mutual trust (Firth-Cozins 1998), team vision, task orientation (the commitment of team members to perform as well as possible), support for innovation (West 1990), and participative safety (how much the team participates in making decisions and whether team members feel

psychologically safe in proposing new ideas). Structural factors, such as team size and composition, can also be relevant. Effective clinical teams can improve the safety, effectiveness, and efficiency of patient care (West et al. 2002).

For our hand hygiene and diabetes examples, this approach means that an improvement program should aim to encourage team collaboration to tackle these problems. Also, professionals with specific expertise may be added to the team to enhance its performance (e.g. pharmacist, nurse practitioner). The team should define a clear goal and set targets – for example, the maximum number of infections on a ward or the number of diabetes patients followed up – and regularly review whether these targets are met as well as roles and responsibilities in meeting them.

2.3.5 Theories on Professionalization

Professionals (such as physicians and nurses) have a body of knowledge not easily accessible to non-professionals and highly valued by society because of its practical relevance to citizens. *Sociological theories on professionalization* describe a number of factors which may influence change in professional behavior (Freidson 1970, 2001). The health professions have usually succeeded in obtaining a certain degree of autonomy in their decisions. Access to the professions is based on training and examination, controlled by members of the profession. Information is disseminated via professional journals or similar electronic communication channels. Professionalization can influence behavior change in different ways. The development of "professional standards," which may or may not be in line with innovations, have the potential to significantly hinder or facilitate the implementation of specific innovations.

The fact that professions have a strong internal orientation means that members' main loyalty often tends to be to their profession, specialty, or discipline rather than to the healthcare organizations in which they practice. *Organizational science theories* have elaborated on the position of professionals in organizations (Mintzberg 1996). Professions also produce, assess, and transfer new knowledge in their field by being involved in research, theory, and knowledge transfer. Many healthcare organizations are professional bureaucracies, in which professionals (individually and collectively) possess a high degree of autonomy and authority (Mintzberg 1996). Rather than the organization or its management, specific professionals are responsible for the implementation of innovations. Most decision making takes place within organizational units. For instance, decisions on technological innovations are often dominated by a small group of professionals (e.g. radiologists, pathologists, anesthesiologists).

Innovations which are consistent with the developing body of knowledge in a profession are more likely to be implemented than other innovations. For our examples in hand hygiene or diabetes care, this theory particularly emphasizes the importance of using professional pride, professional standards, and professional loyalties to transfer the idea that something needs to be done about poor care. National guidelines should at least be endorsed by a profession or specialty as the professional standard and adapted to local practices if needed.

2.3.6 Theories on Leadership

Formal or informal leaders can be very influential in changing clinical practice or a healthcare organization. A "clinician leader," for example, may be a full-time manager but may also have informal influence, for example in the role of a respected senior physician or nurse (Øvretveit 2004). While the top management takes strategic decisions that determine the conditions, the implementation of innovations in practice is highly dependent on leaders of teams and organizational units (Aarons et al. 2014).

Therefore, it is important to involve middle management in implementation programs.

Theories on leadership have elaborated on the role of leaders in organizations. Effective leadership is assumed to promote, guarantee, or (in some circumstances) impede an innovation. Such power or influence can be based on different sources: on formal authority; on control over scarce resources; on possession of information, expertise, or skills needed to achieve specific, valued aims; on being part of a strong social network; or on belonging to a dominant culture (Donaldson 1995). Leaders can influence the organizational climate by the way they allocate attention, respond to incidents, allocate resources and rewards, show exemplary behavior, offer coaching, and select new staff (Aarons et al. 2014). Quality improvement can be stimulated by leaders by involving physicians, training staff members, delegating responsibilities, showing personal commitment, showing a good example, and demonstrating a vision for change (Øvretveit 2004).

Specific types of leadership are probably effective for specific innovations in specific settings. For instance, in changing the culture and mission of a hospital on the prevention of infections, a different leader may be required than for implementing a new operating technique or new imaging equipment. Ross and Offerman (1997) make a distinction between two types of leadership: transactional and transformational leadership (Aarons et al. 2014). The first type of leader provides support in achieving concrete targets, while the second type is particularly effective in changing the culture in the organization and the ambitions of the individuals who work there.

The effective implementation of guidelines on infection prevention or hand hygiene requires a clear understanding of who in the organization are the formal and informal leaders, how they use their power or influence, and how this can be used optimally within a plan aimed at specific changes in patient care. Inadequate hand hygiene could at least in part be traced to a lack of interest and commitment in this area by the managers and leaders in teams and hospitals. In this case, they would need to make the active prevention of infections part of the mission and policies of the hospital, support it intellectually, provide resources for it, and set up monitoring and tracking systems on infections (Teare et al. 2001).

2.4 Theories on Organizational Systems

These theories find the opportunity for change in patient care particularly in organizational factors and processes, such as better organization of care processes, a different division of tasks and roles, a change in the culture in the work setting, or collaboration between professionals. The following theoretical approaches are explored in this section:

- Theories of effective organizations
- Theory of quality and safety management
- Theory of operations management
- Theory of complex systems
- Theory of organizational learning
- Theories of organizational culture.

2.4.1 Theories of Effective Organizations

This approach focuses on the characteristics of organizations which determine whether and to what extent they are able to implement innovations (Wolfe 1994). Some organizations adopt innovations more quickly and easily than other organizations. Specific characteristics of organizations such as hospitals may be associated with innovativeness. A review of studies found that innovativeness was predicted by a high level of specialization, functional differentiation, a high level of professionalism, decentralized decision making, better technical knowledge, good internal and external communication, a positive attitude to change among leaders and managers, and, finally, the ability to overcome problems financially (Damanpour 1991). No associations were found between the extent of formalization, management tenure, and vertical differentiation and innovation. Associations between organizational characteristics and innovation differed however between commercial and not-for-profit organizations, between industry and service organizations, and between single and multifaceted innovations. It can be concluded that (static) characteristics of organizations may be related to the uptake of innovations, but it remains uncertain whether these associations are consistent or predictable.

2.4.2 Theory of Quality and Safety Management

Quality and safety management approaches argue that improvement of outcomes requires continuous attention, and that audit and feedback of performance measures to decision makers, followed by planned improvement, are key drivers. Total quality management (TQM), or continuous quality improvement (CQI), is a theory stressing the importance of the continuous improvement of multidisciplinary processes in healthcare with the aim of better meeting the needs of customers (Shortell et al. 1998). While this is more a theory of change than a theory of practice, we briefly summarize it, as it puts emphasis on specific types of determinants of practice and has been highly influential in healthcare across the world.

Quality management was introduced in healthcare by Berwick (1989), Berwick et al. (1990), Batalden and Stoltz (1993), and Laffel and Blumenthal (1989) after successful use in other industries. Quality management has become widely adopted, particularly in hospitals. It emphasizes the importance of a thorough understanding and improvement of work processes and systems of healthcare delivery. Inadequate performance is not seen as an individual problem but as a system failure, and real change can only be achieved by changing the system (Berwick 1989). Safety management also emphasizes the systems and processes of healthcare delivery. Organizational changes, strong leadership, and team building are important components of this approach.

Basic principles of quality management are (Plsek et al. 2003): a comprehensive, organization-wide effort to improve quality (activities at all levels of the organization); a patient- and customer-centered focus; continuous improvement and redesign of care processes; alternating periods of change with periods of relative stability; and management by objective information (continuously monitoring data, evidence-based guidelines, and protocols). A positive view of individuals is central to TQM: performance gaps are related to organizations rather than to individual professionals. The use of Plan–Do–Study–Act cycles (PDSA cycles; Langley et al. 2009) is an important tool in improving care (see Box 2.2; Langley et al. 2009). Finally, as for other approaches, the need for effective and visionary leadership is a central theme in TQM. Leaders must be actively involved in the initiation of and support for all improvement activities.

The implementation of quality improvement and safety management is a challenge in itself. Determinants of successful execution include the participation of clinicians, the provision of feedback to individual clinicians, and a supporting organizational culture (Shortell et al. 1998). An investment in quality improvement is also needed; gaining professional expertise costs time and money (Øvretveit 2004). Quality management is an intensive approach for both individuals and organizations, with its focus on an open culture, continuous leadership, training and support of staff, continuous monitoring, and well-functioning data systems (Gustafson and Hundt 1995).

When we apply this theory to our examples of diabetes care and hand hygiene, the focus of an improvement program should be less on changing individual behavior and more on understanding processes that are associated with optimal disease management. Starting with a sound insight into these processes, one could set ambitious goals for improvement (such as a reduction in the number of complications by 25%) and encourage

---

Box 2.2   The Plan–Do–Study–Act Cycle

The PDSA cycle to change healthcare processes uses continuous learning by introducing and reflecting on changes (Langley et al. 2009). Generally, one cycle is considered inefficient; improvements in a system usually require gradual changes made in various cycles. This contrasts with changes that are implemented in one single large change effort. Before starting a PDSA cycle, three crucial questions need to be asked:

- *What are we trying to accomplish?* For this, the formulation of specific, ambitious goals to meet external needs and expectations is required. Leaders have the responsibility to help formulate and clarify these goals.
- *How will we know that a change is an improvement?* This encompasses measuring or monitoring of the change to guide the process and support change; not for incentive, punishment, and selection purposes. Leaders have to ensure the correct purpose of monitoring.
- *What changes can we make that will result in improvement?* This means selecting optimal strategies for change. Leaders have to challenge the status quo, show it is unacceptable to continue in the old way, and enable a vision of truly innovative care.

multidisciplinary teams to work toward these goals via PDSA cycles, while continuous evaluation and monitoring of care outcomes take place to show possible improvements. The entire process must be actively supported and shared by formal and informal leaders in the organizations involved.

2.4.3 Theory of Operations Management

Like quality management, the *theory of operations management* focuses on the design and functioning of healthcare delivery processes, covering both incremental changes and disruptive redesign. Approaches such as business process redesign (BPR), integrated care, and disease management aim to better organize and manage care processes, in particular for specific patient populations (e.g. people with diabetes or cancer), in such a way that optimal care is provided, patients' needs are better met, and costs are maintained when possible. BPR and related processes usually include top-down, management-driven approaches, in which current practices and processes are analyzed, reconsidered, and subsequently redesigned. Most of the time these approaches include the organization of new collaborations between care providers, a different allocation of tasks, the efficient transfer of information, the efficient scheduling of appointments, and the use of new types of health professionals (such as nurse case managers). The patient and his or her disease are central to these processes, not the interests of the care providers and professionals involved in their care (Hunter 2000). Typically, one person coordinates the process. Specific guidelines (called care pathways) are developed and used to determine exactly what care should be provided by whom at what time, and in what setting, for each part of the care process. This should lead to reducing traditional boundaries between disciplines and fragmentation of care processes.

Some research supports operations management approaches. For instance, successful intervention programs for chronic patients proved to share specific characteristics (Wagner et al. 1996; Casalino et al. 2003), such as case management and performance feedback to individual care providers; the use of explicit protocols and pathways; disease registries, electronic chart-based reminder systems; and practice reorganization to better meet the needs of patients. This type of approach would view optimal diabetes care as a process with interconnected activities. The process should be thoroughly analyzed, and – if needed – redesigned. The use of explicit protocols, task division, coordination of activities, and monitoring and feedback of both the process and the outcomes can all contribute to improvements in management. Enhancing patients' self-management is another important component of structured diabetes care.

2.4.4 Theory of Complex Systems

The *theory of complex systems* is a theoretical perspective on the behavior of individuals and organizations, starting from the assumption that the world of healthcare has become increasingly complex and that it is important to observe and improve systems as a whole instead of focusing on separate parts or components (Braithwaite 2018). The complex systems view assumes that systems consists of many elements, which are interconnected and facilitate processes that have random variation, resulting in unpredictable outcomes that include self-organization as well as chaos (Brainard and Hunter 2016). There is a substantial body of basic research on complex systems in the quantitative social sciences, but applications of a quantitative complex systems approach in healthcare are rare.

Complexity theory has informed both improvement strategies and their evaluation in healthcare settings (Churruca et al. 2018), but a review of the research literature remained overall inconclusive regarding its added value (Brainard and Hunter 2016). These applications tend to use a qualitative approach. For instance, the NASSS (nonadoption, abandonment, scale-up, spread, and sustainability) framework has been developed to encourage a complex systems approach to the implementation of technologies (Greenhalgh et al. 2017). It distinguishes factors in seven domains: the health condition, the technology, the value proposition, adopters, the organization, the wider system, and embedding/adapting over time. These domains can be used to guide the design and evaluation of implementation strategies.

The theory sees most systems in healthcare – hospitals, primary care teams, or the care organized around a specific disease – as "complex adaptive systems" (Lanham et al. 2013). These are defined "as a collection of individual agents (i.e., components or elements) with the freedom to act in ways that are not always totally predictable, and whose actions are interconnected, so that one agent's actions change the context for the other agents" (Plsek and Greenhalgh 2001). One of the claims of the theory is that, in order to improve patient care, comprehensive plans with detailed targets for parts of the system will seldom be very effective. The focus should be the system as a whole, using simple goals and actions with potentially large impact, as small influences can have a large impact on other parts of the system and even outside the system. The theory on complex systems may explain why specific events have large-scale impacts. For instance, in the UK one scandal in healthcare (the Bristol case) and the subsequent analysis of this case (the Bristol Inquiry) had a nationwide effect on quality improvement policies.

Likewise, infection control in a hospital, including hand hygiene routines, may be seen as a complex system with many components and agents influencing each other. In its turn, the infection control system can be seen to be part of other wider systems in the hospital.

According to complexity theory, it is important not to focus on single parts of this system, such as the hand-washing routines of individual nurses. Rather, it is important to set broad targets for change, observe the system as a whole, consider unexpected outcomes due to random variations, and find the key factors or events which can make changes to the system.

2.4.5 Theory of Organizational Learning

Not only individuals learn, organizations can also learn, according to the *theory of organizational learning.* A "learning organization" has been defined as one "skilled at creating, acquiring and transferring knowledge, and at modifying its behavior to reflect new knowledge and insights" (Garvin 1993). Individuals learn as agents for the organization and the knowledge acquired is stored in the memory of the organization (e.g. embedded in routines; Örtenblad 2002). Learning is seen as a characteristic of the organization because knowledge and expertise are retained even when individuals leave the organization (DiBella et al. 1996).

The boundaries between the concepts of "organizational learning" and "knowledge management" are unclear. A review of the organizational literature on both concepts showed that learning organizations are mostly associated with training, organizational development, and human resources development, while knowledge management is most frequently associated with information technology, intellectual capital, and the use of information systems (Scarbrough and Swan 2001). Both theories stress that it is only through the learning of individuals that organizational routines are changed. Therefore, improving organizational learning ability would primarily include the creation of favorable conditions for learning by professionals and others within the system (Senge 1990).

Effective learning organizations can be characterized by an external orientation; an experimental mindset; curiosity about trying new things; a climate in which openness, debate, and conflict are acceptable; ongoing commitment to education, growth, and development at all levels of the organization; and committed leadership.

We may hypothesize on the basis of these theories that improving hand hygiene routines will be more successful in a learning organization in which effective infection control belongs to the collective expertise of the hospital. Individuals at different levels are eager to acquire the knowledge about best practices in infection control and how to solve the problem of poor hand hygiene, experiences and information about better hand hygiene are shared and exchanged between different units and teams, and conditions for this type of change are present.

2.4.6 Theories of Organizational Culture

The interest in *theories of organizational culture* is based on the assumption that culture is related to performance and that a given culture can or should be altered to change that performance (Scott et al. 2003a). There is little consensus about the precise meaning of "organizational culture," as many competing definitions exist. According to Schein (1985), culture gradually develops when a group of individuals or an organization becomes stable, having developed shared experiences and history. Over time, the organization learns to cope with the problem of external demands and internal integration. Values and norms are passed on to the members and are embedded in routines ("this is the way we do things here"). Culture, therefore, is not merely something one can "observe" (e.g. company clothing), but a body of shared knowledge, norms, and values of which individuals may not be particularly aware.

Although definitions vary considerably, most authors in healthcare emphasize that, to achieve real change in patient care, organizations have to develop a "quality culture" in which continuous learning, teamwork, and patient focus are central (Ferlie and Shortell 2001). Likewise, organizational culture is crucial for the implementation of evidence-based practice (Aarons et al. 2014). For an organizational culture to develop, systems require leaders who clearly present the mission and vision of the organization, involve all staff members actively in quality improvement, and value a focus on continuous learning. Research on the relation between organizational culture, quality improvement, and outcomes showed that a flexible, innovation-centered culture was associated with quality improvement activities, in turn associated with better outcomes (Shortell et al. 1995). A systematic review by Scott et al. (2003b) partly confirmed the effect of culture on outcomes.

A relatively frequently used conceptual model to describe different types of organizational culture is "the Competing Values Framework" (Quinn and Rohrbaugh 1981), characterized by a two-dimensional space that reflects different value orientations. The first dimension is the flexibility–control axis, demonstrating the degree to which the organization emphasizes either change or stability. The second is the internal–external axis, addressing the organization's focus on activities occurring within the organization or outside in the external environment. This typology leads to four ideal cultural orientations (Stock and McDermott 2001):

- *Group or clan culture*, characterized by strong human relations, affiliation, and a focus on the internal organization.
- *Developmental culture*, focused primarily on growth, creativity, and adaptation to the external environment.

- *Rational culture*, emphasizing competition, productivity, and achievement.
- *Hierarchical culture*, with the focus on the internal organization, and characterized by stability, uniformity, and a close adherence to rules and regulations.

For improving diabetes care or hand hygiene routines, this theory emphasizes the importance of creating a flexible, innovation-centered culture that stimulates improvement of this aspect of healthcare delivery. Optimal care needs to become an element of the mission of the organization. Individuals and teams need to perceive prevention and monitoring of infections or diabetes care as a priority, and as part of the organization's quality culture.

2.5 Theories on Economic and Societal Structures

Theories on the influence of the societal context of changes include theories on regulation, competition, reimbursement, and financial incentives. These may be changed by policy makers and high-level managers of healthcare organizations, and usually not by healthcare providers or patients. Even if these factors are out of reach for specific individuals, it is important to identify them when implementing changes in healthcare. We briefly introduce two categories of theories, those related to economics and those on contracting.

2.5.1 Economic Theories

Economic theories have as their basis the assumption that individuals aim for optimization of their goals and avoid risks. In addition to rational considerations, such as benefits, costs, and risk, there is increasing attention to the behavioral factors associated with decision making in economics (Rice 2013). Economic theories on implementation of innovations primarily concern market regulation, in which aspects such as competition, reimbursement, transparency, and price setting are included. For instance, the type of reimbursement system in healthcare is considered to be relevant to reaching financial goals and avoiding financial risks. Both healthcare providers and patients are sensitive to prices and the financial risks that are associated with them. Changes in the reimbursement of providers can therefore be used to influence professional or organizational performance and to implement innovations (Barnum et al. 1995).

Different reimbursement systems exist, each of which has a specific impact. For instance, co-payment by patients is an incentive to reduce healthcare utilization (Rice and Morrison 1994). Reimbursement systems for care providers may be prospective (capitation, salary, budgets) or retrospective (fee-for-service, case-based payment). Fee-for-service systems generally lead to increased volume, so providing an extra fee is an option when one is trying to influence a particular behavior. This has been successful in increasing the uptake of yearly flu vaccinations in general practices in the Netherlands or in reducing waiting lists. Prospective systems place the financial risk with care providers and appear to reduce the volume of care (e.g. prescriptions, admissions to hospital, etc.; Chaix-Couturier et al. 2000). However, there are disadvantages: such systems may lead to reduced attention to patients, waiting lists, selection of low-risk patients, or use of cheaper, less effective treatments.

In improving hygiene routines in hospitals, the financial cost due to hospital infections may be used as a motivator to induce change. For example, a financial bonus may be provided to teams that succeed in improving their hygiene routines and in reducing the number of infections. Alternatively, a fixed budget for infection control or budgets to cover several materials such as soap, alcohol, and new sinks may be provided to wards.

2.5.2 Theories on Contracting

Contracts are legally binding arrangements between two or more parties, which often describe activities to be done and transfers of money. Fundamentally, they specify benefits and sanctions in transactions between two or more parties. This is done to enhance mutual trust, which can be key to the uptake of innovations. For instance, some health insurers in Germany use contracts to promote continuity of primary care and a coordinating role of primary care physicians, a healthcare delivery model with proven positive impacts on quality of care and population health (Wensing et al. 2016). For physicians and patients, participation in these contracts is voluntary, but is associated with additional work and a reduction of autonomy (e.g. physicians are expected to prescribe specific medication). There is a financial benefit for both patients and physicians, which aims to compensate for these aspects.

Game theory conceptualizes the decision to join in specific practices, such as adherence to clinical practice guidelines, as a prisoner's dilemma (or a variation of it) (Gächter and Thöni 2011). In this type of dilemma, the outcome is best for all if all join in, but worst for any party if it collaborates but others do not. The probability of joining a practice is positively influenced by factors such as repeated interactions, presence of rewards and sanctions for cooperation behaviors, visibility of behaviors and impact on individuals' reputations, and the possibility of sorting out of non-cooperators (Gächter and Thöni 2011). The relevance of these factors for changes in patient care is a topic of ongoing research.

In summary, if the uptake of recommendations for diabetes care or hand hygiene practices is better reimbursed, then their uptake is expected to be higher. Contracts may be seen as instruments to compensate for lack of trust. The role of network-related determinants of cooperation behavior is currently under investigation.

2.6 Conclusions

A number of theories on the implementation of innovations and change in practice have been presented in this chapter. Lessons for change derived from these theories are summarized in Table 2.1. Although this overview is far from exhaustive, it is clear that many of the theories described are not totally distinct, but build on others and sometimes overlap considerably. It is also clear that the different theories are often based on different assumptions about human behavior and behavioral or organizational change. The empirical evidence behind these assumptions is, for most of these approaches, limited, in particular with regard to their relevance for healthcare (Wensing and Grol 2019). In addition, it is challenging to determine which theories are particularly valid for use in implementing change in healthcare; possibly all of them can usefully contribute to understanding change processes (Grol and Grimshaw 2003).

Planners of implementation programs should make their assumptions and hypotheses explicit in order to avoid a narrow perspective on change, which is not well supported by research and experience. In most situations, a wide range of factors is relevant (Grol 1997). It can be useful to apply a conceptual framework of implementation science, which summarizes factors from a range of theories (Damschroeder et al. 2009; Flottorp et al. 2013). This will be elaborated in subsequent chapters.

For those individuals responsible for developing and implementing change programs, it is particularly important to express ideas and hypotheses explicitly and to present a broad vision of changing patient care. In most situations, a wide range of different factors will influence change processes (Grol 1997; Ferlie and Shortell 2001), which implies that hypotheses regarding effectiveness would also be derived from a variety of theories.

Table 2.1 Lessons from theory for planned improvement in healthcare.

Theory	Lessons for change	Lessons for hand hygiene or diabetes care
Individual professionals		
Cognitive theories	Implementation needs to take into account professionals' decision processes; they need good information and methods to support their decisions in practice	Provide convincing and timely information to professionals on desired care, and support their decision making on hand hygiene routines or diabetes management
Educational theories	Implementation should be linked to professionals' needs and motivation; intrinsic motivation is crucial; individuals change on basis of experienced problems in practice	Involve professionals in finding solutions for the problem; define personal targets for improvement as well as individual "learning plans" related to desired performance
Motivational theories	Implementation needs to focus on attitudes, perceived social norms, and experienced control related to desired performance	Convince professionals of importance of better hand hygiene or diabetes care; show that they can do it and that others find it important that they do it
Social interactions		
Social learning theory	Changing performance takes place through demonstration and modeling and through positive feedback (reinforcement) by others	Have hand hygiene or best practices in diabetes care modeled by "leaders" and desired routines reinforced by respected peers, provide feedback on performance
Theories on communication	Importance of the source of the innovation (credibility), the framing and rehearsal of messages, and the characteristics of the messages' recipient	Develop very convincing messages, have credible persons present them, and adapt messages to receiver's competence and motivation
Social network theories	Change demands local adaptation of innovations and use of opinion leaders in local networks for dissemination	Study the interaction in the team; determine the opinion leaders; and use these to improve infection control or diabetes management
Theories on teamwork	Effective teams are able to make necessary changes to improve care because they share goals and are able to share knowledge	Create teams in which roles are defined and individuals encourage one another to work on the common goal of fewer infections or complications in diabetes patients
Theories on professionalization	Professional loyalty, pride, and consensus, and "reinvention" of change proposal by professional body are important	Use professional pride and define professional standards for the desired performance. Appoint a hygienist or diabetes nurse
Theories on leadership	Involvement and commitment of formal and informal leaders in change process are important, particularly in institutional boards	Have top management or informal leaders initiate activities and provide continuous support and monitoring aimed at changing routines in diabetes care or hand hygiene
Organizational context		
Theory of innovative organizations	Implementation should take into account the type of organization; professionalizing and decentralized decision making about innovation is important	Create broad coalitions of clinicians from different wards to change the systems for infection control or diabetes care; increase responsibilities for the wards and create communication between the wards

Table 2.1 (Continued)

Theory	Lessons for change	Lessons for hand hygiene or diabetes care
Theory of quality and safety management	Improvement is a continuous cyclic process, with plans for change continually adapted on the basis of previous experience; organization-wide measures are aimed at improving culture, collaboration, customer focus, and processes	Reorganize work processes around diabetes care or infection control; develop primary care or hospital-wide system for optimal diabetes care or for prevention of infections; monitor progress and continually adapt plans for change on the basis of data. Leaders support these processes
Operations management theory	Change multidisciplinary care processes and collaboration instead of individual decision making	Analyze and redesign the work processes related to diabetes care or hand hygiene, and make these more effective and efficient
Theory on complex systems	Focus on system as a whole, find patterns in behavior (attractors) and link change plan to these, and test and improve the plan	See infection control or diabetes management as a system with many agents; find patterns/attractors; define crucial (minimum) specifications for change; and test them
Theory of organizational learning	Creation or availability of conditions in the organization for continuous learning at all levels can lead to successful changes	Offer continuous learning and exchange of information and experiences about diabetes management and better hygiene at all levels of the organization
Theories on organizational culture	Changes in culture are a prerequisite for changes in performance, particularly a culture of teamwork, flexibility, and external orientation	Work on improving the general culture in the hospital or the practice in which infection control and integrated care for diabetes patients are seen as priorities and make a connection to infection control or disease management policies
Societal context		
Economic theories	Attractive rewards and (financial) incentives can influence the volume of specific activities	Reward the decrease of infections or achievement of diabetes care targets with non-material or material/financial incentives (extra budget, staff, sabbatical leave)
Theories on contracting	Contractual arrangements can guide professional and organizational performance	Provide contractual arrangements of purchasers (insurance companies, government) and care providers related to diabetes control or meeting of infection targets

References

Ajzen, I. (1988). *Attitudes, Personality and Behaviour*. Milton Keynes: Open University Press.

Ajzen, I. (1991). The theory of planned behaviour. *Organ. Behav. Hum. Decis. Process.* 50: 179–211.

Aarons, G.A., Ehrgart, M.G., Farahnak, L.R., and Sklar, M. (2014). Aligning leadership across systems and organizations to develop a strategic climate for evidence-based practice implementation. *Annu. Rev. Public Health* 35: 255–274.

Bandura, A. (1986). *Social Foundation of Thought and Action: A Social Cognitive Theory*. New York: Prentice Hall.

Barnum, H., Kutzin, J., and Saxenian, H. (1995). Incentives and provider payment methods. *Int. J. Health Plann. Manag.* 16: 23–45.

Batalden, P.B. and Stoltz, P.K. (1993). A framework for the continual improvement of health care. *Jt. Comm. J. Qual. Improv.* 19: 424–452.

Berwick, D.M. (1989). Continuous improvement as an ideal in health care. *N. Engl. J. Med.* 320: 53–56.

Berwick, D.M., Godfrey, A.B., and Roessner, J. (1990). *Curing Health Care*. San Francisco: Jossey-Bass.

Brainard, J. and Hunter, P.R. (2016). Do complexity-informed health interventions work? A scoping review. *Implement. Sci.* 11: 127.

Braithwaite, J. (2018). Changing how we think about healthcare improvement. *BMJ* 361: k2014.

Brehaut, J.C. and Eva, K.W. (2012). Building theories of knowledge translation interventions: using the entire menu of constructs. *Implement. Sci.* 7: 114.

Casalino, M.D., Gillies, R.R., Shortell, S.M. et al. (2003). External incentives, information technology, and organised processes to improve health care quality for patients with chronic diseases. *JAMA* 289: 434–441.

Chaix-Couturier, C., Durand-Zaleski, I., Jolly, D. et al. (2000). Effects of financial incentives on medical practice: results from a systematic review of the literature and methodological costs? *Int. J. Qual. Health Care* 12: 133–142.

Churruca, K., Pomare, C., Ellis, L.A. et al. (2018). The influence of complexity: a bibliometric analysis of complexity science in healthcare. *BMJ Open* 9: e027308.

Damanpour, F. (1991). Organizational innovation: a meta-analysis of effects of determinants and moderators. *Acad. Manag. J.* 34: 555–590.

Damschroeder, L.J., Aron, D.C., Keith, R.E. et al. (2009). Fostering implementation of health services research findings into practice: a consolidated framework for advancing implementation science. *Implement. Sci.* 4: 50.

DiBella, A.J., Nevis, E.C., and Gould, J.M. (1996). Understanding organizational learning capability. *J. Manag. Stud.* 33: 361–379.

Dijkstra, J. (2004). *Implementing diabetes guidelines at outpatient clinics*. Thesis. Nijmegen: Radboud Universiteit.

Dijkstra, J. and Van Assen, M.A.L.M. (2017). Explaining cooperation in the finitely repeated simultaneous and sequential prisoners' dilemma game under incomplete and complete information. *J. Math. Sociol.* 41: 1–25.

Donaldson, L. (1995). Conflict, power, negotiation. *BMJ* 310: 104–107.

Doumit, G., Wright, F.C., Graham, I.D. et al. (2011). Opinion leaders and changes over time: a survey. *Implement. Sci.* 6: 117.

Evans, J.S.B.T. and Stanovich, K.E. (2013). Dual-process theories of higher cognition: advancing the debate. *Perspect. Psychol. Sci.* 8: 223–241.

Ferlie, E. and Shortell, S. (2001). Improving the quality of health care in the United Kingdom and the United States: a framework for change. *Milbank Q.* 79: 281–315.

Festinger, L. (1954). A theory of social comparison processes. *Hum. Relat.* 7: 117–140.

Firth-Cozins, J. (1998). Celebrating teamwork. *Qual. Health Care* 7: S3–S7.

Fishbein, M. and Ajzen, I. (1975). *Belief, Attitude, Intention and Behavior*. New York: Wiley.

Flottorp, S., Oxman, A.D., Krause, J. et al. (2013). A checklist for identifying determinants of practice: a systematic review and synthesis of frameworks and taxonomies of factors that prevent or enable improvements in healthcare professional practice. *Implement. Sci.* 8: 35.

Fox, R.D. and Bennett, N.L. (1998). Learning and change: implications for continuing medical education. *BMJ* 316: 466–468.

Francis, J.J., O'Connor, D., and Curran, J. (2012). Theories of behavior change synthesized into a set of theoretical groupings: introducing a thematic series on the theoretical domains framework. *Implement. Sci.* 7: 35.

Freidson, E. (1970). *Profession of Medicine*. New York: Doddds Mead.

Freidson, E. (2001). *Professionalism, the Third Logic*. Chicago, IL: University of Chicago Press.

Gächter, S. and Thöni, C. (2011). Micromotives, microstructure, and macrobehavior: the case of voluntary cooperation. *J. Math. Sociol.* 35: 26–65.

Garvin, D.A. (1993). Building a learning organization. *Harv. Bus. Rev.* 71: 78–91.

Graham, I.D., Logan, J., Harrison, M.B. et al. (2006). Lost in knowledge translation: time for a map? *J. Cont. Educ. Health Prof.* 26: 13–24.

Greenhalgh, T., Wherton, J., Papoutsi, C. et al. (2017). Beyond adoption: a new framework for theorizing and evaluating nonadoption, abandonment, and challenges to the scale-up, spread, and sustainability of health and care technologies. *J. Med. Internet Res.* 19: e367.

Greer, A.L. (1988). The state of the art versus the state of the science. The diffusion of new medical technologies into practice. *Int. J. Technol. Assess. Health Care* 4: 5–26.

Grol, R. (1992). Implementing guidelines in general practice care. *Qual. Health Care* 1: 184–191.

Grol, R. (1997). Beliefs and evidence in changing clinical practice. *BMJ* 315: 418–421.

Grol, R. and Grimshaw, J. (2003). From best evidence to best practice: effective implementation of change in patients' care. *Lancet* 362: 1225–1230.

Grol, R. and Wensing, M. (2004). What drives change? Barriers to and incentives for achieving evidence-based practice. *Med. J. Aust.* 180: S57–S60.

Grumbach, K. and Bodenheimer, T. (2004). Can health care teams improve primary care practice? *JAMA* 291: 1246–1251.

Gustafson, D.H. and Hundt, A.S. (1995). Findings of innovation research applied to quality management principles for health care. *Health Care Manag. Rev.* 20: 16–33.

Handwashing Liaison Group (1999). Handwashing: a modern measure with big effects. *BMJ* 318: 686.

Hobus, P. (1994). *Expertise van huisartsen.* [Professional competence of primary care physicians]. Thesis. Maastricht: Universiteit Maastricht.

Holm, H.A. (1998). Quality issues in continuing medical education. *BMJ* 316: 621–624.

Hunter, D.J. (2000). Disease management: has it a future? It has a compelling logic, but it needs to be tested in practice. *BMJ* 320: 530.

Jones, E.E., Kannouse, D.E., Kelley, H.H. et al. (eds.) (1972). *Attribution: Perceiving the Causes of Behavior*. Morristown, NJ: General Learning Press.

Koele, P. and van der Pligt, I. (eds.) (1993). *Beslissen en beoordelen. Besliskunde in de psychologie. [Judge and Assess. Decision Making in Psychology]*. Amsterdam/Meppel: Boom.

Kok, G., de Vries, H., Mudde, A.N., and Strecher, V.J. (1991). Planned health education and the role of self-efficacy: Dutch research. *Health Educ. Res.* 6: 231–238.

Laffel, G. and Blumenthal, D. (1989). The case for using industrial quality management science in health care organization. *JAMA* 262: 2869–2873.

Langley, G., Nolan, K., Nolan, T. et al. (2009). *The Improvement Guide: A Practical Approach to Enhancing Organizational Performance*, 2e. San Francisco, CA: Jossey-Bass.

Lanham, H.J., Leykum, L.K., Taylor, B.S. et al. (2013). How complexity science can inform scale-up and spread in healthcare: understanding the role of self-organisation in variation across local contexts. *Soc. Sci. Med.* 93: 194–202.

Lewis, A.P. and Bolden, K.J. (1989). General practitioners and their learning styles. *J. R. Coll. Gen. Pract.* 39: 187–189.

Mammen, J., Fischer, D., Anderson, A. et al. (2007). Learning styles vary among general surgery residents: analysis of 12 years of data. *J. Surg. Educ.* 64: 386–389.

Mann, K.V. (1994). Educating medical students: lessons from research in continuing education. *Acad. Med.* 69: 41–47.

Manojlevic, M., Squires, J.E., Davies, B., and Graham, I.D. (2015). Hiding in plain sight:

communication theory in implementation science. *Implement. Sci.* 10: 58.

May, C. (2013). Towards a general theory of implementation. *Implement. Sci.* 8: 18.

McKevoy, R., Ballini, L., Maltoni, S. et al. (2014). A qualitative systematic review of studies using the normalisation process theory to research implementation processes. *Implement. Sci.* 9: 2.

Merriam, S.B. (1996). Updating our knowledge of adult learning. *J. Contin. Educ. Heal. Prof.* 16: 136–143.

Michie, S., Johnston, M., Abraham, C. et al. (2005). Making psychological theory useful for implementing evidence-based practice: a consensus approach. *Qual. Saf. Health Care* 14: 26–33.

Michie, S., Richardson, M., Johnston, M. et al. (2013). The behaviour change technique taxonomy (v1) of 93 hierarchically clustered techniques: building an international consensus for the reporting of behaviour change interventions. *Ann. Behav. Med.* 46: 81–95.

Michie, S., Van Stralen, M.M., and West, R. (2011). The behaviour change wheel: a new method for characterising and designing behaviour change interventions. *Implement. Sci.* 6: 42.

Mintzberg, H. (1996). *Organisational Structures*. Englewood Cliffs, NJ: Prentice Hall: Academic Service.

Mittman, B.S., Tonesk, X., and Jacobson, P.D. (1992). Implementing clinical practice guidelines: social influence strategies and practitioner behaviour change. *QRB* 18: 413–422.

Nilsen, P. (2015). Making sense of implementation theories, models, and frameworks. *Implement. Sci.* 10: 53.

Norman, G. (2002). Research in medical education: three decades of progress. *BMJ* 324: 1560–1562.

Norman, G.R. and Schmidt, H.G. (1992). The psychological basis of problem-based learning: a review of the evidence. *Acad. Med.* 67: 557–565.

Nylenna, M., Aasland, O.G., and Falkum, E. (1996). Keeping professionally updated: perceived coping and CME profiles among physicians. *J. Contin. Educ. Heal. Prof.* 16: 241–249.

Örtenblad, A. (2002). A typology of the idea of learning organization. *Manag. Learn.* 33: 213–230.

Øvretveit, J. (2004). *The Leader's Role in Quality and Safety Improvement: A Review of Research and Guidance*. Stockholm: Association of County Councils (Lanstingsforbundet).

Plsek, P.E. and Greenhalgh, T. (2001). Complexity science: the challenge of complexity in health care. *BMJ* 323: 625–628.

Plsek, P., Solberg, L., and Grol, R. (2003). *Total quality management and continuous quality improvement*. In: *Oxford Textbook of Primary Medical Care* (eds. R. Jones, N. Britten, L. Culpepper, et al.), 490–495. Oxford: Oxford University Press.

Pratt, R.J., Pellowe, C., Loveday, H.P. et al. (2001). The EPIC project: developing national evidence-based guidelines for preventing healthcare associated infections. Phase I: guidelines for preventing hospital-acquired infections. Department of Health (England). *J. Hosp. Infect.* 47: S3–S82.

Quinn, R. and Rohrbaugh, I. (1981). A competing values approach to organizational effectiveness. *Public Product. Rev.* 5: 122–140.

Rice, T. (2013). The behavioural economics of health and healthcare. *Annu. Rev. Public Health* 34: 431–437.

Rice, T. and Morrison, K.R. (1994). Patient cost sharing for medical services: a review of the literature and implications for health care reform. *Med. Care Rev.* 51: 235–287.

Rogers, E.M. (2003). *Diffusion of Innovations*. New York: Simon & Schuster.

Ross, S.M. and Offerman, L.R. (1997). Transformational leaders: measurement of personality attributes and work group performance. *Personal. Soc. Psychol. Bull.* 23: 1078–1086.

Rossi, P., Freeman, H., and Lipsey, M. (1999). *Evaluation: A Systematic Approach*. Thousand Oaks, CA: Sage.

RWJF (2011). *Teamwork and Collaborative Decision-Making Crucial to Health Care of the*

Future. Princeton, NJ: Robert Wood Johnson Foundation.

Scarbrough, H. and Swan, J. (2001). Explaining the diffusion of knowledge management: the role of fashion. *Br. J. Manag.* 12: 3–12.

Schein, E.H. (1985). *Culture and Leadership*. San Francisco, CA: Jossey-Bass.

Scott, T., Mannion, R., Davies, H., and Marshall, M.N. (2003a). Implementing culture change in health care: theory and practice. *Int. J. Qual. Health Care* 111-8: 15.

Scott, T., Mannion, R., Marshall, M., and Davies, H. (2003b). Does organisational culture influence health care performance? A review of the evidence. *J. Health Serv. Res. Policy* 105-17: 8.

Senge, P.M. (1990). *The Fifth Discipline. The Art and Practice of the Learning Organization*. London: Random House.

Shortell, S.M., Bennett, C.L., and Byck, G.R. (1998). Assessing the impact of continuous quality improvement on clinical practice: what it will take to accelerate progress. *Milbank Q.* 76: 593–624.

Shortell, S.M., Marsteller, J.A., Lin, M. et al. (2004). The role of perceived team effectiveness in improving chronic illness care. *Med. Care* 42: 1040–1048.

Shortell, S.M., O'Brien, J.L., Carman, J.M. et al. (1995). Assessing the impact of continuous quality improvement/total quality management: concept versus implementation. *Health Serv. Res.* 30: 377–401.

Smith, F., Singleton, A., and Hilton, S. (1998). General practitioners' continuing education: a review of policies, strategies, and effectiveness, and their implications for the future. *Br. J. Gen. Pract.* 48: 1689–1695.

Smits, P.B.A., Verbeek, J.H.A.M., and de Buisonjé, C.D. (2002). Problem based learning in continuing medical education: a review of controlled evaluation studies. *BMJ* 324: 153–156.

Stock, G.N. and McDermott, C.M. (2001). Organizational and strategic predictors of manufacturing technology implementation success: an exploratory study. *Technovation* 21: 625–636.

Stone, S. (2001). Hand hygiene – the case for evidence based education. *J. R. Soc. Med.* 94: 278–281.

Striffler, L., Cardoso, R., McGowan, J. et al. (2018). Scoping review identifies significant number of knowledge translation theories, models, and frameworks with limited use. *J. Clin. Epidemiol.* 100: 92–102.

Tassone, M.R. and Heck, C.S. (1997). Motivational orientations of allied health care professionals participating in continuing education. *J. Cont. Educ. Health Prof.* 17: 97–105.

Teare, L., Cookson, B., and Stone, S. (2001). Hand hygiene. *BMJ* 323: 411–412.

Thomas, A., Menon, A., Boruff, J. et al. (2014). Applications of social constructivist learning theories in knowledge translation for healthcare professionals: a scoping review. *Implement. Sci.* 9: 54.

Valente, T.W. (1996). Social network thresholds in the diffusion of innovations. *Soc. Networks* 18: 69–89.

Wagner, E.H., Austin, B.T., and van Korff, M. (1996). Organizing care for patients with chronic illness. *Milbank Q.* 74: 511–544.

Walker, A. and Leary, H. (2009). A problem based learning meta analysis: differences across problem types, implementation types, disciplines, and assessment levels. *Interdiscipl. J. Prob. Based Learn* 3: 6–28.

Walker, A.E., Grimshaw, J.M., and Armstrong, E.M. (2001). Salient beliefs and intentions to prescribe antibiotics for patients with a sore throat. *Br. J. Health Psychol.* 6: 347–360.

Wensing, M., Bosch, M., and Grol, R. (2010). Developing and selecting interventions for translating knowledge to action. *CMAJ* 182: E85–E88.

Wensing, M. and Grol, R. (2019). Knowledge translation in health: how could implementation science could contribute more. *BMC Med.* 17: 88.

Wensing, M., Szecsenyi, J., Stock, C. et al. (2016). Evaluation of a program to strengthen general practice care for patients with chronic disease in Germany. *BMC Health Serv. Res.* 17: 62.

West, M.A. (1990). *The social psychology of innovation in groups*. In: *Innovation and*

Creativity at Work: Psychological and Organizational Strategies (eds. M.A. West and J.L. Farr), 3–36. Hoboken, NJ: Wiley.

West, M.A., Borrill, C., Dawson, J. et al. (2002). The link between the management of employees and patient mortality in acute hospitals. *Int. J. Hum. Resour. Manag.* 13: 1299–1310.

Wieringa, S. and Greenhalgh, T. (2015). 10 years of mindlines: a systematic review and commentary. *Implement. Sci.* 10: 45.

Wolfe, R.A. (1994). Organizational innovation: review, critique and suggested research directions. *J. Manag. Stud.* 31: 405–431.

3

Effective Implementation of Change in Healthcare: A Systematic Approach

Richard Grol[1,2] and Michel Wensing[3,4,5]

[1] *Radboud University, Nijmegen, The Netherlands*
[2] *Maastricht University, Maastricht, The Netherlands*
[3] *Faculty of Medicine, University of Heidelberg, Heidelberg, Germany*
[4] *Department of General Practice and Health Services Research, Heidelberg University Hospital, Heidelberg, Germany*
[5] *Department IQ healthcare, Radboud Institute for Health Sciences, Radboud University Medical Center, Nijmegen, The Netherlands*

SUMMARY

- The effective implementation of innovations, new procedures, clinical guidelines, and best practices requires a systematic approach with good preparation and planning.
- The following steps are important in a systematic approach to the implementation of change:
  - Formulating a concrete, well-developed, and attainable proposal or recommended practice with clear targets.
  - Assessing the actual performance and mapping the problems in using the new procedures.
  - Analyzing the target group and the setting: what factors are stimulating or hampering the process of change.
  - Selecting and developing a set of strategies for change: strategies for the effective dissemination, implementation, and maintenance of change.
  - Developing and executing an implementation plan containing activities, tasks, and a time schedule.
  - Integrating the improvement within the normal practice routines.
  - Evaluating and revising the plan: continuous monitoring on the basis of indicators.
- While many implementation processes do not follow these exact steps, most still benefit from a systematic, well-planned approach.

3.1 Elements of Effective Implementation

In the previous chapter, we presented a number of theories and frameworks on the determinants of effective change and improvement ("impact theories"). In this chapter, we present different theories and frameworks that can be used for planning and managing change ("process theories"). Several crucial elements or principles for successful implementation recur through most publications of theories and models (e.g. Lomas and Haynes 1988; Kotler and Roberto 1989; Green and Kreuter 1991; Grol 1992; Mittman et al. 1992; Grol et al. 1994; Langley et al. 1996; Robertson et al. 1996; Davis and Taylor-Vaisey 1997; Grol 1997; Cretin 1998; Kotter et al. 1998; Feder et al. 1999; Moulding et al. 1999; NHS 1999; Ovretveit 1999; Ferlie and Shortell 2001; Grol and Grimshaw 2003; Greenhalgh et al. 2004;

Improving Patient Care: The Implementation of Change in Health Care, Third Edition. Edited by Michel Wensing, Richard Grol, and Jeremy Grimshaw.

Grol and Wensing 2004; Grol and Buchan 2006; Lomas 2007; Graham and Tetroe 2009; May et al. 2009; Straus et al. 2009). The research evidence for these models is still sketchy, but they provide a framework for developing an implementation plan. These elements (summarized later in Box 3.6) are as follows:

- Most importantly, it is critical to consider the complexity of the usual patient care in changing routines in clinical practice and in the implementation of innovations; a large number of factors can hinder or facilitate change (Box 3.1 provides an example). To manage this complexity and to achieve change, *a systematic approach and careful planning* of the implementation activities are needed. One single action is seldom effective. There is a clear need for a well-planned process of change in which all factors are addressed, progress is evaluated regularly, and the plan is adapted to respond to experiences and challenges. Even in instances in which implementation programs do not follow a linear process, a well-planned approach is helpful. Based on regular checks on progress, one can decide to go back in the process or to prepare for later steps. The model introduced in this chapter is not meant to be used in a rigid way, but as flexible guidance and support.

- In preparing the change process, attention needs to be paid to the *resources and practical aspects* of the implementation on the one hand (for example, is there sufficient expertise, budget, and a clear time or schedule?) and to *social and organizational aspects* on the other hand. (Is the target group motivated to start with the process? Are specific organizational conditions in place?)

- For the target group of care providers and teams, implementation usually means that

---

Box 3.1   Implementation of the "Ottawa Ankle Rules" in an Emergency Department

The "Ottawa Ankle Rules" have been an important guideline for the diagnosis of acute ankle trauma. The use of the rules contributed to a large (>25%) reduction in unnecessary X-rays. Nevertheless, the recommendations in this guideline are often not followed at emergency departments. A project at two emergency departments in Adelaide, Australia, focused on the implementation of the ankle rules by providing feedback, education, reminders, the use of a special X-ray order form, and approval of the test by experienced persons at the radiology department (Bessen et al. 2009). This intervention was developed on the basis of an analysis of the implementation problems. Barriers proved to be related to the physicians (lack of knowledge, concerns about missing a fracture, lack of self-confidence in own expertise), to the patients (pressure to perform an X-ray), and to the organization of care (changes in staff, X-rays as part of a process to control the flow of patients). After the intervention, 9–12% fewer X-rays were ordered, and those that were performed increased their sensitivity (7–12% more fractures were diagnosed). The largest improvements were seen for nurse practitioners and trainees, who appeared to profit most from clear guidelines. The study indicated the positive effects of such a systematic approach, but it also noted a difference in preparedness to change among the professionals involved. It also proved to be more difficult to change existing behavior than to introduce new behavior. In a further analysis of this study (Thomson 2009), the moderate effects were explained by the lack of a solid theoretical framework for the intervention elements. A more in-depth qualitative analysis of the implementation problems was recommended.

a *step-by-step process* is followed: the factors that one must tackle successively in order to move forward in that process follow an iterative, progressive process. Different problems are surmounted in each step and different measures or strategies called for. Before attempting actual change, the target end-users of an innovation need an awareness of the need for change; a concept of what the improvement includes; and the belief that such an improvement is both desirable and possible. Furthermore, in order to successfully make the next step in the change process, new problems usually need to be tackled. Different models for such a step-wise approach are presented in the literature (see for example Boxes 3.2 and 3.3); an integrated model is discussed in detail in this book.

- Specific attention should be given to the *innovation, guideline, or new routine itself.* This concerns both the process of development (Who are the developers? What is their status?), the scientific basis of the innovation, its format or presentation, and its content. A well-designed and attractive "product" (e.g. a good change proposal) is more readily accepted and adopted than one that is less well thought out and presented. This often means that any innovation – for example an evidence-based guideline, an integrated care protocol, or an information technology application – is tailored to the local setting.

Box 3.2   Planned Change or Planned Action Theories

Planned action refers to deliberately aiming at change. Theories, frameworks, and models in this area are numerous. These should help change agents responsible for organizing improvement to control the factors increasing or decreasing the chance of change. For instance, Graham and Tetroe (2009) identified 60 theories and models, most comprising similar features and steps:

- Identification of a problem in healthcare.
- Identification and analysis of the knowledge or scientific findings relevant for solving the problem (such as clinical guidelines).
- Adaptation of these insights to the local setting.
- Analysis of barriers to using the insights.
- Selection and tailoring interventions to stimulate the use of the insights and to implement change.
- Monitoring the use of the insights.
- Evaluation of the outcomes of the use of the insights.
- Maintenance of the change.

Box 3.3   Some Models for Planning or Managing Change

- Precede–proceed model (Green and Kreuter 1991)
- Marketing theory (Kotler and Roberto 1989)
- Continuous improvement, Plan–Do–Study–Act (PDSA) cycles (Langley et al. 1996; Ovretveit 1999)
- Stages of change theories (Grol 1992; Prochaska and Velicer 1997; Rogers 2003)
- Persuasion–communication models (McGuire 1981; Kok 1983; Rogers 2003)
- Intervention mapping (Bartholomew et al. 2001; van Bokhoven et al. 2003)
- Organizational development (Garside 1998)
- Planned action model (Graham and Tetroe 2009)
- Normalization theory (May et al. 2009)

- A solid and credible *analysis of actual performance* in practice relative to the use of the proposed routine or innovation is needed before the implementation process commences. This is important for various reasons. It makes it possible to focus the implementation actions on those aspects of the new way of working that are most in need of improvement. Further, it demonstrates to the target group strong as well as weak aspects of their performance, thus contributing to a sense of urgency or need – a feeling that change is necessary. Further, it provides a baseline measure for the assessment of change at a later stage. Finally, valid and acceptable quality measures and indicators, as well as accessible data sources, are crucial to the analysis of the actual performance, both before and after the change.

- Before embarking on any implementation plan, it is essential to know as much as possible about its various target groups. It is advisable to begin the implementation process with a *diagnostic or problem analysis.* This step provides insights on the characteristics of the target group and, if applicable, subgroups within it; the setting in which the implementation is to take place; the most important factors which can hamper or stimulate the change in performance; the wider context (for example social, regulatory, or organizational) of the healthcare setting; and finally the important parties involved in the process of implementing the innovation.

- Individuals or groups within the implementation's target group may be in different *phases of a process of change.* Thus, awareness, needs, experiences, and willingness to change may vary between these groups. For this reason, it is important when introducing change to differentiate properly between subgroups. So-called *segmentation* may be practiced. Different groups may demand different approaches. Health professionals may be at one time aware of the

guideline, aware but not agree with it, agree and have adopted it albeit irregularly, or adhere to it at all times. Different models for categorizing these groups can be distinguished (see Table 3.1).

- *Commitment from the target group* to the entire process will ultimately contribute to successful implementation. Planning an implementation strategy requires an understanding of the perceptions, needs, worries, and realities of the working situation of those individuals or groups who must ultimately carry it out. The target group should ideally be involved in the development of a proposal for change. If national guidelines or prevention programs are involved, it is possible to adjust or adapt them to local needs in order to suit the situation and the specific needs of the healthcare setting. Ideally, the target group will also be active participants in the implementation plan and in developing and testing the measures and strategies that will be used in that plan before applying them on a large scale.

- *The choice of strategies* to bring about change is linked, as far as possible, to the measurement of actual performance and to the results of the diagnostic or problem analysis and to the array of facilitating or impeding factors already identified (see Boxes 3.4 and 3.5 for examples). On the basis of this an efficient mix can be devised of, for instance, education, rewards, feedback, and organizational or practical measures. This approach will have to be tailored to the needs and situations of various subgroups within the larger target group.

- A single method is usually insufficient to cause change. Subgroups within the target group are most often at various stages in terms of their willingness to change and experience different problems in realizing change in practice. Therefore, successful strategies most often need to be *multifaceted*, a feature which carries with it the following caveat. First, multifaceted interventions come at a price: necessary resources must

Table 3.1 Steps in the process of change.

	1	2	3	4	5	6	7	8	9
Zaltman and Duncan (1977)	Knowledge/awareness	Knowledge/awareness		Attitude formation	Decision	Initial implementation		Sustained implementation	
McGuire (1981)	Exposure/interest	Comprehension	Skills	Attitude change/agreement	Decision	Behavior change	Reinforcement	Consolidation	
Kok (1983)	Attention	Understanding		Attitude change	Intention to change	Behavior change		Sustained change	
Orlandi 1987		Seeking information		Persuasion about relevance	Decision to adopt	Change of practice		Sustained change	
Cooper and Zinud (1990)		Initiation			Adoption	Acceptance/use		Incorporation	Infusion (wide use)
Grol (1992)	Awareness/interest	Knowledge	Insight into own performance	Positive attitude	Intention to change	Implementation (trial)		Maintenance of change	
Spence (1994)	Awareness/interest			Evaluation		Trial		Adoption	
Pathman et al. (1996)	Awareness			Agreement		Adoption		Routine adherence	
Prochaska and Velicer (1997)	Precontemplation			Contemplation	Preparation	Action		Maintenance	
Rogers (2003)		Knowledge		Persuasion	Decision	Implementation		Confirmation	

Box 3.4 The Precede–Proceed Model

The precede–proceed model, developed by Green et al. (1988), is a theory of behavioral change which can be used both for planning and for explaining change in patient care. The model distinguishes nine planning steps to be taken in a process of change. The first three steps are "social diagnosis," "epidemiological diagnosis," and "behavioral and environmental diagnosis" – all aimed at determining important factors influencing the behavior. A distinction is made between *predisposing factors* for a specific behavior (e.g. the knowledge, attitudes, and values held by the target group), *enabling factors* (such as capacity, availability, and accessibility of services), and *reinforcing factors* (opinions and behaviors of others). Steps 4 and 5 of the model outline the best approach to influence performance; step 6 is the actual implementation; while steps 7–9 are the evaluation of process, impact, and effect.

Green describes a number of important principles underlying effective change of behavior. First, strategies for the implementation of change should be based on an analysis of crucial determinants of the behavior, called the diagnostic principle. The theory considers a "hierarchical principle" here: there is a natural order in the factors influencing change, first predisposing, then enabling, and finally reinforcing factors. Implementation strategies should be structured in that order. Another principle is that of "cumulative learning": to influence the performance of professionals, a series of learning experiences needs to be planned in such a way that earlier experiences are optimally used in later experiences. A further principle

is called "participation": a target group defining both its own need for change and the preferred method for change increases the chance of success. The principle of "situational specificity" comprises the idea that no strategy is uniformly superior or inferior for achieving change. The ultimate impact always depends on the specific circumstances, the characteristics of the target group, the timing, the commitment of opinion leaders and change agents in the setting, and so on. The next principle is that of "multiple methods": because existing performance is determined by a variety of factors, a suitable strategy for each of these factors needs to be selected. The principle of "individualization" emphasizes the importance of tailoring the implementation of change to the needs and experiences of individuals in the target group. And finally, the "feedback principle" identifies the necessity of direct feedback to individuals on the progress of the desired change.

This model has frequently been used in healthcare, particularly in the field of health promotion. Two systematic reviews on the implementation of guidelines and change found combined interventions focusing on all three types of factors to be more effective than interventions focusing on only one type of factor (Davis et al. 1992, 1999; Solomon et al. 1998). Green's model offers a comprehensive understanding and a perspective on planning the implementation of change (Weir et al. 2011). Elements are employed in this chapter as well as in the framework used to structure this book.

---

be available for a plan to be implemented: just as in clinical practice, a balance must be sought between effectiveness and costs incurred in implementation activities. Second, deploying more interventions does not automatically lead to greater success (Squires et al. 2014). A large, complex program with scores of activities will not always be the most efficient approach. Further, it may not be accepted by the sponsors,

---

Box 3.5   Improving the Diagnosis and Treatment of Depression

Depression is highly prevalent among patients in primary care. Many depressed patients do not receive optimal care, reflected in both diagnosis and treatment with anti-depressants. In this context, Baker et al. (2001) conducted a randomized controlled study of an intervention based on psychological theories: 34 physicians participated in the intervention group and 30 in the control group that only received clinical guidelines for the management of depression in primary care. Six weeks after receiving treatment guidelines, the intervention group participants were interviewed about perceived obstacles to use the guideline recommendations. For each obstacle, a psychological hypothesis was formulated to explain the problem and to select a suitable improvement strategy. For instance, when a physician indicated problems in assessing suicide risk or in asking diagnostic questions, the self-efficacy theory was used and a concrete list of questions was offered as the implementation strategy. Thus, strategies tailored to the problems of each individual doctor were offered six weeks after the interviews. To measure effect, the participants identified patients with depression; both adherence to the guidelines and the proportion of patients with a Beck Depression Inventory (BDI) score under 11 at 16 weeks after the diagnosis were assessed. In the intervention group, there was a significant increase in the number of patients who received an assessment of suicide risk and a BDI score under 11. The study authors concluded that the tailored approach based on an analysis of obstacles to change was effective, but that its cost-effectiveness needs further research.

---

funders, or the target group itself; they may feel that too many resources are being spent on a specific improvement.

- When selecting suitable strategies to support the implementation of change, it is useful to distinguish between *dissemination* (spreading the information, keeping individuals informed, getting the innovation accepted) and *implementation* (actual adoption, and integration into normal routines or care processes). For both steps, different methods and measures are suitable and effective. In addition, one must ask oneself at what level the measures can best be deployed. Some can be tackled optimally at national or state level (for instance, financial compensation for extra work), while others are best deployed at a professional, practice, or team level (for instance, feedback on current performance).
- It is crucial that the new ways of working are *integrated as well as possible in the normal care routines* in practice: the innovation

needs to be "institutionalized" or "normalized" in order to prevent relapse or decay to old routines (May et al. 2009). Programs meant for introducing innovations need to become an integral part of existing structures for professional development, quality control, and quality improvement. It is important to be constantly aware of the proposed change to avoid regression or diversification. Ultimately, the success criterion for an implementation is its long-term sustainability.

- Each systematic attempt to change clinical practice should be accompanied by a plan in order to monitor progress and to *evaluate* to what extent the intended changes are achieved. Such monitoring is an important component of every implementation strategy. In doing so, it is important to use appropriate indicators and easily accessible data sources in an interactive fashion. On the basis of this information one can adjust the plan or, if it fails, reanalyze the problems

---

Box 3.6   Elements of Effective Implementation of Change

- *Systematic approach*: sound planning of the implementation activities.
- *Conditions of change*: consider resources, practicalities, as well as social and organizational context for the process of change.
- *Step-wise process*: undertake a sequenced, logical process leading to the implementation of the plan and its impact on target groups.
- *Evidence for and format of the innovation*: sound evidence supporting the innovation, attractive format and presentation.
- *Analysis of performance*: mapping the actual performance and use of the proposed innovation or new practice by target groups.
- *Diagnostic analysis*: a study of the target group and setting before the start of the implementation.
- *Segmentation of the target group*: consideration of different stages of the change process and different needs of subgroups.

- *Engagement of the target group* in the development, adaptation, and planning of the innovation.
- *Alignment*: matching the choice of implementation activities to the results of the diagnostic analysis.
- *Multifaceted strategy*: consideration of multiple interventions in the strategy for change, aiming for a cost-effective mix of methods tailored to the obstacles and incentives to change identified.
- *Staging*: distinguishing between the phases of implementation (dissemination, implementation, integration); different strategies are effective at different stages.
- *Level of change*: take the correct measures at various levels: national, local, team, practice, and professional.
- *Sustainable change*: integrating the new practice into existing routines and structures ("normalization").
- *Continuous evaluation*: ongoing assessment of the impact of the implementation process and its result.

---

involved in its introduction. Feedback is provided to the target group on the (lack of) progress made to enhance their motivation.

The elements of effective implementation of change described here are summarized in Box 3.6.

3.2 The Implementation of Change Model

According to Kotter et al. (1998), the most generic lesson learned from successful cases of change is that the change process goes through a number of steps that, in total, can take quite some time. Neglecting steps creates the illusion of speed, but seldom leads to good results. A second general lesson

is that critical mistakes in one of the steps can have a very negative impact. A process of implementation of change may be initiated for different reasons. First, new scientific information or new technologies may become available that indicate that patient care can be provided more effectively, safely, or efficiently. Ideally, the innovation is supported by a systematic analysis of research. Such new information may be incorporated into guidelines for practice, in care protocols, or care pathways, in which the desired care is described for a department, team, or practice.

Second, the starting point for the implementation may arise from dissatisfaction with current routines within a work setting among one or more stakeholders. Examples of this are the occurrence of critical or undesired incidents in an institution, or data from "audits" or patient questionnaires showing that care could be improved. In many cases, a search of published research will identify relevant studies of improvement strategies, because many problems in healthcare have been the topic of research. There may also be ideas or experiences from one's own or other work settings on how patient care could be better organized or made more efficient ("best practices"), and from these experiences proposals are developed to improve care processes. In the latter cases, evaluation is recommended, because initial or local experiences with improvement strategies may not be transferable to other settings.

Both situations, the one more "guided" and the other more "participatory," can start a process of change that should subsequently be tackled in a *planned and systematic fashion*, in so far as this is possible. "Planned and systematic" does not mean that there is a final plan that permits no deviations. On the contrary, an incremental process is often optimal; here, lessons are learned from previous steps and the approach is adapted continuously and when necessary. Such an iterative or incremental change process demands planning, rigorous preparation, and a number of logical steps. Most authors in this field describe more or less similar steps to be taken in such a change process (e.g. Boxes 3.2–3.4 and 3.8); several examples in this chapter illustrate this phenomenon (see Boxes 3.1 and 3.5).

The *implementation of change model* presented in this chapter represents a summary of this literature and follows the actual practice of improving patient care as closely as possible. The model is shown in diagrammatic form in Figure 3.1 and is used to structure this book in the next few chapters. Beware, however: a model is always a simplification of reality. The actual practice of improving care may demand a different sequence of steps, a rehearsal of steps, or supplementary steps. We will outline the different steps in the model here briefly and will go into more detail in the rest of the book.

3.3 Developing a Proposal and Targets for Change

The first step in the model is the development and determination of a concrete and feasible proposal, or recommended practice, and targets for desired improvement in existing practice. Such a proposal may include new routines for practice, guideline recommendations for effective or efficient care, the introduction of new valuable techniques or procedures into existing clinical work, the use of new information technologies, or insights concerning the organization of patient care processes. Just like other innovations, these must be developed carefully and with an eye to their quality, meet the needs of the target group, be usable and easily available, and be attractively designed (see also Box 3.7). The development of clinical guidelines is discussed in Chapter 6. The ultimate adoption and success of the change strategy require a solid understanding of the characteristics of an innovation and the plan for change. Relevant characteristics include:

- The methods used for its development.
- The quality and credibility of the proposed or recommended practice.
- The credibility of the developers.
- The degree of support for the innovation.
- The accessibility and attractiveness of the proposed improvement.
- The scope for adapting the proposed improvement to suit local situations and needs.

Communication theories emphasize the importance of messages that are understandable and easy to recall. Gladwell (2002) uses the term "sticky message" – a message that is easily retained in the memory. Some authors claim that innovations are a sort of "half-product" that develop their final form by use in practice. An important question is whether these adapted versions of the proposed innovation or guideline are still effective and safe. Many authors have discussed features of

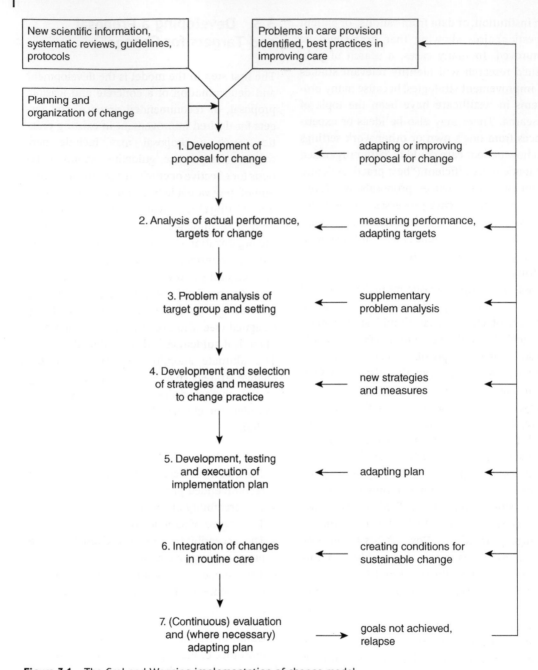

Figure 3.1   The Grol and Wensing implementation of change model.

innovations that facilitate or hinder use in practice. These features are discussed in more detail in Chapter 5. Rogers (1995), for example, highlights the following crucial features of a successful innovation. Such an innovation:

- Conveys more advantages than disadvantages for the user.
- Is consistent with existing values regarding the provision of patient care.
- Is understandable and the implementation is seen as possible and not too difficult.

Box 3.7   Social Marketing Theory

Social marketing theory relates to the process of understanding and satisfying the needs and culture of a target group; the theory provides crucial insights into the process of inducing change. Good "marketing" (the implementation of an innovation) does not start with a ready "product" (a guideline, a new procedure, or best practice). Target group needs and perceptions relative to the optimization and improvement of patient care require systematic collection and analysis. In social marketing, a change agent has different tasks to perform as part of the implementation efforts (Kotler and Roberto 1989; Dickinson 1995):

- Exploring the setting: what are the problems, the strengths and weaknesses? Who is influential in the process of change? Can they be involved in that process?
- Diagnosing the target group: exploring their needs and identifying "segments" in the target population with different needs and different routes for change.
- Identifying competitive messages and their attractiveness for the target group.
- Developing a change strategy optimally suited to the target group and setting. The theory uses seven "Ps" to describe

important elements to be taken into consideration: product (quality, name, style, format, etc.), price (necessary investments), place (dissemination channels, service, and help desk functions), promotion (public relations, advertising, special events), personnel (who will disseminate, source of information), presentation (how and where the innovation will be introduced), and process (phases that a target group needs to complete to adopt the innovation).

- Planning (another "P"), involving the preparation of the implementation plan and its actual implementation, organizing, controlling, and evaluating of activities.

Various researchers (e.g. Dickinson 1995) have applied the framework of social marketing theory to the implementation of guidelines in healthcare. The approach of "moving knowledge to practice" should, in their view, be replaced by an approach in which professionals are central in implementing change. They should be involved in developing both the plans and the actual execution of new practice routines, rather than being the target of information or warnings when they deviate from guidelines.

- Is able to be experienced without risk before starting the implementation.
- Displays its results in a highly visible and accessible manner.

3.4   Assessment of Performance

Before beginning the implementation of an innovation or new routine, the actual care provided should be assessed: What type of care is given? Is the care provided in line with the proposal for change and to what extent? What are the most important deviations of the proposed or recommended way of working? Which

aspects of the proposed performance have been implemented and which have not?

Most proposals for change include a variety of specific recommendations for professional performance and healthcare delivery. Some of these may have been adopted, others not. An efficient approach is to focus mainly on the most important deviations from the recommendations, and on those problems where change is possible and will lead to better outcomes for patients. Since a target group can address only a few targets at the same time, it is important to select the most relevant ones.

A detailed assessment of the actual performance in practice and deviations from the desired care will also help to create a sense of urgency in the target audience – a feeling that care provision should be improved and a feeling of responsibility for that change. Various theories point to the importance of insight into the discrepancy between optimal and actual performance as a motivator of change. These issues are addressed in Chapter 7. Most care providers overestimate the quality of their work and are usually (often unhappily) surprised when they see the "facts," the actual metrics describing their performance (Davis et al. 2006). For a reasonable assessment of actual performance that may stimulate improvement, one needs:

- Indicators to measure actual performance in a valid and reliable way, preferably employing a systematic method used in the development of such indicators.
- Reliable methods for collecting performance data.
- Understandable, acceptable, and motivational feedback for the target group, which encourages participation in a process of improving patient care.

- The formulation of concrete targets for change.

3.5 Analysis of the Target Group and Setting

The analysis of the context in which improvement of routines is to take place, the characteristics of the target group, and the factors stimulating and hampering change are the next step in our model (Box 3.8). The factors that determine whether the implementation of an innovation is successful or not are many and varied (Wensing et al. 2010). Success factors may be connected to the setting in which one wants to implement the innovation, the relationship between individuals within the setting, the goals of the implementation, the actual care provision proposed, the professionals who will have to carry out the innovation, the patients who will have to cooperate with the implementation, the resources available, and the organizational or structural conditions for its effective introduction. Each target

---

Box 3.8 Continuous Quality Improvement in Teams

Ovretveit (1999) proposes a model for quality improvement to be carried out in teams, in which a clear distinction is made between a diagnostic phase and a solution or therapeutic stage. The author suggests that

individuals are often inclined to skip the analysis of the problem and its causes, and move on too quickly to plans for solution. The model has nine steps:

Investigation:

1. Choosing the problem or improvement

2. Formulating the problem and forming the team

3. Guessing the causes of the problem

4. Gathering data to find the cause

5. Deciding on the real cause

Solution:

6. Planning the solution

7. Implementing the change

8. Evaluating the results

9. Finishing or continuing

group or setting will be in some sense unique. Not everyone in the target group can be placed in the same category. Some members or subgroups will be further advanced in the process of acceptance and adoption of an innovation than others. Thus, effective implementation cannot take place without an analysis of the setting and the target group in which the implementation is to take place. One must, as it were, get inside the heads of the individuals and the institution that must change. This type of *diagnostic or problem analysis* may relate to:

- The aims and settings of the implementation: Who wants what change? In what areas? For what reasons?
- Segments within the target group: What phase of change are they now in?
- Facilitators of and barriers to the change.

We discuss each of these aspects briefly here; more details can be found in Chapters 8 and 9.

3.5.1 Aims and Settings of the Implementation

First, it is important to consider the aims of the implementation, the individuals involved, and the roles played by those involved in the process. For example, it makes a sizable difference whether a regional health insurer is planning on introducing the rational use of antibiotics to reduce the costs of antibiotic use; a national multiprofessional commission on antibiotic use has launched guidelines to combat antibiotic resistance in institutions; or a local hospital committee wants to improve antibiotic prescribing because of increasing antimicrobial resistance. The players and their interests are different, as is the impact of the innovation. These differences influence the level of acceptance that might be anticipated when the innovation is introduced. This information is important when formulating an implementation plan, particularly if one is to make decisions about the tasks of those involved. Furthermore, it is important to have an overview, a "social map" of the individuals and

organizations that play a role or have an interest in the implementation. This information is also required for developing a successful, feasible plan.

3.5.2 Segments within the Target Group and Stages of Change

In the varying theories on change (see Chapter 2), attempts have been made to identify specifically recognizable subgroups within a target group that have different features and therefore require a different approach. The most familiar classification is that provided by Rogers (2003), which divides individuals into:

- "Innovators": a small group that is very keen on new ideas.
- "Early adopters": an active group that often carries a good deal of status within the target group and that functions as a point of reference for most innovators.
- "Early majority": a group that does not consist of leaders, but that has close contact with "early adopters" and lets them lead the way.
- "Late majority": a group that is skeptical about change and not susceptible to information sources, that has more faith in public opinion, or is more influenced by pressure from colleagues.
- "Laggards": a conservative group that offers resistance to change.

Rogers also describes that change takes place through social networks within the target group and that this is the means whereby various subgroups influence one another. Within this social network, the availability of "innovators" and "change agents" is of great importance for effective implementation within the total group. "Educationally influential" physicians are identified by their colleagues as professionals who encourage learning and sharing knowledge, are clinically up to date, and treat their peers as equals (Wright et al. 2004).

3.5.3 Phases in a Process of Change: A Summary of the Literature

A number of theories in the field of implementation of innovations take the *perspective of the target group* as their starting point. These theories describe change or implementation as a step-wise *process* that individuals, groups (teams), or organizations (institutions, practices) must follow to ultimately arrive at the desired practice. Even though they originate from different disciplines and domains (organization studies, marketing, communication sciences, health information services, management sciences, and psychology), the similarity in steps which play a role in these sorts of processes is striking. Despite varying terms, a number of steps emerge that should be kept in mind when introducing improvements in clinical practice. Within each of these steps, important problems or bottlenecks can arise which must be solved before the next step can be taken. In this sense, they follow a set sequence (Kotter et al. 1998). See Table 3.1 for a summary of a number of models. Examples of steps in the change process can be found in Rogers' diffusion of innovation theory (Rogers 2003), Pathman's models of adherence to guidelines (Pathman et al. 1996), and Prochaska's transtheoretical model (Prochaska and Velicer 1997; Prochaska et al. 2008; see Box 3.9).

If we summarize the different step-by-step models on the implementation of change described in the literature, different phases can be distinguished (Box 3.10). These phases – based on the planning model proposed in this book – represent those which most individuals pass through if an innovation, clinical routine,

---

Box 3.9   Transtheoretical Model

One of the theories of change with a central role for different phases of change is the transtheoretical model of change in healthy behavior (Prochaska and Velicer 1997; Prochaska et al. 2008). Prochaska outlines six distinct motivational stages:

- *Precontemplation*: a person does not have the intention to change in the near future. Reading or thinking about change is avoided. Change can be stimulated in this phase by increasing awareness and involvement, and by discussing the consequences of current behavior for others.
- *Contemplation*: a person considers that he or she might change within the next six months. Advantages and disadvantages are considered; however, the person is not yet ready for concrete actions. Change is promoted in this phase by discussing the attitude toward the proposed new behavior and the barriers to adopting the change.
- *Preparation*: a person has the intention to change in a more timely fashion and seeks interventions or support for the new behavior. Change is stimulated by enhancing the self-efficacy and beliefs of the actor or target group and by overt commitment to the change planned.
- *Action*: a person manages to adopt visible changes in behavior. This is facilitated by learning of new skills, social support, and incentives for the new behavior.
- *Maintenance*: a person aims at preventing relapse into old routines; this may take from several months to years. This can be promoted by organizational measures and support that reinforce the new behavior (such as continuous monitoring and feedback).
- *Termination*: relapse is impossible.

The theory is partly supported by research in the clinical and behavioral area, such as smoking cessation and alcohol addiction, but the findings are not consistent. The model is criticized for the overlapping nature of the phases and the difficulty in distinguishing between them.

Box 3.10   Phases in the Process of Change for Individuals

Orientation:	Awareness of the innovation
	Interest and involvement
Insight:	Understanding the proposed change
	Insight into own routines
Acceptance:	Positive attitude, motivation to change
	Positive intention or decision to change
Change:	Actual adoption in practice
	Confirmation of benefit or value of change
Maintenance:	Integration of new practice into routines
	Embedding of new practice in the organization

Source: Grol and Wensing (2004); Grol and Buchan (2006).

---

or desired change in patient care is to be integrated into practice routines (Grol and Wensing 2004; Grol and Buchan 2006). The phases may also apply to change in teams and organizations, which is often characterized by additional complexities. Not all steps are always taken or taken in the order presented, but the model can help to differentiate between groups with different degrees of preparedness to change.

3.5.4   Orientation

This phase aims at making the healthcare setting – the "soil," to use an agricultural analogy – ready to make change possible. The target group needs to become aware, interested, and involved in the innovation or new way of working. Actions should be focused on:

- *Awareness of the innovation*: first and foremost, care providers, teams, or institutions must be aware of an innovation, even if they are unaware of its details. It should be made available in such a way that as many individuals from the target group (professionals, patients, managers, policy makers, etc.) as possible are aware of the proposed or recommended practice.
- *Interest and involvement*: curiosity about the innovation is aroused. New working methods and techniques are presented in such a way that relevant individuals think: "this is interesting or possibly useful and relevant to my work. I would like to find out more about this."

3.5.5   Insight

This phase aims at informing the target group about the innovation and about actual performance in relation to the innovation. It should lead to a sense of urgency – a belief that it is unacceptable to continue with current routines. Implementation focuses on:

- *Understanding*: the target group, particularly clinical professionals, must know exactly what recommended care involves and what is expected in terms of new behavior. The transfer of information in this phase must be such that individuals have a clear understanding of what the innovation entails.
- *Insight into own routines*: equally important, the target group needs to develop clear insight into their own performance and know which features differ from the new proposals.

3.5.6   Acceptance

In this phase the emphasis is on the motivation needed for behavior change. The target group needs to develop the feeling that change is important and feasible. Actions are focused on:

- *Positive attitude or a motivation to change*: the targeted care providers, the team or the institution, including all individuals involved, must weigh the advantages and disadvantages of the new working method and be convinced that it is valuable, effective, or useful, and/or that it will lead to savings in time or money or to better healthcare outcomes.

- *Positive intention or decision to change*: the target group resolves to work differently in the short term. If they are to live up to this decision they need to have a good idea of how the innovation can be applied to their own work setting, what problems may arise in so doing, and how these can be solved. The feeling must grow that they are capable of carrying through the change and that applying it to their own work setting is feasible.

3.5.7 Change

This phase aims at making a start with the change in practice. The target group needs to experiment with the new routines and begin to believe that it is effective and feasible. Implementation in this phase focuses on:

- *Actual adoption in practice*: an opportunity to try out the new working method on a small scale is provided in order to allow the target group to gain experience in using it, to learn the skills involved, and to carry out practical and organizational adaptations.
- *Confirmation of benefit or value of change*: having begun to implement the new routines, the care provider or team concludes whether it works or has begun working, whether it is satisfactory, and whether it can be further implemented without major problems, costs, or harm.

3.5.8 Maintenance

In this phase the new way of working becomes part of the normal routines and processes in practice or in the institution. Implementation focuses on:

- *Integration of new practice into routines*: the new way of working will have to be integrated with existing care protocols or care plans. Reverting to old routines or forgetting

the guideline or innovation should be avoided.
- *Embedding of new practice in the organization*: finally, the new routines must be embedded and supported by the care organization to such an extent that continuous implementation is possible. Organizational, financial, and structural conditions for maintaining implementation are fulfilled.

3.5.9 Barriers and Facilitators to Changing Practice

Different factors may be important at each phase or step in the change process. Both stimulating and impeding factors may play a role in determining the success of the implementation. Insight into these factors is of great importance in order to inform how improvement strategies should be designed and understand what kind of activities should be developed (Grol and Wensing 2004). Factors may be related to the following:

- Individual care providers: their knowledge, skills, attitudes, values, self-confidence, habits, and personalities.
- Social factors: patients (their knowledge, attitude, behavior, expectations, needs, experiences, and priorities); attitude and behavior of colleagues; the culture in the social network; the opinion of leaders and key figures; and the presence of innovators.
- Healthcare organization: financial resources, organization of care processes, qualified staff, institutional policies, task divisions, logistics processes, electronic health records and information systems, and leadership.
- Healthcare system: reimbursements, contracts, rules, regulations, and laws.
- Various barriers and facilitators may play a role in the different phases of a process of change and may thereby activate the need for diverse strategies and interventions. Indicators for evaluating the success of the

implementation activity can also be derived from this process.

3.6 Selection and Development of Improvement Strategies

By linking the factors identified in the previous stages and any other relevant information, a cost-effective mix of measures, methods, and strategies for improving patient care may be selected, developed, and then tested out in the targeted population. Different phases of the implementation process usually require different strategies:

- *Dissemination*: increasing interest in, and understanding of the innovation and encouraging a positive attitude and a willingness to adapt existing routines.
- *Implementation*: encouraging its actual adoption and ensuring that the recommended performance becomes a set part of daily routines.

The literature identifies a great number of strategies that can be used when introducing innovations and changes. Examples include continuing education programs, audit and feedback, reminders, computerized decision support, patient education, financial incentives, enhanced interprofessional teams, and redesign of care processes. The Cochrane Effective Practice and Organization of Care Group (EPOC) has categorized strategies according to mode of delivery into:

- Interventions directed at individual or groups of health professionals, for instance continuing medical education (CME) or continuing professional development (CPD), outreach visits, audit and feedback, or reminders, use of opinion leaders.
- Interventions directed at patients, focused on better care provision and implementation of knowledge.

- Financial interventions, directed at care providers or patients.
- Organizational interventions, structural measures and interventions directed at organizational changes.
- Laws and formal regulations.

The selection and tailoring of strategies for improving healthcare practice are expanded in more detail in Chapter 10. The published body of research evidence on such strategies is substantial and has been summarized in many literature reviews (e.g. Wensing et al. 1998). Chapters 11–18 provide summaries of the available research evidence on a wide range of strategies for implementation and improvement in healthcare. A mix of activities and tailoring to local settings are usually needed in line with the results of the diagnostic analysis (see Section 3.5 and the example in Box 3.11). In practice, a balance must be reached between, on the one hand, the possibility of achieving the desired effects and, on the other, the amount of money, time, effort, and personal commitment invested and the disruption the innovation may cause.

3.7 Development, Testing, and Execution of an Implementation Plan

When developing an implementation plan, it is important to pay attention to the effective dissemination of information (in order to arouse interest and to promote sufficient knowledge about the guideline) and encouragement of its acceptance (to foster a positive attitude and willingness to bring about real behavioral change), as well as to promoting actual implementation and integration into normal working routines and care processes. Various strategies may be effective in different phases of the process of change. These steps are covered in more detail in Chapter 19. In planning

---

Box 3.11 Prevention of Infections

In Chapter 2, we discussed the problem of hospital infections and hand hygiene before and after contact with patients. This is one of the major causes of morbidity and mortality. Many theories offer different opinions on how best to address this problem. To implement a national evidence-based guideline on prevention of hospital infections, we selected a number of key recommendations on hand hygiene. In a written survey (Hopman and Grol 1991), 120 physicians and nurses were asked to rate problems with using these recommendations in normal hospital practice. Problems proved to be related to the professionals, the social context, and the organizational context.

	Experienced as problem in implementation of guideline (%)
Problems related to professional	
I hardly see any complications	61
I easily fall back in old routines	49
Hard evidence for guideline is lacking	43
Frequent washing gives damage and irritation to hands	81
Problems related to social context	
Nobody controls hand hygiene	50
Management is not interested	45
Problems related to organizational context	
I forget it during rush hours	65
Impossible in normal work	61
Costs more time that is not available	50
We do not have hygiene guidelines in our hospital	49
Insufficient equipment in our hospital	42

On the basis of this diagnostic analysis, a detailed plan for implementation of the guideline can be developed with, for instance, the following strategies:

- A brochure with the most important recommendations and the relevant scientific evidence.
- Team meetings to discuss the guideline, the problems with adoption, and a plan for implementation.
- A protocol for the hospital developed by the teams involved, but authorized by the Executive Board and disseminated to all wards.
- Regular reminders, regular monitoring of hand hygiene performance.
- Observation and feedback by team leaders.
- Continuous monitoring of infections; comparison of results of different wards with feedback.
- External support for teams to achieve their targets.

A discussion is needed about which mix of strategies is feasible and affordable and will lead to the largest improvements. The literature on improving hand hygiene suggests that a program with a variety of strategies will have the most effect (Pittet et al. 2000; Naikoba and Hayward 2001; WHO 2009; Pronovost et al. 2010; Sawyer et al. 2010).

improvement activities, it is helpful to consider the following points:

- Start on a small scale with a limited number of motivated individuals, teams, or institutions. The implementation plan and the various interventions may be tested on them for suitability and feasibility, and may be modified or adjusted in the light of this experience.
- Plan according to the different phases of the change process: What must still be done to inform and interest specific subgroups? What must be done to overcome resistance? What is needed to incorporate a change into existing care processes?
- Establish at what level interventions and measures can best be planned. This will be different for national programs, institution-directed programs, ward or team projects, and projects aimed at local groups or practices.
- Involve the target group: it is critically important to engage this group in the development of an innovation or protocol and/or in analyzing problems in implementation. Representatives of the target group can play an important part in designing and testing the implementation plan. They may often know best what is possible and can think creatively about suitable interventions.
- Plan activities over time: develop and distribute a timetable and a logical sequence of planned activities.
- Distribute tasks, procedures, and responsibilities: issues such as who does what, where, and who checks it has been done must be clearly established.
- Build the implementation plan into the existing structures and channels for contacting or training the target group.
- Identify the plan's long-term aims; these are used to guide ongoing evaluation.
- Plan for and identify adequate structures, resources, and personnel: depending on whether it is a small-scale ward or practice implementation project or a large-scale

implementation project, it will need appropriate resources and suitable expertise.
- Finally, attend to the organizational culture in the setting in which the implementation is to take place. Clear leadership, good collaboration between professionals, and a culture in which continuous learning and improvement of care can occur are all desirable; they most often represent a prerequisite to achieving change.

3.8 Sustainable Change: Integration of Change into Practice Routines

It is crucial that the planned improvements are integrated into normal practice routines and embedded in organizational processes in order to prevent relapse and arrive at the stage of "normalization" (Box 3.12). When the implementation of an innovation or new routine is no longer actively supported by a project or an improvement team, the chance of relapse is considerable. To guarantee the sustainability of an improvement, specific measures are needed – for example additional resources, new skilled staff, health information technology, or system changes. Alternatively, specific parts of the implementation program can be continued on a structural basis. For example, continuous monitoring of the proposed new performance or regular training on the new behavior may be required. The issue of sustainable improvement is discussed in more detail in Chapter 19.

3.9 Evaluation and (Possible) Adaptations to the Plan

The final step in the implementation of innovations in care is the evaluation of the results, responding to the question: Have the goals been achieved? This is a crucial step which often fails to receive the attention it deserves. Evaluation shows whether the energy that has been invested has led to the desired degree of change and, where this is not the case,

---

Box 3.12 Normalization Process Theory

Normalization process theory (May et al. 2009) is a sociological theory on the integration of new routines and organizational innovations within normal patient care. The theory provides a framework for studies of complex interventions. In such interventions, one has to deal with three interacting components:

- *Actors*: individuals and groups that play a role in the implementation.
- *Objects*: procedures, protocols, and resources that should make adoption possible.
- *Contexts*: physical, organizational, and legal structures that hinder or facilitate change.

In order to arrive at the stage of "normalization," a change strategy should meet the following criteria:

- *Interactional workability*: all stakeholders have the same expectations with regard to the targets that should be achieved.
- *Relational integration*: the implementation strategy enhances the target group's knowledge about the proposed change, and achieves a better understanding of the performance of others in the social network.
- *Skill-set workability*: the change strategy influences the way in which patient care is defined, divided, and conducted.
- *Contextual integration*: the change strategy promotes the integration of the new way of working within existing structures and procedures and the resources available.

---

considers what can be done to ensure greater success (see the example in Box 3.13). In addition, rigorous evaluation studies add to the accumulation of scientific knowledge, which supports future initiatives to improve patient care. The evaluation may result in (Figure 3.1):

- Adaptation of the proposal for change.
- Repeated assessment of actual performance, and revision of the goals if these prove to be unrealistic.
- Supplementary analyses of enabling factors and barriers or impediments to success.
- Further strategies and measures to bring about change and more potentially effective change strategies being developed.
- Revision of the plan and execution of the implementation, including the manner by which it has been introduced or the way in which the process of change has been organized.
- Measures to support the sustainability of the improvements and prevent relapse.

Evaluation is not the final step in an implementation project, however. Ideally,

implementers continuously assess whether and how activities reach and impact on the target group, revising procedures on the basis of these findings. How the evaluation is tackled depends on the type of project: a small-scale improvement project (Box 3.13), a scientific study of implementation (Box 3.14), or a nationwide implementation program. The aims of these different projects vary, as do the populations and the evaluation designs. In all cases, one really wants to know if the goals formulated beforehand have been attained in the project or program:

- *Short-term aims*: have the conditions for implementation been met; does the target group know about the change and has it been accepted?
- *Intermediate aims*: is the proposed change in performance actually being applied?
- *Long-term goals*: what is the effect in terms of health benefits, greater well-being and patient satisfaction, or cost reduction?

Further information about many of these issues is available throughout the book. In

---

Box 3.13   Improvement of Hospital Care for Patients with Head and Neck Cancer

To improve care for patients with head and neck cancer in an academic hospital, professionals of all wards involved in and responsible for the care pathway started by formulating indicators for effective multidisciplinary care (Ouwens 2007). Cancer patients were interviewed about their opinions and needs concerning optimal management. The indicators created were used to assess actual performance. This process revealed that the time to diagnosis and treatment was too long for most patients, that many patients were not discussed in multidisciplinary team meetings, and that patients did not receive appropriate information about their condition and treatment. In turn, this process led to an improvement project with all wards involved, aimed at better collaboration and improved workflow processes. An assessment 1 year after the intervention demonstrated that receiving a diagnosis within 10 days increased from 35 to 70%, and the percentage of patients who had contact with a case manager increased from 50 to 85%. The percentage of patients receiving counseling on food intake improved from 0 to 42%. Care providers particularly valued the feedback on their performance and saw the discussion of this feedback in a safe, moderated setting as crucial for the change process.

Box 3.14   Improving the Treatment of Urinary Tract Infections and Sore Throat

In a randomized trial of 142 primary care practices in Norway, half of the practices received a series of interventions aimed at evidence-based management of urinary tract infections, and the other half got the same interventions aimed at better management of sore throat (Flottorp et al. 2003). The groups thus served as each other's controls. The project aimed at improving the use of antibiotics, to reduce laboratory testing and to increase telephone consultations. The project started with an analysis among physicians, staff, and patients of barriers and facilitators related to the proposed changes. Based on this analysis, specific interventions and measures were selected to stimulate change:

- A summary of the recommendations on a poster and in a computerized tool
- Educational materials for patients
- Computerized decision support and reminders
- Incentives for telephone consultations
- Interactive education for doctors and staff
- Recognition (such as credits or continuing professional development points) for participation in the education.

The changes in performance were, for both topics, very small and not significantly different between the intervention group and the control group. The reasons for this lack of effect were unclear. One hypothesis is that practices need more intensive personal support in order to change clinical care. Another is that inadequate attention was paid to the context and culture of practice affecting both patients and professionals: it was a well-established practice to prescribe antibiotics for all infections. A more rigorous analysis of the barriers to improvement was suggested.

order to determine whether implementation goals have been reached, they must be made measurable. For this purpose, "indicators" or metrics and criteria for goal attainment should be formulated and selected; this is described in Chapter 7. The question of how the evaluation of the "effects" can best be established and which study design and methods can be used for this are described in more detail in Chapters 20 and 21. "Process evaluation" – determining whether the implementation plan has been carried out as intended, and which factors influenced its success or failure – is described in greater detail in Chapter 22. Finally, the evaluation of the costs and efficiency of implementation strategies is discussed in Chapter 23.

3.10 Planning of the Implementation Process

After introducing the cyclic model for the implementation of change in patient care (Figure 3.1), we return to the start of this model: planning and preparation for the change process. Successful implementation of innovations or changes requires careful preparation and planning of all of the steps in the implementation process represented in the cyclical model (see Table 3.2 for an example). This is as true for introducing an evidence-based guideline, a new procedure, or a best practice into clinical practice as it is for remedying shortcomings in patient care. The shape of this planning varies according to whether the implementation program is large-scale, national, regional, or a smaller-scale project aimed at improving care in a single ward or practice. There will also be differences between a controlled study design on the one hand and an improvement project with simple monitoring of goal attainment on the other. Nevertheless, on the basis of experience from a wide range of implementation projects, there are a number of common points that require attention:

- *Create a team* that has both sufficient expertise and motivation to coordinate and stimulate the project. Depending on the scale and the budget, the team may need expertise in the fields of *leadership* (someone who plays a central role in communicating the aim and involving the target group in the implementation); *coordination* (the daily organization of activities); *technical expertise* (specific knowledge and skills in the area of, for instance, literature analysis, data gathering, or computer use); and *administrative support* (for example, in order to organize meetings, to plan social activities, or to develop products). The team needs to develop a plan in which different tasks and responsibilities are confirmed and for which members have accountability.

- Explore whether there is enough *support for the improvement activities* in the target setting. The target audience may have a negative attitude toward quality improvement, knowledge transfer, or implementation of innovations in general, or may lack a firm understanding of change processes in their work. In addition, leaders in the setting may lack the motivation needed for the project or important organizational conditions for project management may be lacking, such as the availability of team meetings, data, or computers. Financial interests, such a fear for a loss of income or earlier investments that have not yielded benefit, may play a role as well. In such cases, it is necessary first to work on a "positive context for change" and prepare the target setting for a change process.

- Guarantee clarity about the nature of the *target group* and ensure that in all stages of the project members of the group are involved in the implementation process. The group of individuals who experience the consequences of an implementation is often far larger than one imagines beforehand (Lomas 1997). It is worth compiling a list of those individuals, groups, units, and

Table 3.2 A step-by-step approach to implementation of a blood transfusion protocol in the Royal Melbourne Hospital is described on the basis of a number of questions.

Steps	Blood transfusion
1. What is the aim, what do you want to achieve?	Reduction in the use of incorrect blood products
2. Who can help me to do this?	Team was formed with head of hematology as coordinator and doctors from the transfusion committee
3. What is the existing care practice, does it differ from elsewhere or from guidelines?	Use of blood products was incorrect for 16% of red cell transfusions, 13% of platelet transfusions, and 31% of "fresh frozen plasma" transfusions
4. Who should be involved in the improvement?	Hematology ward, medical staff, hospital managers
5. What are the key messages and recommendations?	Follow the blood transfusion protocol to the letter
6. Which concrete goals are being aimed at?	Reduction of the number of incorrect blood transfusions to an acceptable level (<5%)
7. Is the information about the improvement suitable for the target group(s)?	Draft protocol was produced based on the literature and presented to the transfusion committee for comments. The subsequent draft was distributed throughout the hospital for comment. Final recommendations were printed on the application form
8. What are the bottlenecks in terms of its introduction?	Doctors are not used to having to make decisions according to protocols nor to being required to check them; it takes extra time
9. What are the possible suitable interventions and measures?	Audit and feedback; using opinion leader; educational materials; reminders; administrative measures (application form); feedback if guideline not adhered to
10. Is there sufficient support for the change?	Transfusion committee with all members involved continuously supporting the process
11. What does the change cost and is it worth it?	(Not calculated)
12. Did it work?	Incorrect red cell transfusion rates fell from 16 to 3%; incorrect platelet transfusion rates from 13 to 2.5%. For fresh frozen plasma incorrect transfusion rates fell, from 34 to 15%, but this was still not thought to be acceptable

Source: Metz et al. (1995); Tuckfield et al. (1997); NHMRC (2000).

organizations whose opinions are important and whose cooperation is desirable. One might form one or more brainstorming groups made up of a variety of individuals involved who can look at it from their viewpoint and thus provide useful input. These may be different individuals at various stages in the process. Different inputs are required in the phase when a proposal for improvement in care practice is being developed from those at the stage of defining indicators or the analysis of the target group and setting. They may be different again from those at the stage of planning and introduction of an implementation strategy (Hall and Eccles 2000).

- *Involve the leaders* of the practice, clinic, hospital, or other health setting. This is important for both the formal leaders (e.g. executive board members and managers need to support the program or project) and the informal, often front-line leaders who need to "sell" the project to the target group.

- Ensure *sufficient budget and support staff* for the project or program. As difficult as this is, even in the case of small projects, individuals need to be able to free up their time for extra work. In addition, books, instruments, or computers may be required. The collection and analysis of data to evaluate performance changes bear costs and human resources. A calculation of the necessary budget as well as an estimation of individuals' time to be invested is therefore very important, as is the authorization for the budget by the appropriate organization.
- Finally, develop a realistic *timetable*: What is happening when? One should take into consideration that most implementation paths and change processes take a certain amount of time and that the time required is often underestimated beforehand (Evans and Haines 2000; Wye and McClenahan 2000).

3.11 Conclusions

In the first three chapters of this book, we have provided a description of what "implementation of change" involves in practice, which theoretical points of view exist regarding changes in care practice, and how – in general terms – a program or project aimed at the introduction of new working methods or improvements in practice could be set up. We have seen that – regardless of whether it is a large-scale or small-scale project and no matter whether it involves the introduction of new care procedures or best practices, or aims to solve problems in care practice – good preparation and planning are always important. All the steps in the implementation process must be given the necessary amount of attention. Precisely what this may mean and what science and experiences in practice can teach us will be discussed in the remainder of the book.

References

Baker, R., Reddish, S., Robertson, N. et al. (2001). Randomised controlled trial of tailored strategies to implement guidelines for the management of patients with depression in general practice. *Br. J. Gen. Pract.* 51: 737–741.

Bartholomew, L., Parcel, G., Kok, G., and Gottlieb, N. (2001). *Intervention Mapping. Designing Theory and Evidence Based Health Promotion Programmes*. Mountain View, CA: Mayfield.

Bessen, T., Clark, R., Shakib, S., and Hughes, G. (2009). A multifaceted strategy for implementation of the Ottawa ankle rules in two emergency departments. *BMJ* 339: b3056.

van Bokhoven, M., Kok, G., and van der Weijden, T. (2003). Designing a quality improvement intervention: a systematic approach. In: *Quality Improvement Research* (eds. R. Grol, R. Baker and F. Moss), 147–164. London: BMJ Books.

Cooper, R. and Zinud, R. (1990). Information technology implementation research: a technological diffusion approach. *Manag. Sci.* 36: 123–129.

Cretin, S. (1998). *Implementing Guidelines: An Overview*. Santa Monica, CA: RAND.

Davis, D.A., Mazmanian, P.E., Fordis, M. et al. (2006). Accuracy of physician self-assessment compared with observed measures of competence: a systematic review. *JAMA* 296 (9): 1094–1102.

Davis, D.A., O'Brien, M.A., Freemantle, N. et al. (1999). Impact of formal continuing medical education: do conferences, workshops, rounds, and other traditional continuing education activities change physician behaviour or health care outcomes? *JAMA* 282: 867–874.

Davis, D.A. and Taylor-Vaisey, A. (1997). Translating guidelines into practice: a systematic review of theoretic concepts, practical experience and research evidence in the adoption of clinical practice guidelines. *CMAJ* 157: 408–416.

Davis, D.A., Thomson, M.A., Oxman, A.D. et al. (1992). Evidence for the effectiveness of CME: a review of 50 randomized controlled trials. *JAMA* 268: 1111–1117.

Dickinson, E. (1995). Using marketing principles for health care development. *Qual. Health Care* 4: 40–44.

Evans, D. and Haines, A. (2000). *Implementing Evidence-Based Changes in Health Care*. Abingdon: Radcliffe Medical Press.

Feder, G., Eccles, M., Grol, R. et al. (1999). Using clinical guidelines. *BMJ* 318: 728–730.

Ferlie, E. and Shortell, S. (2001). Improving the quality of health care in the United Kingdom and the United States: a framework for change. *Milbank Q.* 79: 281–315.

Flottorp, S., Havelsrud, K., and Oxman, A. (2003). Process evaluation of a cluster randomised trial of tailored interventions to implement guidelines in primary care. Why is it so hard to change practice? *Fam. Pract.* 20: 333–339.

Garside, P. (1998). Organisational context for quality: lessons from the fields of organisational development and change management. *Qual. Health Care* 7 (Suppl): S8–S15.

Gladwell, M. (2002). *The Tipping Point*. Boston: Little, Brown.

Graham, I.D. and Tetroe, J. (2009). Getting evidence into policy and practice: perspective of a health research funder. *J. Can. Acad. Child Adolesc. Psychiatry* 18: 46–50.

Green, L.W., Eriksen, M.P., and Schor, E.L. (1988). Preventive practices by physicians: behaviorial determinants and potential interventions. *Am. J. Prev. Med.* 4 (Suppl): 101–107.

Green, L.W. and Kreuter, M.W. (1991). *Health Promotion Planning: An Educational and Environmental Approach*. Palo Alto, CA: Mayfield Publishing.

Greenhalgh, T., Robert, G., Macfarlane, F. et al. (2004). Diffusion of innovations in service organizations: systematic review and recommendations. *Milbank Q.* 82: 581–629.

Grol, R. (1992). Implementing guidelines in general practice care. *Qual. Health Care* 1: 184–191.

Grol, R. (1997). Beliefs and evidence in changing clinical practice. *BMJ* 315: 418–421.

Grol, R. and Buchan, H. (2006). Clinical guidelines: what can we do to increase their use? *Med. J. Aust.* 185: 301–302.

Grol, R. and Grimshaw, J. (2003). From best evidence to best practice: effective implementation of change in patients' care. *Lancet* 362: 1225–1230.

Grol, R.T.P.M., van Everdingen, J.J.E., and Casparie, A.F. (1994). *Invoering van richtlijnen en veranderingen. Een handleiding voor de medische, paramedische en verpleegkundige praktijk. [Implementing Guidelines and Changes. A Manual for Medical, Allied Health and Nursing Practice]*. Utrecht: De Tijdstroom.

Grol, R. and Wensing, M. (2004). What drives change? Barriers to and incentives for achieving evidence-based practice. *Med. J. Aust.* 180: S57–S60.

Hall, L. and Eccles, M. (2000). Case study of an interprofessional and inter-organisational programme to adapt, implement and evaluate clinical guidelines in secondary care. *Br. J. Clin. Gov.* 5: 72–82.

Hopman, J. and Grol, R. (1991). Preventie van infecties in het verpleeghuis. [Prevention of infections in the nursing home]. In: *Kwaliteitsbewaking in de Verpleeghuisge-Neeskunde. [Monitoring of Quality in Nursing Home Medicine]* (ed. R. Grol). Den Haag: VUGA.

Kok, G. (1993). Theorieen over verandering (Theories on change). In: *Gezondheidsvoorlichting en -opvoeding. [Health Promotion]* (eds. V. Damoiseaux, H.T. van der Molen and G.J. Kok, pp. 221–235. Assen/Maastricht: Van Gorcum.

Kotler, P. and Roberto, E.L. (1989). *Social Marketing: Strategies for Changing Public Behavior*. New York: Free Press.

Kotter, J.P., Collins, J., Porras, J. et al. (1998). *Harvard Business Review on Change*. Boston, MA: Harvard Business School Press.

Langley, G., Nolan, K., Nolan, T. et al. (1996). *The Improvement Guide*. San Francisco, CA: Jossey-Bass.

Lomas, J. (1997). *Beyond the Sound of Hand Clapping: A Discussion Document on Improving Health Research Dissemination and Uptake*. Sydney: University of Sydney.

Lomas, J. (2007). The in-between world of knowledge brokering. *BMJ* 334: 129–132.

Lomas, J. and Haynes, R. (1988). A taxonomy and critical review of tested strategies for the application of clinical practice recommendations: from "official" to "individual" clinical policy. In: Battista, R. and Lawrence, R. (eds.) Implementing preventive services. *Am. J. Prev. Med.* 4: 77–95.

May, C.R., Mair, F., Finch, T. et al. (2009). Development of a theory of implementation and integration: normalization process theory. *Implement. Sci.* 4: 29.

McGuire, W. (1981). Theoretical foundation of campaigns. In: *Public Communications Campaigns* (eds. R. Rice and W. Paisley), 43–66. Beverley Hills, CA: Sage.

Metz, J., McGrath, K.M., Copperchini, M.L. et al. (1995). Appropriateness of transfusions of red cells, platelets and fresh frozen plasma. An audit in a tertiary care teaching hospital. *Med. J. Aust.* 162: 572–577.

Mittman, B.S., Tonesk, X., and Jacobson, P.D. (1992). Implementing clinical practice guidelines: social influence strategies and practitioner behaviour change. *QRB Qual. Rev. Bull.* 18: 413–422.

Moulding, N.T., Silagy, C.A., and Weller, D.P. (1999). A framework for effective management of change in clinical practice: dissemination and implementation of clinical practice guidelines. *Qual. Health Care* 8: 177–183.

Naikoba, S. and Hayward, A. (2001). The effectiveness of interventions aimed at increasing handwashing in healthcare workers – a systematic review. *J. Hosp. Infect.* 47: 173–180.

NHMRC (2000). *How to Put the Evidence into Practice: Implementation and Dissemination Strategies*. Canberra: Commonwealth of Australia.

NHS (1999). Centre for reviews and dissemination. Getting evidence into practice. *Eff. Health Care* 5: 1–15.

Orlandi, M. (1987). Promoting health and preventing disease in health care settings: an analysis of barriers. *Prev. Med.* 16: 119–130.

Ouwens, M.M.T.J. (2007). Integrated care for patients with cancer. Thesis. Nijmegen: Radboud Universiteit.

Ovretveit, J. (1999). A team quality improvement sequence for complex problem. *Qual. Health Care* 8: 239–246.

Pathman, D.E., Konrad, T.R., Freed, G.L. et al. (1996). The awareness-to-adherence model of the steps to clinical guideline compliance. The case of pediatric vaccine recommendations. *Med. Care* 34: 873–889.

Pittet, D., Hugonnet, S., Harbarth, S. et al. (2000). Effectiveness of a hospital-wide programme to improve compliance with hand hygiene. Infection control programme. *Lancet* 356: 1307–1312.

Prochaska, J.O., Redding, C.A., and Evers, K.E. (2008). The transtheoretical models and stages of change. In: *Health Behavior and Health Education*, 4e (eds. K. Glanz, B.K. Rimer and K. Viswanath), 99–120. San Francisco, CA: Jossey-Bass.

Prochaska, J.O. and Velicer, W.F. (1997). The transtheoretical model of health behavior change. *Am. J. Health Promot.* 12: 38–48.

Pronovost, P.J., Goeschel, C.A., Colantuoni, E. et al. (2010). Sustaining reductions in catheter related bloodstream infections in Michigan intensive care units: observational study. *BMJ* 340: c309.

Robertson, N., Baker, R., and Hearnshaw, H. (1996). Changing the clinical behaviour of doctors: a psychological framework. *Qual. Health Care* 1: 51–54.

Rogers, E. (1995). Lessons for guidelines from the diffusion of innovation. *Jt Comm. J. Qual. Improv.* 21: 324–328.

Rogers, E.M. (2003). *Diffusion of Innovations*. Simon and Schuster: New York.

Sawyer, M., Weeks, K., Goeschel, C.A. et al. (2010). Using evidence, rigorous measurement, and collaboration to eliminate central catheter-associated bloodstream infections. *Crit. Care Med.* 38: S292–S298.

Solomon, D.H., Hashimoto, H., Daltroy, L., and Liang, M.H. (1998). Techniques to improve physicians' use of diagnostic tests: a new conceptual framework. *JAMA* 280: 2020–2027.

Spence, W. (1994). *Innovation. The Communication of Change in Ideas, Practices and Products*. London: Chapman and Hall.

Squires, J.E., Sullivan, K., Eccles, M.P. et al. (2014). Are multifaceted interventions more effective than single-component interventions in changing health-professionals' behaviour? An overview of systematic reviews. *Implement. Sci.* 9: 152.

Straus, S., Tetroe, J., and Graham, I.D. (2009). *Knowledge Translation in Health Care. Moving from Evidence to Practice*. London: Wiley-Blackwell/BMJ Books.

Thomson, R. (2009). Evidence based implementation of complex interventions. *BMJ* 339: b3124.

Tuckfield, A., Haeusler, M.N., Grigg, A.P. et al. (1997). Reduction of inappropriate use of blood products by prospective monitoring of transfusion request forms. *Med. J. Aust.* 167: 473–476.

Weir, C., McLeskey, N., Brunker, C. et al. (2011). The role of information technology in translating educational interventions into practice: an analysis using the PRECEDE/PROCEED model. *J. Am. Med. Inform. Assoc.* 18: 827–834.

Wensing, M., Bosch, M., and Grol, R. (2010). Developing and selecting interventions for translating knowledge into action. *CMAJ* 18: E85–E88.

Wensing, M., van der Weijden, T., and Grol, R. (1998). Implementing guidelines and innovations in general practice: which interventions are effective? *Br. J. Gen. Pract.* 48: 991–997.

World Health Organization (2009). *WHO Guidelines on Hand Hygiene in Health Care First Global Patient Safety Challenge: Clean Care Is Safer Care*. Geneva: World Health Organization.

Wright, F.C., Ryan, D.P., Dodge, J.E. et al. (2004). Identifying educationally influential specialists: issues arising from the use of "classic" criteria. *J. Contin. Educ. Heal. Prof.* 24: 213–226.

Wye, L. and McClenahan, J. (2000). *Getting Better with Evidence*. London: King's Fund.

Zaltman, G. and Duncan, R. (1977). *Strategies for Planned Change*. New York: Wiley.

4

Planning and Organizing the Change Process

Richard Grol[1,2] and Michel Wensing[3,4,5]

[1] Radboud University, Nijmegen, The Netherlands
[2] Maastricht University, Maastricht, The Netherlands
[3] Faculty of Medicine, University of Heidelberg, Heidelberg, Germany
[4] Department of General Practice and Health Services Research, Heidelberg University Hospital, Heidelberg, Germany
[5] Department IQ healthcare, Radboud Institute for Health Sciences, Radboud University Medical Center, Nijmegen, The Netherlands

---

SUMMARY

- Careful planning of improvement activities (when, where, how, and by whom?) is of great importance to the successful introduction of new procedures in practice.
- Minimum requirements include:
  - A motivated team comprising all relevant expertise.
  - The development of a context which is positive to change.
  - Involvement of the target group in the plan.
  - The commitment of leaders and key stakeholders.
  - Good planning and time management.
  - Adequate resources and support.

4.1   Introduction

In the previous chapters we described general principles of effective implementation of improvements in patient care. A generic implementation model based on these principles was introduced in Chapter 3 and is shown again in Figure 4.1. This chapter discusses how this model can be used in practice, as suggested by experience and some research.

How best to design this entire process and what exactly should be done in each of the steps is not always clear in advance. In many cases, what is required is *careful preparation* and *planning of the implementation process*. Successful implementation of new procedures

in patient care also appears to be a question of involving all relevant stakeholders and good management of the improvement activities (Box 4.1 illustrates this). Using systematic methods does not mean that deviations from the plan are impossible. On the contrary, implementation is often an "incremental" and iterative process in which individuals learn in each of the steps and in which the approach is adjusted as necessary. Such a process requires systematic, sound preparation and a step-by-step approach.

The scope and setting of an implementation project are also important. Planning to implement the recommendations of a national multidisciplinary guideline on stroke is markedly

Improving Patient Care: The Implementation of Change in Health Care, Third Edition. Edited by Michel Wensing, Richard Grol, and Jeremy Grimshaw.
© 2020 John Wiley & Sons Ltd. Published 2020 by John Wiley & Sons Ltd.

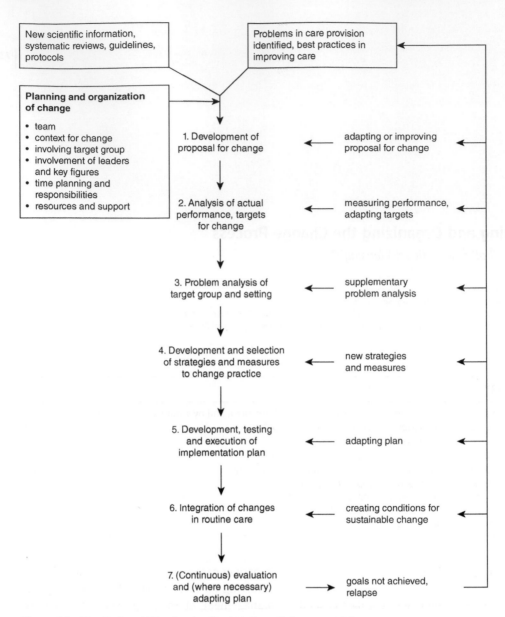

Figure 4.1 The Grol and Wensing implementation of change model.

Box 4.1 Determinants Influencing the Implementation of Breakthrough Collaboratives

As part of a national program for improvement in healthcare in the Netherlands, "breakthrough collaboratives" attempted to improve care in 24 hospitals for a number of issues such as pressure ulcers, medication safety, infection of wounds, and patient throughput. A research team (Dückers 2009) studied whether certain preconditions for success, mentioned in the literature, had a positive influence on the implementation of breakthrough collaboratives and the results achieved. The study showed that the subjective experience of success was related to:

- The composition and organization of the team.
- Leadership, support, and involvement of the hospital's management.
- Support by an external advisor and/or change agent.
- Team training.

Fewer obvious links existed between these factors and actual outcomes on a patient level (for example, the percentage of patients suffering from pressure ulcers).

different from that for optimizing antibiotic policy or medication safety in a hospital, or introducing a new care pathway for an outpatient clinic for breast cancer or vascular diseases. It differs from a situation in which a group of physicians or a community-based nursing care team wants to bring treatment more in agreement with a local protocol. It is dissimilar from the situation of a practice wanting to implement a new appointment system that has been tested elsewhere. While each of these cases concerns the implementation of potentially valuable innovations requiring changes in daily patient care, the scale on which one or another occurs, the ambitions involved, and the investment of time, staff involved, and materials differ greatly.

Nevertheless, the principles of planning and preparation are generally the same and are illustrated below. They address:

- Organizing a motivated team comprising all relevant expertise.
- Creating a context which is positive to change.
- Involving the target group and stakeholders in all phases of the process.
- Ensuring the involvement of leaders and key stakeholders.
- Sharing responsibilities and time planning.
- Organizing adequate resources and support.

These aspects will be elaborated in this chapter.

4.2 A Motivated Team Comprising All Relevant Expertise

To carry out the implementation activities effectively, a *team or small group* is usually required to steer, coordinate, and communicate the activities, and, where necessary, provide support (Kotter and Rathgeber 2006). A well-functioning improvement team can be a key factor in the success of quality improvement collaboratives (Schouten 2010).

The composition of such a team for improvement, innovation, or change depends largely on the scale of the implementation project (national, local, team, or practice), the type of innovation, and the budgetary possibilities. It is generally preferable to include different kinds of expertise and backgrounds in such a group:

- *Leadership*: an individual acknowledged by the target group as an authority, someone who provides a good example of the change, who performs a central role in communicating the message, and who involves the target group in the implementation. Frequently, in the implementation of innovations in clinical practice, a clinician will assume, or be asked to assume, this role in order to effect a change in clinical practice.
- *Coordination expertise*: someone who establishes goals, responsibilities, and timelines of the project and who monitors their progress, directs others, and provides feedback.
- *Technical expertise*: one or more individuals who have specific knowledge or skills that are advantageous to the process of implementing change, such as familiarity with data collection, data analysis, and evaluation research.
- *Administrative expertise*: one or more individuals who prepare materials, send invitations, prepare meetings, and plan social activities.

Once formed, such a team develops a plan in which the concrete implementation targets and the tasks and responsibilities that go with those targets have been carefully developed, and clearly communicated and documented. Since many interests often play a role in the implementation of changes, it is important for the improvement team to find support among the stakeholders. Apart from its content expertise, an effective team is also characterized by reflecting the multidisciplinary working environment in which the innovation is to be adopted (Greenhalgh et al. 2004). Furthermore, it is important to include key managers (representatives of a management team or directorate, for example), representatives of governance structures (e.g. a member of the board of directors), and the clinical staff (medical, nursing, and related health professions) in the team.

The success of an improvement team can depend on two, somewhat contradictory competencies. On the one hand, a successful team should function (semi-)autonomously and with some flexibility within the organization. On the other hand, it also requires formal approval and representation by the management, which is often also the "sponsor." The latter sets an example, frequently propagating the implementation plan, and assuming a crucial role in achieving success (Dückers 2009).

Studies and practical experience show that participation of at least one nurse or other health professional and at least one physician in the improvement team helps to acquire credibility with all parties involved (Wagner 2000). Increasingly, involving patients or clients in the improvement team is seen as important (Gagliardi et al. 2008).

4.3 Creating a Context for Change

In achieving change in patient care, an organizational culture aimed at innovation and change in an institute or within a professional group can be highly beneficial. Although this does not directly lead to changes, a favorable culture provides such an advantage to effective improvement that specific attention to it may be a part of the implementation plan itself (Weiner 2009). For example, Zahra and George (2002) demonstrated that the "ability to absorb" new knowledge in an organization can contribute to the success of implementation initiatives. A study by Shortell et al. (1995) in 61 hospitals revealed that a flexible, risk-taking organizational culture was strongly related to a successful implementation of quality care activities. This appeared to have more influence than the available number of formal quality-of-care structures. Other studies showed the association between a favorable organizational culture with well-functioning teams (Strasser et al. 2002), patient satisfaction (Meterko et al. 2004), and the quality of the care delivered (Shortell et al. 2000).

Many authors mentioned a "culture of change" and a "receptive environment" as conditions for realizing a process of change (Greenhalgh et al. 2004). It is not, however, always clear what this means, nor how it should be measured. In this chapter, we will limit our study to a smaller, discrete number of aspects of organizational culture that could be connected with the effective implementation of new procedures.

While some individuals consider culture as a characteristic of organizations, others consider it as the essential nature of an organization (i.e. the organization is the culture). Culture concerns not only observable characteristics, but also the implicit knowledge and attitudes of healthcare professionals. This makes it difficult to quantify and measure "culture." For example, in a review of 12 studies of different instruments to measure "safety culture," Flin et al. (2006) concluded that the majority of the instruments lack grounding in both a theoretical and a psychometric sense. When analyzing 48 instruments to measure organizational culture, Jung et al. (2009) found that most instruments were still in the early stages of development and validation, while an "ideal" instrument was lacking. Box 4.2 describes a study of organizational culture in healthcare organizations.

4.3.1 The Central Role of Physicians

In many clinical settings and improvement projects, the central and leading role of physicians has been emphasized in achieving change in patient care (Ovretveit 1996; Weiner et al. 1997; Berwick 1998). In many countries, nurses increasingly control their own work

---

Box 4.2   Organizational Culture in Hospitals, Nursing Homes, and Primary Care Practices

One of the instruments to measure organizational culture in healthcare is the competing values framework (Scott et al. 2003). This instrument distinguishes four idealized cultures, based on five questions about culture in general, style of leadership, relationship with the organization, strategic vision, and system of reward. By scoring the organization using the instrument, a respondent can indicate which aspects of culture are the most representative for his/her own organization:

- *Group culture*: an emphasis on internal orientation, cohesion, loyalty to the group, and interpersonal relations.
- *Innovation culture*: an emphasis on creativity, entrepreneurship, innovation, and risk taking.
- *Hierarchic culture*: an emphasis on rules, uniformity, clear agreements, stability, and predictability.
- *Rational culture*: an emphasis on goal attainment, competition, production, and market orientation.

The theory states that, to some extent, all elements of culture should be present and balanced, but innovation and external orientation are necessary to improve quality. Bosch (2009) studied the occurrence of the various types of culture in different settings, with the following results:

	Hospitals (n = 37 wards)	Nursing homes (n = 67 wards)	Primary care practices (n = 30)
Group culture	29%	32%	51%
Innovation culture	18%	19%	17%
Hierarchic culture	32%	29%	20%
Rational culture	21%	20%	12%
Total	100%	100%	100%

The strong presence of the hierarchic component in hospitals is noticeable, while in primary care practices group culture appears dominant. The latter group's cultural characteristics appear to lack elements of innovation, rationality, task focus, and competition. Innovations and implementation strategies thus need to be handled differently in each setting.

---

and take responsibility for improving their own performance. This implies that they can also hold leading roles in improvement. As *opinion leaders*, physicians and nurses can be an important and influential factor for the success of the implementation (Locock et al. 2001; Fitzgerald et al. 2002; see Box 4.3). However, some physicians and nurses may remain unfamiliar with or skeptical about quality improvement, for instance because they did not read about it in clinical journals and did not discuss at the educational courses they attend; and quality improvements are frequently initiated by managers (Berwick 1998; Blumenthal and Kilo 1998; Shortell et al. 1998; Provonost et al. 2009).

According to Blumenthal and Kilo (1998), the high degree of autonomy of healthcare professionals to design essential processes in patient care themselves also plays a role. Often pressed for time themselves, they are not easily motivated to take part in time-consuming projects of change. Despite being positively disposed toward it, individuals often lack the knowledge and skills needed to successfully engage in an improvement project (Solberg et al. 1998). Finally, many physicians and other health workers are untrained in the language and science of quality improvement, safety management, and implementation science. While quality, patient safety, and implementation science are increasingly taught to health

---

Box 4.3   Involving Physicians in Improving Safety

In order to involve physicians in improving quality and safety, the Beth Israel Deaconess Medical Center, Harvard Medical School, Boston, has put into action a number of sequential activities using the collection of data on quality and safety in gynecology and obstetrics (Mann and Pratt 2010). Leaders in healthcare and improvement at this center have encouraged and facilitated physicians and others to:

- Create a quality team with a broad representation.
- Agree on which quality indicators will be used to monitor care and encourage care

providers to participate in measurements via anonymous data collecting.
- Look for suitable data sources to gather relevant data for the indicators.
- Write feedback reports and submit these at monthly quality meetings.
- Train those involved whenever necessary.
- Present relevant and instructive quality cases at study groups, refresher courses, and postgraduate meetings.
- Define care processes and find out if improvements are needed.
- Formulate annual reports on quality and safety.

---

professionals, they are yet to become embedded as structural elements of the curricula for future healthcare professionals (Baker et al. 2005b).

Ovretveit (1996) argues that it is untrue that physicians are disinterested in improving procedures in practice. Most of them strive to introduce useful improvements in their management of health problems and to attend courses. To be more successful, Ovretveit suggests that improvement programs must provide an answer to the actual worries and problems of the clinicians and their practice. They must see that the programs actually generate something of value for the patients and the care providers. In addition, they need or appreciate support with respect to performance measurement.

Training in quality improvement often best occurs during participation in improvement activities and adjusted to time limitations, preferably when professionals are beginning to work on an improvement project. It avoids jargon and an over-zealous approach to management (Reinertsen et al. 2007; Ovretveit 2009). Training should be anchored in the kinds of problems that are relevant for the target group (Ovretveit 1996). An example of this is "cascade

training," in which individuals who are higher in the organizational hierarchy train those in the next level down in the organization, a concept which implies that top management receives the same training. Cascade training is a form of "train-the-trainer" methodology, a long-standing concept of adult education (Meneses and Yarbro 2008). However it is delivered, the measurement and analysis of data should be part of such quality training – frequently the most difficult part of many quality improvement projects (Ovretveit 1996; Solberg et al. 1998; Geboers et al. 1999a,b).

In summary, the central role of physicians and nurses in improving the quality of care and patient safety is important (Heenan and Higgins 2009). Several strategies have been developed for involving and training professionals in improving quality (Reinertsen et al. 2007; Reinertsen 2008; Ham and Dickinson 2009).

4.3.2   Collaboration in Teams for Patient Care

Achieving good results in healthcare is partly dependent on individual attitudes, expertise, and performance. However, many care providers work in groups and teams and partly depend on others for the effectiveness of their own performance, a process which also applies to the implementation of innovations, guidelines, and new procedures. To improve processes in care, it is often necessary to first improve interaction and communication between those involved in these processes (Clemmer et al. 1998; Firth-Cozins 1998). Disciplines such as sociology and psychology have studied collaboration in teams and networks, which provided important insights for patient safety and clinical effectiveness. A large percentage of airplane accidents appear to be partly the result of communication errors in the cockpit, a phenomenon strongly related to healthcare quality and safety (Oriol 2006). In healthcare, human errors often lead to near accidents or near misses with preventable damage or worse (de Bruijne et al. 2007). The basic assumption here is that, by definition, individuals by themselves do not work impeccably; thus a team can function as a safety net (Baker et al. 2005a).

Teams in which all individual members are continuously focused on quality and the improvement of quality make fewer mistakes and provide better care (Shortell et al. 2004; Clancy 2007). To create a culture focusing on improvement, members of multidisciplinary care teams need crucial knowledge, skills, and behavior in the field of teamwork (see Boxes 4.4 and 4.5). Research and practical experience show that these teamwork competencies can be practiced well in care teams, even those

with divergent characters (Baker et al. 2005a,b; Salas et al. 2008). Using, for instance, the Team Climate Inventory (TCI; West 1990) or the Safety Climate Survey (Kho et al. 2005, Pronovost and Sexton 2005), teams can check whether they really do work well together, whether targets are clear, whether everyone feels safe in the team, and whether the team is really focused on achieving the best possible result. In a review article, Clemmer et al. (1998) describe how leaders in healthcare can stimulate cooperation in teams. They can:

- Develop a joint objective (e.g. to improve a certain important part of the care provided).
- Provide an open, safe atmosphere in which everyone can participate.
- Involve everyone who has something to do with achieving the goal.
- Encourage the expression of diverse opinions.
- Learn how to manage and yet achieve consensus.
- Urge honesty and equality between participants.

Therefore, prior to starting the actual implementation of innovations, positive attitudes to quality and safety improvement require support and encouragement across an institution, within teams, and within the health professions involved. In addition, professionals need to have sufficient skills to perform the implementation of changes (see Box 4.6; Bosch 2009). In

---

Box 4.4   Improving Teamwork Including Patients

In a project aimed at improving teamwork at a new 30-bed medical unit in an acute hospital, the Interprofessional Teamwork Innovation Model (ITIM) was implemented (Li et al. 2018). This comprises a daily bedside clinically focused round, including not only physicians and nurses, but also the patient, family caregivers, pharmacist, and case manager. A structured approach was used in the implementation. The study was designed as a quality improvement project (with Plan–Do–Study–Act cycles), with statistical process control charts for monitoring performance. ITIM use was associated with reduced readmissions to the hospital (odds ratio of 0.56), but not with reduced visits to the Emergency Department or reduced costs. However, team members reported enhanced communication in teams and overall time savings.

Box 4.5   Improvement through Team Training

In 2006 in the USA, the national rollout began of the program Team Strategies and Tools to Enhance Performance and Patient Safety (TeamSTEPPS; www.ahrq.gov; Clancy 2007; AHRQ 2010). TeamSTEPPS offers:

- Support for care institutions in improving communication between care professionals and other teamwork competencies.
- A combination of didactic materials, workshops, and practical instruments for the purpose of team training.
- An extensive strategy for organizational change and program management, with divergent measuring and evaluation instruments and methods to involve professionals in change processes and to sustain the improvements.

"Tailor-made" applications of this program combine process improvement with multidisciplinary team training. The goal is to create a culture in which care professionals are more receptive to proposed improvements in procedures. Since 2006, TeamSTEPPS has been applied in a large number of healthcare institutions (Deering et al. 2009). Studies showed positive outcomes of the team approach, for instance on attitudes regarding teamwork, patient safety, culture, and communication in multidisciplinary teams (Stead et al. 2009). Within multidisciplinary education, significantly positive outcomes have been noted on knowledge and attitude in relation to teamwork with medical and nursing students (Hobgood et al. 2010).

Box 4.6   Organizational Culture, Team Climate, and Healthcare Delivery

As described in Box 4.2, Bosch (2009) studied the relation between organizational culture, team climate, quality management, and the occurrence of pressure ulcers in hospitals (n = 37) and nursing homes (n = 67). Organizational culture was measured by the competing values framework (Scott et al. 2003) and team climate with the TCI (West 1990). Quality management, for the purpose of preventing pressure ulcers, was measured at the level of both department (8 items) and institution (11 items). No relationship was found between the prevalence of decubitus and other variables. Still, quality management at the level of institutions was strongly connected with quality management at the level of the department.

In a different study, Bosch (2009) examined the relation between organizational culture and team climate and diabetes care and diabetes outcomes. Here, the same instruments (competing values framework and TCI) were used. Diabetes care was measured with a set of valid indicators. No relation was found between clinical indicators such as HbA1C and blood pressure and organizational measures of culture and team climate. However, a higher score on group culture (internal orientation) was related to a better score on diabetes indicators. A good balance between the various culture types was connected with a better quality of diabetes care.

---

some instances, resistance to change or improvement can be high, making the development of a receptive culture for the whole institution somewhat futile. In such cases, it is better to focus on a limited group of highly motivated professionals and to start on a small scale by setting examples and providing role models. Further, it is also important to focus on and support active professionals and teams (*champions*) who devote themselves enthusiastically to a certain improvement or innovation initiative. In summary, change teams would do well to find such individuals in their organization and, moreover, to combine active support from top management (the *sponsor*) and the effort of clinicians of distinction (*opinion leaders*) with the enthusiasm of these champions (Greenhalgh et al. 2004). Box 4.6 describes empirical studies that demonstrate that the impacts are not necessarily straightforward.

4.4 Involving the Target Group and Stakeholders in the Plan

Since it is difficult for external observers to fully understand a given setting in advance, it is important to involve representatives of the target group in the analysis of the problem, the selection of strategies to accomplish the change, and developing a plan for its introduction. This can be done by methods described in this book, such as interviews or group meetings (Chapter 9). Individuals from the target group are asked, among other questions, what kind of innovations and implementation strategies are attainable, will be accepted, and are likely to work best. The involvement of certain representatives or key individuals from the target group in actually introducing the implementation can also be discussed.

Usually, the range of targeted individuals – that is, those for whom the implementation has consequences – is much greater than initially imagined (Lomas 1997). Often, implementation is found to affect not only clinicians but also patients, the management or directors of the institution, colleague care providers, insurers, politicians, and policy makers, and sometimes individuals from the business world who provided materials for implementation. It is desirable to draw up a list of all those individuals and organizations who, in one way or another, are involved. This list would include those who are able to take stock

of the bottlenecks in implementation and for whom a separate strategy must be developed and introduced. In this setting, the example of a *sounding board* composed of different kinds of concerned individuals empowered to discuss the development of an effective plan can be considered (NHMRC 2000).

Although formal research evidence is scarce, practical experience in many projects suggests that it is best to start with a *small group* of enthusiastic care providers, practices, or institutions (Evans and Haines 2000); this means seeking individuals or organizations who are prepared to start an improvement and who meet certain conditions. For example, a project to implement guidelines for the prevention of cardiac and vascular diseases in primary care first searched for motivated practices with a satisfactory electronic health record and enough practice nurses, since these aspects were considered preconditions for the implementation. These motivated individuals or organizations next functioned as examples for others (Lobo 2002). In the introduction of small local quality collaboratives of primary care physicians in the 1980s, efforts were first made with teachers involved in training for primary care practice. Next, the program was offered to "average" physicians and was implemented widely, with the help of participants in the early groups serving as models for a wider rollout (Grol 1987).

4.5 Leaders and Key Figures

Involvement of directors, top management, and key figures in institutions and professional groups in the implementation of improvements is also seen as critical when introducing changes in care (Berwick 1989; Berwick et al. 1990; Berwick and Nolan 1998), stressing the importance of having the "board on board."

Leaders of an institute or professional group are frequently seen as enthusiastic at the beginning of a project, taking the initiative to start the changes, but then delegating the actual implementation. A reduction of enthusiasm may well undo the introduced change. In contrast, leadership requires a consistent viewpoint and messaging about the change proposal, establishing realistic and appropriate goals, the ability to manage strict deadlines, and setting an example (Schellekens 2000). Directors of an institution or practice must make quality policy and improving care provision a central item of their daily work and direct this item themselves. They need to educate themselves about the concepts and methods of improvement, and arrange for proper information and set up preconditions within their own organization.

In a study of over 2000 hospitals in the USA, when top managers assumed a clear leadership role, greater success was noted in the formation of improvement teams and projects on the work floor. Further, if physicians assumed leadership, more projects were undertaken to improve quality (Weiner et al. 1997). A study in Dutch hospitals showed that specialists became much more active in improving quality of care when it was apparent that the board of directors of their institution were stimulating quality initiatives more (Dückers 2009). Another study (Leistikow 2010) indicated that hospital executives can contribute to safe care if they establish favorable preconditions, assess care processes and monitor them, and ratify accepted outcomes and embed them in the organization. Leadership walkrounds were found to be positively associated with patient safety climate and risk reduction in a study across 49 hospitals in the USA (Schwendimann et al. 2013). A survey of the literature (Ovretveit 2009) revealed that leaders in care organizations can have important – both positive and negative – influences on improvement. Because of their position, leaders are able to develop structures, systems, and processes that will pave the way to a successful implementation of new procedures.

4.5.1 Medical Leadership

Leadership is an important part of the work of physicians and other clinicians, regardless of their specialty or the location of their work.

To an increasing extent, good care provision depends on the pace and efficiency with which several care providers collaborate within the care system surrounding the individual patient. Physicians (and occasionally also nurses) play a unique role, most frequently bearing the final responsibility for the care process. Because of their crucial role, involving physicians in leadership is an important point of interest in change processes (Ferlie and Shortell 2001). The physician is not only an expert with respect to content, but also a partner in and often the leader of the care team. This leading role has specific competencies in which physicians must be skilled in order to contribute optimally to continuous improvements in the quality of care (Ham and Dickinson 2009).

A practical understanding of leadership does not come easily. Physicians primarily focus on individual patients, whereas managers – along with their improvement programs – often assume an approach focused on populations and systems (Reinertsen et al. 2007). Table 4.1 outlines key competencies in the area of medical leadership, emphasizing its influence on improvement processes.

4.6 Project Management: Time Schedule and Responsibilities

The preparation of an implementation project also contains a number of practical activities, among which is a *timeline* or *plan*: a concrete schedule for the various parts of a project or plan, assigning the tasks and responsibilities to the various persons involved. For this purpose, the project is divided into parts. The actual work involved in each part, who will perform the various tasks, and who will have the ultimate responsibility for the outcome are described. It is important to record this process, distributing (in paper or electronic format) the resulting project document among all those involved, consulting it consistently during project meetings and using it to evaluate

Table 4.1 The competencies of medical leadership.

1 Orientation	*2 Personal qualities*
Being able to assess the impact of changes	Working from integrity
Taking decisions	Aimed at continuous personal development
Applying practical experience and evidence	Self-management
Analyzing the context (of change)	Developing self-awareness
3 Working with others	*4 Managing care provision*
Working in teams	Managing performances
Stimulating participation of others	Managing humans
Building on and keeping relationships	Managing means
Developing networks	Planning
5 Improving the provision of care	
Facilitating transformation (lasting development)	
Stimulating improvement and innovation	
Guaranteeing patient safety	

Source: Data from Clark and Amit (2010).

progress. Regular periods of evaluation and feedback will be incorporated into the plan, allowing it to function as a *checklist* in which the activities performed can be monitored. This process also enables planners to anticipate problems during progress, and to assess new priorities or the needs of the target group.

To avoid frustration, it should be accepted that the full course of most change processes often requires a long time period in order to meet goals: "Progress is not linear, but three steps forward and two steps back" (Wye and McClenahan 2000). At the same time, while changes proceed slowly, a certain speed and boldness are necessary to prevent a loss of momentum and a return to former habits. Those in the target group, especially the directors, generally want quick success, once they have committed themselves to a new way of working.

Another factor to consider is *innovation fatigue* within organizations undertaking widespread improvements. Improvements are mostly taken on thematically, sometimes resulting in overburdening staff who participate in project after project. Too many improvement projects in a short time can make it difficult for change teams to continue

implementations in a successful way. Steering improvements in the right direction, juggling and prioritizing them, requires continuous attention.

4.7 Resources and Support

Only a few implementation or change plans will be successful when they depend completely on the voluntary, unpaid efforts of everyone involved. A precondition for success usually involves an adequate *budget*, differing in amount depending on the scope (national, local, institution based, or practice based), the nature of the project, and staffing needs. Such a budget needs to be negotiated with sponsors – government, insurers, granting organization, the board of an institution, or the management of a team or practice. Mostly, a good estimate of profits and costs is required to convince investors of the relevance of the plan. Depending on the objective and the scale, the budget will contain certain facilities, for example for:

- Coordination
- Auxiliary staff

- Computers, instruments, and materials
- Reimbursements for extra work of the performers.

4.8 Conclusions

Adequate planning and preparation of implementation activities are often preconditions for the successful introduction of new procedures and changes in the practice of healthcare. Furthermore, an enthusiastic team comprising all relevant expertise is needed to support the activities. Prior to introducing changes, it is often necessary to first "prepare the ground," which means creating a positive attitude among those involved and teaching them how best to set about change. Involving the target group, most notably the physicians and the top management of the institution, forms a crucial step in this process. Also, a plan needs to be developed and communicated that describes the tasks and responsibilities as well as there being sufficient means and staff to carry out the activities. Progress should be studied regularly and where necessary adjusted, recognizing that often more time is needed for real changes in patient care than was anticipated beforehand.

References

AHRQ (2010). *TeamSTEPPS™: National Implementation*. Rockville, MD: Agency for Healthcare Research & Quality.

Baker, D.P., Gustafson, S., Beaubien, J. et al. (2005a). *Medical Teamwork and Patient Safety. The Evidence-Based Relation*. Rockville, US: Agency for Healthcare Research & Quality.

Baker, D.P., Salas, E., King, H. et al. (2005b). The role of teamwork in the professional education of physicians: current status and assessment recommendations. *Jt. Comm. J. Qual. Patient Saf.* 31: 185–202.

Berwick, D.M. (1989). Continuous improvement as an ideal in health care. *N. Engl. J. Med.* 320: 53–56.

Berwick, D.M. (1998). Developing and testing changes in delivery of care. *Ann. Intern. Med.* 128: 651–656.

Berwick, D., Godfrey, B., and Roessner, J. (1990). *Curing Health Care*. San Francisco, CA: Jossey-Bass.

Berwick, D.M. and Nolan, T.W. (1998). Physicians as leaders in improving health care. *Ann. Intern. Med.* 128: 289–292.

Blumenthal, D. and Kilo, C.M. (1998). A report card on continuous quality improvement. *Milbank Q.* 76: 625–648.

Bosch, M. (2009). *Organizational determinants of improving health care delivery*. Thesis. Nijmegen: Radboud University Nijmegen.

de Bruijne, M.C., Zegers, M., Hoonhout, L.H.F., and Wagner, C. (2007). *Onbedoelde schade in Nederlandse ziekenhuizen: dossier-onderzoek van ziekenhuisopnames in 2004. [Adverse Events in Dutch Hospitals: File Study of Hospital Admissions in 2004]*. Amsterdam/Utrecht: EMGO/NIVEL.

Clancy, C.M. (2007). TeamSTEPPS: optimizing teamwork in the perioperative setting. *AORN J.* 86: 18–22.

Clark, J. and Amit, K. (2010). Leadership competency for doctors: a framework. *Leadersh. Health Serv.* 23: 115–129.

Clemmer, T., Spuhler, V., Berwick, D. et al. (1998). Cooperation: the foundation of improvement. *Ann. Intern. Med.* 128: 1004–1009.

Deering, S., Rosen, M.A., Salas, E., and King, H.B. (2009). Building team and technical competency for obstetric emergencies: the mobile obstetric emergencies simulator (MOES) system. *Simul. Healthc.* 4: 166–173.

Dückers, M.L.A. (2009). *Changing hospital care*. Thesis. Utrecht: Utrecht University.

Evans, D. and Haines, A. (2000). *Implementing Evidence-Based Changes in Health Care*. Abingdon: Radcliffe Press.

Ferlie, E. and Shortell, S. (2001). Improving the quality of health care in the United Kingdom and the United States: a framework for change. *Milbank Q.* 79: 281–315.

Firth-Cozins, J. (1998). Celebrating teamwork. *Qual. Health Care* 7: S3–S7.

Fitzgerald, L., Ferlie, E., Wood, M., and Hawkins, C. (2002). Interlocking interactions, the diffusion of innovations in health care. *Hum. Relat.* 55: 1429–1449.

Flin, R., Burns, C., Mearns, K. et al. (2006). Measuring safety climate in health care. *Qual. Saf. Health Care* 15: 109–115.

Gagliardi, A.R., Lemieux-Charles, L., Brown, A.D. et al. (2008). Barriers to patient involvement in health service planning and evaluation: an exploratory study. *Patient Educ. Couns.* 70: 234–241.

Geboers, H., Grol, R., van den Bosch, W. et al. (1999a). A model for continuous quality improvement in small scale practices. *Qual. Health Care* 8: 43–48.

Geboers, H., van der Horst, M., Mokkink, H. et al. (1999b). Setting up improvement projects in small scale primary care practices: feasibility of a model for continuous quality improvement. *Qual. Health Care* 8: 36–42.

Greenhalgh, T., Robert, G., Macfarlane, F. et al. (2004). Diffusion of innovations in service organizations: systematic review and recommendations. *Milbank Q.* 82: 581–629.

Grol, R. (1987). *Kwaliteitsbewaking in de huisartsgeneeskunde.* Effecten van onderlinge toetsing. [Quality Improvement in General Practice. Effect of Peer Review]. Thesis. Nijmegen: Radboud University Nijmegen.

Ham, C. and Dickinson, H. (2009). *Engaging Doctors in Leadership: What We Can Learn from International Experience and Research Evidence?* Warrick: NHS Institute for Innovation and Improvement.

Heenan, M. and Higgins, D. (2009). Engaging physician leaders in performance measurement and quality. *Healthc. Q.* 12: 66–69.

Hobgood, C., Sherwood, G., Frush, K. et al. (2010). Teamwork training with nursing and medical students: does the method matter? Results of an interinstitutional, interdisciplinary collaboration. *Qual. Saf. Health Care* 19: e25.

Jung, T., Scott, T., Davies, H. et al. (2009). Instruments for exploring organizational culture: a review of the literature. *Public Adm. Rev.* 69: 1087–1096.

Kho, M., Carbone, J., Lucas, J. et al. (2005). Safety climate survey: reliability of results from a multicenter ICU-survey. *Qual. Saf. Health Care* 14: 273–278.

Kotter, J. and Rathgeber, H. (2006). *Our Iceberg Is Melting: Change and Success under Adverse Conditions.* New York: St. Martin's Press.

Leistikow, I.P. (2010). *Patiëntveiligheid, de rol van de bestuurder. [Patient Safety, the Role of the Director].* Amsterdam: Elsevier.

Li, J., Talari, P., Kelly, A. et al. (2018). Interprofessional Teamwork Innovation Model (ITIM) to promote communication and patient-centered coordinated care. *BMJ Qual. Saf.* 27: 700–709.

Lobo, C. (2002). *Improving the Quality of Cardiovascular Preventive Care in General Practice.* Rotterdam: Erasmus University.

Locock, L., Dopson, S., Chambers, D., and Gabbay, J. (2001). Understanding the role of opinion leaders in improving clinical effectiveness. *Soc. Sci. Med.* 53: 745–757.

Lomas, J. (1997). *Beyond the Sound of Hand Clapping: A Discussion Document on Improving Health Research Dissemination and Update.* Sydney: University of Sydney.

Mann, S. and Pratt, S. (2010). Role of clinician involvement in patient safety in obstetrics and gynecology. *Clin. Obstet. Gynecol.* 53: 559–575.

Meneses, K.D. and Yarbro, C.H. (2008). An evaluation of the train the trainer international breast health and breast cancer education: lessons learned. *J. Cancer Educ.* 23: 267–271.

Meterko, M., Mohr, D.C., and Young, G.J. (2004). Teamwork culture and patient satisfaction in hospitals. *Med. Care* 42: 492–498.

NHMRC (2000). *How to Put the Evidence into Practice: Implementation and Dissemination Strategies.* Sydney: Commonwealth of Australia.

Oriol, M.D. (2006). Crew resource management: applications in healthcare organizations. *J. Nurs. Adm.* 39: 402–406.

Ovretveit, J. (1996). Medical participation in and leadership of quality programmes. *J. Manag. Med.* 10: 21–28.

Ovretveit, J. (2009). *Leading Improvement Effectively. Review of Research*. London: Health Foundation.

Provonost, P.J., Miller, M.R., Wachter, R.M., and Meyer, G.S. (2009). Perspective: physician leadership in quality. *Acad. Med.* 84: 1651–1656.

Pronovost, P. and Sexton, B. (2005). Assessing safety culture: guidelines and recommendations. *BMJ Qual. Saf.* 14: 231–233.

Reinertsen, J. (2008). Engaging physicians: how the team can incorporate quality and safety. *Health Expect.* 23: 78–81.

Reinertsen, J.L., Gosfield, A.G., Rupp, W., and Whittington, J.W. (2007). *Engaging Physicians in a Shared Quality Agenda*. Cambridge, MA: Institute for Healthcare Improvement.

Salas, E., Diaz Granados, D., Weaver, S.J., and King, H. (2008). Does team training work? Principles for health care. *Acad. Emerg. Med.* 15: 1002–1009.

Schellekens, W. (2000). Een passie voor patiënten. [A passion for patients]. *Med. Contact. (Bussum)* 55: 412–414.

Schouten, L.M.T. (2010). *Quality improvement collaboratives. Cost-effectiveness and determinants of success*. Thesis. Nijmegen: Radboud University.

Schwendimann, R., Milne, J., Trush, K. et al. (2013). A closer look at association between hospital leadership walkrounds and patient safety climate and risk-reduction: a cross-sectional study. *Am. J. Med. Qual.* 28: 414–421.

Scott, T., Mannion, R., Davies, H.T., and Marshall, M.N. (2003). Implementing culture change in health care: theory and practice. *Int. J. Qual. Health Care* 15: 111–118.

Shortell, S.M., Bennett, C.L., and Byck, G.R. (1998). Assessing the impact of continuous quality improvement on clinical practice: what it will take to accelerate progress. *Milbank Q.* 76: 593–624.

Shortell, S., Jones, R., Rademaker, A. et al. (2000). Assessing the impact of total quality management and organisational culture on multiple outcomes of care for coronary artery bypass graft surgery patients. *Med. Care* 38: 207–217.

Shortell, S.M., Marsteller, J.A., Lin, M. et al. (2004). The role of perceived team effectiveness in improving chronic illness care. *Med. Care* 42: 1040–1048.

Shortell, S., O'Brien, J., Carman, J. et al. (1995). Assessing the impact of continuous quality improvement/total quality management: concept versus implementation. *Health Serv. Res.* 30: 377–401.

Solberg, L., Brekke, M., Kottke, T. et al. (1998). Continuous quality improvement in primary care: what's happening? *Med. Care* 36: 625–635.

Stead, K., Kumar, S., Schultz, T.J. et al. (2009). Teams communicating through STEPPS. *Med. J. Aust.* 190: S128–S132.

Strasser, D.C., Smits, S.J., Falconer, J.A. et al. (2002). The influence of hospital culture on rehabilitation team functioning in VA hospitals. *J. Rehabil. Res. Dev.* 39: 115–125.

Wagner, E.H. (2000). The role of patient care teams in chronic disease management. *BMJ* 320: 569–572.

Weiner, B.J. (2009). A theory of organisational readiness for change. *Implem Sci* 4: 67.

Weiner, B., Shortell, S., and Alexander, J. (1997). Promoting clinical involvement in hospital quality improvement efforts: the effects of top management, board and physician leadership. *Health Serv. Res.* 32: 491–510.

West, M. (1990). The social psychology of innovation in groups. In: *Innovation and Creativity at Work: Psychological and Organizational Strategies* (eds. M.A. West and J. L. Farr), 309–333. Chichester: Wiley.

Wye, L. and McClenahan, J. (2000). *Getting Better with Evidence*. London: King's Fund.

Zahra, A.S. and George, G. (2002). Absorptive capacity: a review, reconceptualization and extension. *Acad. Manag. Rev.* 27: 185–203.

Part II

Guidelines and Innovations

5

Characteristics of Successful Innovations

Richard Grol[1,2] and Michel Wensing[3,4,5]

[1] Radboud University, Nijmegen, The Netherlands
[2] Maastricht University, Maastricht, The Netherlands
[3] Faculty of Medicine, University of Heidelberg, Heidelberg, Germany
[4] Department of General Practice and Health Services Research, Heidelberg University Hospital, Heidelberg, Germany
[5] Department IQ healthcare, Radboud Institute for Health Sciences, Radboud University Medical Center, Nijmegen, The Netherlands

SUMMARY

- Innovations (e.g. clinical guidelines, technologies, proposed or recommended practices) are "products," which have characteristics that make them more or less attractive for potential users.
- Specific characteristics of innovations (e.g. compatibility with existing norms and values, the opportunity to try them out, or a clear and easily accessible format) have a positive influence on adoption by the target population.
- Involving the target group in the development of an innovation or proposal for change and offering them the opportunity to adapt it to their own situation ("co-design") may promote implementation.

5.1   Introduction

The first step in the implementation of innovations or new procedures is the selection and development of a concrete proposal or recommendation for practice (Figure 5.1). As mentioned earlier in this book, we address the implementation of various innovations in patient care and prevention, including clinical guidelines, care protocols, technologies, devices, organizational healthcare delivery models, and health system reforms. Such "innovations" are rarely automatically adopted "as is," since they are frequently inaccessible for users in regular practice and/or it is unclear exactly what performance is expected. A process of implementation should therefore start with a very specific description of the behavior and processes desired, and the changes to be pursued. These changes are preferably very concrete, and both ambitious and feasible within the setting of the implementation. For example, indicating "the reduction of the volume of unnecessary laboratory tests by 15% over a 12-month period" is a better point of reference for improvement than a more general statement, such as "increase the rational use of laboratory tests." This specificity more readily ensures that particular recommendations and proposals are actually implemented in practice.

In the process of defining a proposal or recommendation, features of the innovation that are important for its ultimate adoption by the target group should be taken into account

Improving Patient Care: The Implementation of Change in Health Care, Third Edition. Edited by Michel Wensing, Richard Grol, and Jeremy Grimshaw.

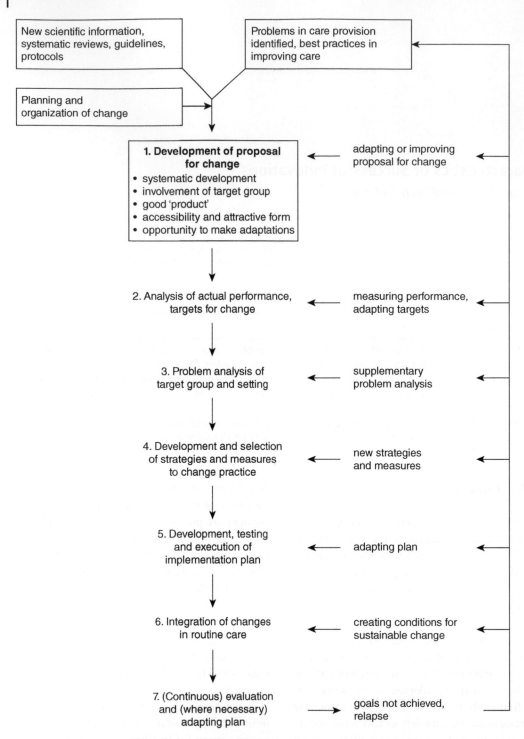

Figure 5.1 The Grol and Wensing implementation of change model.

Box 5.1	**Demands That Users Make on Clinical Guidelines**

The format and presentation of clinical guidelines are crucial for their acceptance and use. In a written survey, almost 400 doctors were asked in which cases they would use clinical guidelines (Watkins et al. 1999). A total of 238 answers were qualitatively analyzed. The results showed the importance of a high-quality product that is comprehensive, easily accessible, and offers solutions to the problems that care providers encounter in everyday patient care. The most commonly

mentioned positive characteristics of guidelines were:

• Sharp delineation, clarity of language, simple to use	24%
• Easy to look up, within reach when needed	18%
• Offer support for complex problems	15%
• Credibility of the guideline	12%

(see Box 5.1). At the same time, many innovations need to be modified – if only slightly – to meet local needs and opportunities, thus translating them into a product adapted to the specific setting. This chapter addresses these issues.

5.2 Various Types of Improvements Require Various Types of Change Proposals

Different types of patient care improvements may require different change proposals (Table 5.1). We discuss each of these types of change proposals briefly.

5.2.1 Scientific Literature, Guidelines, Decision Support, and Decision Aids

Specific knowledge derived from the scientific literature and evidence-based clinical practice guidelines can help care providers and patients make optimal decisions about the most appropriate action to be taken. Such insights are usually primarily published in general scientific or specialist journals, most often located in databases such as Medline (www.pubmed.gov) or the Cochrane Library (www.cochrane-library.com). Also, they are often presented at professional conferences. In many cases, studies have been summarized in systematic reviews. The rate of publication of new insights and techniques is so high that it is not possible for individual care providers to keep up to date

Table 5.1 Implementation of various innovations (Cretin 1998).

Improvement in clinical decision making	Requires, for example, implementation of summary of scientific literature, evidence-based guidelines, risk tables, decision support, decision aids
Continuity and coordination of healthcare	Care protocols/plans, integrated care pathways, disease management programs
Access and efficiency in care provision	Redesigned care processes, "best practices," information technologies

(Mulrow 1994), a phenomenon termed "information overload" (Hemp 2009). Thus, there is an urgent need to collate and summarize the information and to translate it into practical tools that support clinical decision making. Originally, the evidence-based medicine approach aimed to teach care providers the skills required to review the scientific literature critically – how to ask pertinent questions, how to search a database, and how to make critical appraisals of the studies available (Montori and Guyatt 2008). Nowadays, the consensus is that the majority of clinicians lack the time and required skills, and thus need high-quality syntheses of available knowledge (Tomlin et al. 1999; Guyatt et al. 2000).

Most professionals prefer guidelines or practical summaries made by well-informed colleagues (McColl et al. 1998). Well-designed recommendations can be an important aid in the implementation of optimal patient care as long as they are rigorously developed, readily accessible, acceptable, and easily used. Recommendations for practice are increasingly integrated within computerized decision-support systems, either linked to the electronic patient record or as a stand-alone software application. Increasingly they are also integrated in decision aids for patients: paper-based or computerized sources of specific (quantitative) information on options for screening, diagnosis, and treatment. The attempt to better integrate patient preferences and opinions into clinical practice guidelines derives from the larger vision that patients and consumers should be more actively involved in their care (Edwards and Elwyn 1999; Boivin et al. 2009). Often, different options for diagnosis and treatment exist, each with its own advantages and disadvantages in terms of the expected health gain and the risks. Patients attribute different values to these advantages and disadvantages, thus requiring clear presentations of benefits and risks within the framework of shared decision making (Box 5.2).

5.2.2 Clinical Pathways

Actual clinical practice often concerns combinations of actions, decisions, or routines of various healthcare providers that are inter-related and inter-dependent (Van Weel and Knottnerus 1999). In clinical trials, the emphasis usually lies on the internal validity of the study, thus the assessment of intervention efficacy, whereas in daily practice individuals are more often confronted by patient populations with multiple diseases and complicating

---

Box 5.2   Involving Patients in Decisions about IVF Treatment

In vitro fertilization (IVF) for patients with a fertility problem offers at least two options. Employing one embryo in each treatment cycle (eSet) has both advantages (fewer complications for mother and child) and disadvantages (lower probability of pregnancy) compared with deploying two embryos in each cycle (with a higher probability of pregnancy, but substantially more risks). A randomized trial (Van Peperstraten et al. 2010) demonstrated that translating scientific knowledge with an accessible decision aid can help patients with making difficult choices. Patients in the intervention arm received a paper decision aid outlining the advantages and disadvantages of both approaches. An experienced nurse gave support in making the choice, while the costs of an extra cycle of embryo placement were reimbursed. The control group received the usual treatment without the decision aid. In the decision aid intervention group, 52% of the patients chose the single-embryo option, whereas 39% in the control group chose this option. The new approach also proved to be cost-effective, reducing the costs by half.

characteristics and problems that are different from those addressed in scientific studies (Knottnerus and Dinant 1997). Also, many patients receive healthcare from various providers, which needs to be coordinated and tailored to the individual patient.

Clinical pathways, integrated care programs, and disease management systems aim to address these issues. They specify the recommended flow of patients through healthcare, allocation of tasks, and information exchange between providers. The term "integrated care pathway" has been defined by Campbell et al. (1998) as a structured, multidisciplinary care plan in which the actual steps in the care of a patient with a specific clinical problem are described in detail, along with the expected outcomes for the patient. This concerns a structured manner by which evidence-based guidelines are translated into local protocols and decision trees, outlining the roles of the various disciplines, the order in which activities should take place, and time lines.

Clinical and integrated care pathways fit with disease management systems (Hunter and Fairfield 1997). In such systems, the patient with a specific disease state (for example diabetes, heart failure, stroke, or depression) is centrally placed in a care plan built around the treatment process. This care is thus not regarded as a series of separate episodes or fragmentary contacts, but as a continuous process developed for the patient, into which evidence-based guidelines can be integrated. All care becomes the subject of the protocol; all actions, care outcomes, and financial costs are evaluated, and the patient receives tailored information (Wasson et al. 1997). Disease management systems can also facilitate the translation of knowledge into patient care (Rotter et al. 2010).

5.2.3 Improved Care Processes

Many improvements in care are not primarily motivated by published research and clinical guidelines, but by the need to respond to emerging problems that lead to errors, waste, or negative patient experiences. Such problems can be identified from complaints by patients, the experience of care providers, or by monitoring care processes. Scientific knowledge guiding the desired change is often available, but ready-made solutions indicating precisely how the care process should be designed are usually lacking. Therefore, formulating the target of change forms part of the implementation activity. Individuals work step by step to analyze existing processes, search for causes of the undesirable performance, formulate targets for improvement, plan and execute activities, and evaluate their results. This is often an incremental process of learning and improving instead of guided implementation of a defined innovation.

In the case of erroneous, unsafe, or non-patient-centered care processes, professional may have examples of more optimal working methods, often called "best practices." In other institutions or healthcare settings and practices, care providers may have already solved the problem to their satisfaction. Adopting or adapting these solutions to other, local situations can potentially save much time and effort. This approach is integrated into quality improvement collaboratives that have been used in many healthcare systems (Øvretveit et al. 2002). Box 5.3 provides an example of a best practice.

5.2.4 Other Innovations

In addition to systematic reviews, evidence-based guidelines, care protocols, clinical pathways, disease management systems, and best practices, several other innovations can be the subject of implementation, such as healthcare delivery models, preventive programs, and information technologies. Ideally, these have demonstrated effectiveness in well-designed research. Regardless of their effectiveness, the innovations may be neither eagerly awaited nor readily accepted by the target group.

Box 5.3   Safer Surgery Checklists

According to Gawande (2009), one of the major obstacles to increasing safety in medicine is that medical practice has become too complex to leave to the control, memory, and decisions of individual experts. Therefore, he recommended the use of checklists to ensure that all necessary actions have been undertaken. Clinicians and researchers from different countries, in a joint effort, developed the WHO Safer Surgery Checklist for this purpose. This checklist contains 19 "killer items" – actions that, in cases of neglect, may lead to serious complications. The checklist is completed at the start, just before an operation, and after, and involves the entire care team. A pilot study in eight hospitals in eight different countries showed a large reduction in mortality and complications after surgery (Haynes et al. 2009). Similar results were found using another checklist (SURgical PAtient Safety System or SURPASS) in the Netherlands (de Vries et al. 2010). Experiences with such checklists are not uniformly positive: the literature also demonstrates implementation problems (Vats et al. 2010; Walker et al. 2012) related to insufficient preparation and training, hierarchy and lack of leadership in the operating room, and feasibility of using the list; thus some authors have posed questions about the effectiveness of the intervention (Latosinsky et al. 2010). A systematic review of 33 studies on the impact and implementation of surgical checklists (Treadwell et al. 2014) showed, however, that such checklists are overall associated with increased detection of potential safety hazards, decreased surgical complications, and improved communication among operating staff. Strategies for successful checklist implementation included enlisting institutional leaders as local champions and incorporating staff feedback for checklist adaptation.

5.3 Characteristics of Innovations That Promote Implementation

Most importantly, the innovation – a new procedure or technique, a guideline, a care protocol, or a "best practice" – must be of the best possible quality. The target group should have the confidence that using the "product" will lead to the desired goal. In health services, this notion translates, first of all, into better care for patients, leading to better health or better quality of life. Other desirable goals may include better access to healthcare, more affordable or more efficiently organized care, a reduction in work pressure, reduction of drop-out of healthcare workers, or prevention of adverse events in the execution of care tasks. The literature mentions a large number of characteristics of innovations that might promote or hinder their actual application (e.g. Zaltman and Duncan 1977; Orlandi 1987; Spence 1994; Wolfe 1994; Rogers 1995, 2003; Grol et al. 1998; Scott et al. 2008). A summary is provided in Table 5.2. The transferability of these factors across healthcare systems, settings, providers, and patients needs to be assessed critically.

We shall describe in more detail a number of these characteristics, particularly those put forward by Rogers (2003) and frequently cited in publications: benefit, compatibility, complexity, triability, and visibility.

- *Benefit*: the degree to which the innovation can be seen as an improvement on existing practice. In general, a new guideline or procedure is only used if it seems to offer

Table 5.2 Characteristics of innovations that might promote or hinder their implementation.

Characteristic	Description
Relative advantage/utility	It is better than existing or alternative working methods
Compatibility	Consistency with existing norms and values
Complexity	Ease of implementation of the innovation
Costs	Balance between cost (level of investment) and benefits (return on investment)
Risks	Level of uncertainty about result or consequences
Flexibility, adaptability, revisability	Ability of innovation to be adapted to needs/situation of target group
Involvement	Degree to which target group is involved in development
Divisibility	Degree to which parts can be tried out separately and implemented separately
Triability, reversibility	Ability to try, stop, or reverse an innovation if it does not work or causes harm
Visibility, observability	Ability of individuals to observe innovation in a healthcare setting and see results
Centrality	Degree to which the innovation affects central or peripheral activities in daily working routine
Pervasiveness, scope, impact	How much of total work is influenced by innovation, how many persons are influenced, and how much time it takes, what is influence on social relationships
Magnitude, disruptiveness, radicalness	Number of organizational, structural, financial, and personal measures innovation requires
Duration	Time period within which change has to take place
Form, physical properties	Type and nature of innovation or change (material or social, technical or administrative, etc.)
Collective action	Degree to which decision making about innovation has to be performed by individuals, groups, or whole institution
Presentation	Nature of presentation, length, clarity, attractiveness

advantages over the existing situation. Achieving better care outcomes for patients is usually the most important motivation for many care providers. However, other benefits including reduced workload, financial gain, or increased status for the individuals who apply the innovation may also be considerations. Such advantages are weighed against possible disadvantages, such as extra time commitment, money, and disruption of the normal routines that may accompany the innovation. As the balance between the advantages and disadvantages becomes more favorable,

implementation is likely to be more successful. Implementation of an innovation can therefore be promoted by including a clear description in the presentation of the advantages and solutions for any possible disadvantages and limitations.

Different individuals and institutions can have widely varying opinions about the advantages and disadvantages of the same innovation. For example, a hospital may attribute great importance to following a guideline for the prevention of infections, or the appropriate use of antibiotics in the fight against bacterial resistance. In contrast, for individual doctors or nurses, the perceived advantages might be much smaller than those to the hospital or the patient, because they will have to monitor and engage patients more closely, or attend to time-consuming hygiene routines. In addition, patients may be convinced that they should receive antibiotics for their condition, although from a medical point of view those may be of little value.

- *Compatibility*: the degree to which the innovation complies with existing opinions, needs, norms, values, and routines. No matter how great the advantages of a different working method might be, implementation will not be a smooth process if the innovation is not consistent with existing norms and values, or the professional experience of the persons in the target group (Sheldon et al. 1998) Therefore, it is important to involve individuals from the target group (the users) in the development of a proposal to change existing practice, in order that they understand its importance and help ensure that the new procedure or process is consistent with existing views held within the target group. Sometimes an innovation can be linked to other procedures, organizational processes, or routines for which individuals already possess positive perceptions (see the example in Box 5.4).
- *Complexity*: the degree to which a new procedure is considered to be difficult to understand, multifaceted, and/or awkward to use. A complex innovation is obviously more

difficult to implement; users need to spend a great deal of energy in learning to understand it and the intervention itself. The importance of complexity in the implementation of guidelines has been shown in several studies (Grilli and Lomas 1994; Grol et al. 1998; Foy et al. 2002; Burgers et al. 2003; see Box 5.5). As complexity plays such a large role in the implementation of innovations, it is important to pay attention to how users understand and have easy access to the innovation: using summaries, a variety of media, clear text, or dividing complex proposals into more manageable "pieces" so that they are easier to grasp and adopt. The introduction of internet banking provides a less health-related example of the applicability of Rogers' theory of diffusion of innovation. Here the complexities involved in the uptake of a new method of banking were explored in the US context, along with other factors influencing the uptake and spread of the innovation (Nor et al. 2010).

- *Triability*: the degree to which individuals can attempt the innovation on a small scale, without the risk of becoming overwhelmed by its consequences. Trialing an innovation in a limited fashion helps to demonstrate its value in an individual's own setting and to identify what is necessary to make it work. "Trying things out" is of particular importance to early adopters; those who follow can make use of the experience of the group who went before. The effort put in by the

---

Box 5.4 **Physical Exercise Programs for the Elderly**

Physical exercise is known to have a positive effect on health, but the success of physical exercise programs varies in elderly individuals (Wensing et al. 2000). A large proportion of the elderly do not exercise at all, and many effective keep-fit programs do not reach these groups. One explanation is that many elderly individuals do not see themselves as athletic and have a low opinion of sport or having a good physical condition. However, they are interested in social contact with other individuals and participating in enjoyable activities. Therefore, new programs can be developed in which contact with others and enjoyable activities are combined (e.g. dancing lessons).

Box 5.5   Attributes of Guidelines That Influence Guideline Use in Practice

Grilli and Lomas (1994) analyzed recommendations in clinical guidelines and their use in practice as presented in 23 different studies. Of a total of 143 recommendations, Rogers' features of "complexity," "triability," and "visibility" were determined. Adherence to complex recommendations was 42%, and to less complex recommendations 56%. Adherence to recommendations with high triability was 56%; with low triability 37%.

Based on this literature and other studies, Grol et al. formulated 16 attributes of recommendations that could influence the use of guidelines in practice (Grol et al. 1998). A panel of four experts determined the presence of these characteristics in 47 recommendations selected from 10 guidelines developed by the Dutch College of General Practitioners (NHG). Data recorded in primary care were used to determine the extent to which the recommendations were followed. The analysis showed that 17% of the variation in compliance could be explained by the attributes of the recommendations. Attributes with the highest scores were "compatible with existing norms and values," "concrete, specific, and clearly defined," and "demanded no changes in existing routines." Recommendations with these attributes were more often followed in practice.

In a subsequent study, Burgers et al. (2003), using a sample of 96 recommendations selected from 28 guidelines, found that recommendations with high compliance rates were often supported by scientific evidence, were not part of a complex decision tree, and did not require new skills. For diagnostic recommendations, the ease of application and the potential (negative) reactions of patients were more relevant than for therapeutic recommendations.

Another study in 16 gynecology departments in Scotland (Foy et al. 2002) utilized 13 attributes of guidelines to examine compliance with 42 recommendations before and after an audit and feedback intervention. Recommendations compatible with clinical values and recommendations not requiring changes to fixed routines were associated with greater compliance. However, significant changes in compliance were only measured for recommendations seen as incompatible, most likely because there was more scope for improvement in compliance with these recommendations.

---

individuals who have tried out the innovation and the presentation of their experience can form powerful support for broader acceptance of a new practice or routine.

- *Visibility*: the degree to which the results of a new working method are made observable or visible. Demonstrating that the new performance is feasible in practice and quickly accomplishes the desired results can stimulate its widespread implementation. Most individuals are sensitive to the opinions of others when making choices, particularly when they consider the other person to be an example or a role model.

5.4 Format and Presentation

Presentation, appearance, and format are also important aspects of the implementation of an innovation. Which method should be chosen (e.g. written, audio-visual, verbal, online)? How understandable, accessible, and attractive is the final presentation? Different formats can be used for different target users. For example, for self-study or continuing education, texts or online learning formats that deliver extensive information might be useful, whereas for direct instruction in a hospital ward a flow chart or checklist might be more convenient. Decision aids can be designed as print materials,

---

Box 5.6   A Sticky Message

In the book *The Tipping Point*, Gladwell (2005) demonstrates the crucial importance of a powerful, attractive, easily remembered message (the "sticky message"). Individuals are continuously bombarded with information, innovations, interesting ideas, and facts which attract the attention. The average American consumer, Gladwell says, receives over 250 different commercial messages per day. We do not remember most of what we read or hear, unless it is offered as an attractive message that is structured and

packaged in such a manner that it is immediately applicable within our own daily life. Key elements are:

- Method of presentation (packaging) of the message.
- Role of anecdotes (narratives): these help to make the message accessible.
- Rehearsal: presenting the message again and again.
- Use of individuals with special skills to spread the message.

---

stand-alone computer programs, or applications on the internet. The design of technologies (e.g. apps on a smartphone) is equally important for uptake. The issue of formats is made more complicated by the fact that different users have varying opinions and learning styles with regard to formats: some may prefer reading a text or journal article, report, or printed guidelines, while others prefer to search for relevant information on the web. Some innovations, such as software applications and medical devices, may also be learned through trial and error in actual use. The format of such innovations influences their attractiveness and learnability (see Box 5.6).

In addition to "stickiness" and format, issues of the clarity of messages deserve consideration. Here it is important to do the following:

- Use language that is clear and unambiguous, not susceptible to multiple interpretations (Field and Lohr 1990), thus avoiding abstract, jargon-laden, and vague terms; use terminology consistently. The inclusion of a glossary of difficult terms and abbreviations is often helpful.
- Employ logical, easy-to-understand presentations of the recommendations or new routines; keep them as simple as possible to allow rapid understanding and to permit

easy access to information in a variety of situations. Watkins et al. (1999) showed, for example, that the most important demand that doctors made of clinical practice guidelines was that they must be transparent and easily accessible.

- Adapt the form and language of the innovation to everyday problems in care practice and the way in which individuals go about their work. This may mean that a new procedure, guideline, care pathway, or decision aid is presented in the form of a decision tree, or a written plan that gives the chronological order of the activities that care providers have to perform.
- Highlight the most essential elements of the activities of the care providers involved, remaining silent on less important aspects or details. The literature on education shows that a message should be presented in small doses and restricted to the essential information. Important information should be repeated, since individuals can only read and remember a limited number of messages at a time (Grol et al. 1991).
- Provide educational aids to promote understanding and uptake of the innovation or proposed change, for example by offering easily accessible texts or programs for further education, or listing indicators,

Box 5.7   Applicability of Clinical Guidelines
Care providers and patients will make better use of clinical guidelines if these include clinical tools, such as educational materials, summaries, algorithms, patient education leaflets, and indicators for monitoring care provision. Gagliardi and Brouwers (2015) studied the applicability of 137 clinical guidelines in 20 studies, investigating the quality of the guidelines with the AGREE instrument (see Chapter 6). The average score for applicability was 43%, lower than the scores for other aspects of guideline quality, but higher than scores in previous studies. Guidelines from the UK and those developed by non-profit organizations scored higher. In line with the study, Gagliardi et al. (2014) developed a framework of desirable features of clinical guidelines and tools for implementation (Gltools).

quality measures, and criteria for audit or assessment. See also Box 5.7.

- Design an appealing layout. The format of the guideline or proposal for a new working method should immediately attract interest, which may involve:
  - An attractive typographic layout.
  - Selective, appropriate use of bold script and colors.
  - A summary statement.
  - A limited number of literature references.
  - Adequate white space.

5.5 Involvement of the Target Group and Local Adaptation

The preceding sections have emphasized the importance of involving representatives of the target group in the development or selection of a change in procedures, a guideline, a care pathway, or a healthcare delivery model. It may also be necessary to adapt the innovation to the needs, problems encountered, and the work setting of the individuals who are intended to apply the innovation (Kotler and Roberto 1989). Such adaptations are common and take many forms, including changes to the format, content, setting, and targeted patient population (Wiltsey Stirman et al. 2013). In addition, involvement contributes to helping the target group consider that the innovation is their own and encourages them to take responsibility for it.

When considering the question of *who* should be involved in the development process, factors such as recognizability, representativeness, and expertise play a role:

- *Recognizability*: the target group must be able to identify with the developers. In a survey, medical specialists stated, for example, that they seldom used guidelines for primary care physicians (Van Everdingen et al. 2003). An average of less than 25% of the specialists attributed any value to primary care guidelines, as opposed to 80–90% support for the guidelines developed by their own societies.
- *Representativeness*: this is related to the nature of the innovation and whether use is made of the experience and expertise of those stakeholders considered relevant to the clinical state under consideration. These individuals will vary from one innovation to another.
- *Expertise*: the status enjoyed by the developers on the basis of their expertise and authority also influences acceptance. For instance, guidance provided by a healthcare professional with demonstrated clinical competency is more likely to be accepted by colleagues.

5.6 Conclusions

Innovations – such as guidelines, care pathways, decision aids, and best practices – have to meet certain criteria if the target group is to accept them and adopt thém into the normal care routines. To this end, we recommend analyzing the characteristics of the innovation that may promote implementation at an early stage in development. Involvement of the target group, the perceived advantage of the procedure or care process, and an attractive and easy-to-understand presentation affect uptake.

References

Boivin, A., Green, J., van der Meulen, J. et al. (2009). Why consider patients' preferences? A discourse analysis of clinical practice guideline developers. *Med. Care* 47: 908–915.

Burgers, J.S., Grol, R.P.T.M., Zaat, J.O.M. et al. (2003). Characteristics of effective clinical guidelines for general practice. *Br. J. Gen. Pract.* 53: 15–19.

Campbell, H., Hotchkiss, R., Bradshaw, N. et al. (1998). Integrated care pathways. *BMJ* 316: 133–137.

Cretin, S. (1998). *Implementing Guidelines: An Overview*. Santa Monica, CA: RAND.

Edwards, A. and Elwyn, G. (1999). How should effectiveness of risk communication to aid patients' decisions be judged? A review of the literature. *Med. Decis. Mak.* 19: 428–434.

Field, M. and Lohr, K. (eds.) (1990). *Clinical Practice Guidelines: Directions for a New Agency*. Washington, DC: National Academies Press.

Foy, R., MacLennan, G., Grimshaw, J. et al. (2002). Attributes of clinical recommendations that influence change in practice following audit and feedback. *J. Clin. Epidemiol.* 55: 717–722.

Gagliardi, A., Brouwers, M., and Bhattacharyya, O. (2014). A framework of the desirable features of guideline implementation tools (GItools): Delphi survey and assessment of GItools. *Implement. Sci.* 9: 98.

Gagliardi, A. and Brouwers, M. (2015). Do guidelines offer implementation advice to target users? A systematic review of guideline applicability. *BMJ Open* 5: e007047.

Gawande, A. (2009). *The Checklist Manifesto*. New York: Metropolitan Books.

Gladwell, M. (2005). *The Tipping Point*. London: Abacus.

Grilli, R. and Lomas, J. (1994). Evaluating the message: the relationship between compliance rate and the subject of a practice guideline. *Med. Care* 32: 202–213.

Grol, R., van Beurden, W., Binkhorst, T. et al. (1991). Patient education in family practice. The consensus reached by patients, doctors and experts. *Fam. Pract.* 8: 133–139.

Grol, R., Eccles, M., Maisonneuve, H. et al. (1998). Developing clinical practice guidelines. The European experience. *Dis. Manag. Health Out.* 4: 255–266.

Guyatt, G., Meade, M., Jaeschke, R. et al. (2000). Practitioners of evidence based care. *BMJ* 320: 954–955.

Haynes, A.B., Weiser, T.G., Berry, W.R. et al. (2009). A surgical safety checklist to reduce morbidity and mortality in a global population. *N. Engl. J. Med.* 360: 491–499.

Hemp, P. (2009). Death by information overload. *Harv. Bus. Rev.* 87: 82–89.

Hunter, D. and Fairfield, G. (1997). Disease management. *BMJ* 315: 50–53.

Knottnerus, J. and Dinant, G.J. (1997). Medicine based evidence, a prerequisite for evidence based medicine. *BMJ* 315: 1109–1110.

Kotler, P. and Roberto, E. (1989). *Social Marketing Strategies for Changing Public Behaviour*. New York: Free Press.

Latosinsky, S., Thirlby, R., Urbach, D. et al. (2010). CAGS and ACS evidence based reviews in surgery. 32: use of a surgical safety checklist to reduce morbidity and mortality. *Can. J. Surg.* 53: 64–66.

McColl, A., Smith, H., White, P. et al. (1998). General practitioners' perceptions of the route to evidence based medicine: a questionnaire survey. *BMJ* 316: 361–365.

Montori, V.M. and Guyatt, G.H. (2008). Comment on progress in evidence-based medicine. *JAMA* 300: 1814–1816.

Mulrow, C.D. (1994). Rationale for systematic reviews. *BMJ* 309: 597–599.

Nor, K.M., Pearson, J.M., and Ahmad, A. (2010). Adoption of internet banking: theory of the diffusion of innovation. *Int. J. Manage. Stud.* 17: 69–85.

Orlandi, M. (1987). Promoting health and preventing disease in health care settings: an analysis of barriers. *Prev. Med.* 16: 119–130.

Øvretveit, J., Bate, P., Cleary, P. et al. (2002). Quality collaboratives: lessons from research. *Qual. Saf. Health Care* 11: 345–351.

Rogers, E. (1995). Lessons for guidelines from the diffusion of innovation. *Jt Comm. J. Qual. Improv.* 21: 324–328.

Rogers, E.M. (2003). *Diffusion of Innovations*. Simon and Schuster: New York.

Rotter, T., Kinsman, L., James, E.L. et al. (2010). Clinical pathways: effects on professional practice, patient outcomes, length of stay and hospital costs. *Cochrane Database Syst. Rev.* 17 (3): CD006632. https://doi.org/10.1002/14651858.CD006632.pub2.

Scott, S.D., Plotnikoff, R.C., Narunamuni, N. et al. (2008). Factors influencing the adoption of an innovation: an examination of the uptake of the Canadian Hearth Health Kit (HHK). *Implement. Sci.* 3: 41.

Sheldon, T., Guyatt, G., and Haines, A. (1998). Getting research findings into practice: when to act on the evidence? *BMJ* 317: 139–142.

Spence, W. (1994). *Innovation. The Communication of Change in Ideas, Practices and Products*. London: Chapman and Hall.

Tomlin, Z., Humphrey, C., and Rogers, S. (1999). General practitioners' perceptions of effective health care. *BMJ* 318: 1532–1535.

Treadwell, J., Lucas, S., and Tsou, A. (2014). Surgical checklists: a systematic review of impact and implementation. *BMJ Qual. Saf.* 23: 299–318.

Van Everdingen, J., Mokkink, H., Klazinga, N. et al. (2003). De bekendheid en verspreiding van CBO richtlijnen onder medisch specialisten [The acquaintance with and distribution of CBO guidelines among medical specialists]. *Tijdschr. Gezondheidsr.* 81: 468–472.

Van Peperstraten, A., Nelen, W., Grol, R. et al. (2010). The effect of a multifaceted empowerment strategy on decision making about the number of embryos transferred in in vitro fertilisation: randomised controlled trial. *BMJ* 341: c2501.

Van Weel, C. and Knottnerus, J. (1999). Evidence based intervention and comprehensive treatment. *Lancet* 353: 916–918.

Vats, A., Vincent, C.A., Nagpal, K. et al. (2010). Practical challenges of introducing WHO surgical checklist: UK pilot experience. *BMJ* 340: b5433.

de Vries, E., Prins, H., Crolla, R. et al. (2010). Effect of a comprehensive surgical safety system on patient outcomes. *N. Engl. J. Med.* 363: 1928–1937.

Walker, I., Rashamwalla, S., and Wilson, I. (2012). Surgical safety checklists: do they improve outcomes? *Br. J. Anaesth.* 109: 47–54.

Wasson, J., Jette, A., Johnson, D. et al. (1997). A replicable and customizable approach to improve ambulatory care and research. *J. Ambul. Care Manage.* 20: 17–27.

Watkins, C., Harvey, I., Langley, C. et al. (1999). General practitioners' use of guidelines in the consultation and their attitudes to them. *Br. J. Gen. Pract.* 49: 11–15.

Wensing, M., van der Bij, A., and Laurant, M. (2000). *Implementatie van bewegingsprogramma's voor ouderen. Verslag van een literatuurstudie* [Implementation of a training program for the elderly. Report of a literature study]. The Hague: ZON.

Wiltsey Stirman, S., Miller, C.J., Toder, K., and Calloway, A. (2013). Development of a framework and coding system for modifications and adaptations of evidence-based interventions. *Implement. Sci.* 8: 65.

Wolfe, R. (1994). Organisational innovation: review, critique and suggested research directions. *J. Manag. Stud.* 31: 406–431.

Zaltman, G. and Duncan, R. (1977). *Strategies for Planned Change*. New York: Wiley.

6

Clinical Practice Guidelines as a Tool for Improving Patient Care

Jako Burgers[1,2], Trudy van der Weijden[2], and Richard Grol[3,4]

[1] *Dutch College of General Practitioners (NHG), Utrecht, The Netherlands*
[2] *Department of Family Medicine, Care and Public Health Research Institute (CAPHRI), Maastricht University, Maastricht, The Netherlands*
[3] *Radboud University, Nijmegen, The Netherlands*
[4] *Maastricht University, Maastricht, The Netherlands*

SUMMARY

- Clinical practice guidelines are tools for translating research findings and new insights into clinical practice in order to improve quality of care.
- Characteristics of guidelines contributing to their use are:
  - A clear objective and specific target groups are defined.
  - The scope of the guideline is defined by an analysis of barriers in clinical practice involving all relevant stakeholders, including patient representatives.
  - The research evidence supporting the recommendations is clearly described and up to date.
  - The guideline is compatible with the norms and values of the target group(s).
  - The recommendations are specific and unambiguous.
  - The guideline allows flexible use tailored to individual patients.
  - The structure of the guideline is clear and the layout is attractive.
  - The guideline is easy to apply in practice using a summary, flow chart, patient-directed knowledge tools, or electronic applications.
- Guidelines developed within a structured and coordinated program involving the target group are likely to be most effective.
- To promote their implementation, the draft guidelines are sent for review to a random sample of future guideline users, or used in real practice in a pilot implementation study.
- Guidelines can be used as a basis for developing tools and materials targeted to specific groups of professionals and patients.

6.1 Introduction

Clinical practice guidelines summarize research evidence systematically and offer recommendations on a specific clinical topic. They can be defined as follows:

Clinical practice guidelines are statements that include recommendations intended to optimize patient care that are informed by a systematic review of evidence and an assessment of the benefits and harms of alternative care options.

Improving Patient Care: The Implementation of Change in Health Care, Third Edition. Edited by Michel Wensing, Richard Grol, and Jeremy Grimshaw.
© 2020 John Wiley & Sons Ltd. Published 2020 by John Wiley & Sons Ltd.

Box 6.1 Quality Appraisal of Guidelines

Since 2003, the AGREE instrument (Appraisal Instrument for Guidelines, Research, and Evaluation) has been considered as the international standard for guideline quality (AGREE Collaboration 2003). This instrument helps to systematically assess the quality of guidelines. In recent years, several guideline review studies have been conducted using the AGREE instrument. In the review by Alonso-Coello et al. (2010), 42 guideline review studies were found, assessing a total of 626 guidelines published since 1980. In the six domains of the AGREE instrument, the mean domain scores (minimum 0%, maximum 100%) found by the authors were:

- Scope and purpose (three items)   64%
- Stakeholder involvement (four items)   35%
- Methodology (seven items)   43%
- Clarity and presentation (four items)   60%
- Applicability (three items)   22%
- Editorial independence (two items)   30%

The low scores are partly due to lack of information about the development process and the guideline authors. In the last decade the quality of guidelines has improved, which might be explained by the use of the AGREE instrument, the exchange of expertise in conferences such as the Guidelines International Network (G-I-N), and the launch of the GRADE methodology.

They are important tools in defining quality of care and implementing new practices and improvements in patient care. Target users of guidelines are healthcare professionals and patients. Guidelines are reliable sources of information that can be used in the process of shared decision making. Patient decision aids are tools derived from guideline recommendations to support this process (Van der Weijden et al. 2012). However, guidelines – like other innovations – do not implement themselves. If guidelines have specific characteristics, their implementation may be easier and faster. Implementation is not a process that starts after publication of the guideline, but should be considered at all stages of guideline development. This chapter describes the development and presentation of clinical guidelines in anticipation of their implementation.

Since the early 1980s, guidelines have been developed as a tool for improving the quality of healthcare. Initially, they were developed mainly by consensus among a group of experts in a national consensus meeting (Jacoby 1985). However, the quality of published guidelines varies (see Box 6.1). In the 1990s, the principles of evidence-based medicine became more widely adopted in many countries, emphasizing the need for systematic review and assessment of the research literature (Woolf 1990; Grimshaw and Russell 1993; Eccles et al. 1996). Thus, current thinking is that the strength of recommendations in guidelines should be based on an assessment of the best available scientific evidence (considering issues such as methodological risk of bias, consistency and precision of effect estimates, and publication bias), the balance between benefits and harms, societal values and patient preferences, feasibility, equity, and costs (Guyatt et al. 2008; Institute of Medicine 2011a).

6.2 Aims of Guidelines

Clinical guidelines can be developed for different purposes. For effective implementation, the aims of the guideline should be specifically described and be clear for the target users. In general, two main purposes of guidelines can be distinguished:

- *Guidelines as an aid for decision making.* Clinical guidelines provide a description of the current state of knowledge on a specific topic and give recommendations for healthcare practice. In this context, they are a tool for professionals and individual patients in clinical decision making. They can also be used for teaching and continuing professional education and as the basis for interdisciplinary agreements, for instance on participation in a clinical register or a network of training practices.

- *Guidelines as means to external control.* The key recommendations within a guideline can be translated to performance indicators, which can be used for external control and public reporting of healthcare professionals' performance. Other parties, such as healthcare insurers and governmental or federal agencies, may have an interest in clinical guidelines. For insurers, guidelines could be used in contracts or budgetary control. Governments could use guidelines in policy making and coverage decisions. From the policy makers' perspective, cost-effectiveness and efficiency are at least as relevant as quality of healthcare and – in their view – guidelines should primarily aim at preventing unnecessary healthcare and unnecessary costs.

6.3 Potential Benefits and Limitations of Guidelines

Over the past decades there has been a steady increase in guideline development activities. Nowadays, many organizations develop clinical guidelines according to well-established methods and procedures. The Guidelines International Network (G-I-N), founded in 2003 (Ollenschläger et al. 2004), grew from 35 to over 100 member organizations in 2018. In situations in which there is uncertainty about appropriate practice and when scientific evidence can provide an answer, guidelines offer the possibility to define effective and cost-effective care. In other situations, multidisciplinary guidelines may improve the organization of care or cooperation between different disciplines (Woolf et al. 1999).

Guidelines can help to improve both the process and outcome of care (Grimshaw and Russell 1993). The process concerns providing care according to current insights on effective and efficient care, whereas the outcome of care concerns improvement of the health status or quality of life of the patient. It might be assumed that improvement of the process also contributes to improvement of patients' outcomes. However, research does not always confirm this (Box 6.2; Lugtenberg et al. 2009).

Box 6.2 Effects of Evidence-Based Guidelines in the Netherlands

Since 1990, more than 100 national and international articles on the effects of Dutch guidelines have been published. A review of Lugtenberg et al. (2009) included 20 studies in which the changes were examined in designs that involved pre- and post-measurement. The introduction of guidelines was associated with improvements in the process and the structure of care (17 out of 19 studies). Preventive tasks were better performed, for example on diabetes care, cardiovascular risk management, and influenza vaccination. Substantial differences between guideline recommendations were found: some recommendations probably had more impact than others. This might be related to the degree of professional behavioral change or patient compliance that is required to adhere to the recommendation in practice. Also, the implementation strategies used varied widely. Change in outcomes of care after the introduction of guidelines was less often examined (9 out of 20 studies) and showed mixed results. Some studies claimed that diabetes guidelines had an effect on patient outcomes, whereas other studies did not find any effect.

Thus, it is important to examine how guidelines may contribute to relevant outcomes in routine practice.

6.3.1 Potential Benefits

Clinical guidelines can contribute to healthcare improvement in the following ways:

- *Summary of research findings*. The development of an evidence-based guideline includes systematic research into the evidence (Institute of Medicine 2011b). This provides individual care providers with a recent overview of new developments in a particular topic. Guidelines could also highlight gaps in current knowledge, which could be a stimulus for further research (Robinson et al. 2011). Patient versions of guidelines or lay summaries help to inform the public on what they can expect from providers (G-I-N Public Working Group 2015).
- *Transparent information about recommendations for optimal care*. Clinical guidelines summarize the potential benefits and limitations of procedures and interventions for defined health problems in a transparent way. Ideally, guidelines are accompanied by lay-language patient versions, and also by decision aids for specific preference-sensitive recommendations. This provides patients with information which may facilitate shared decision making with healthcare providers (Van der Weijden et al. 2012).
- *Reduction of unwanted variation between healthcare providers*. Using information about optimal care, initiatives could be taken to reduce overuse, underuse, or misuse of healthcare interventions and procedures (Westert and Faber 2011). This could also contribute to cost containment within the healthcare system.
- *Internal and external accountability*. The guidelines can be used as a point of reference for audit and the evaluation of healthcare. Guidelines may be used as a basis for peer review among professionals and for accreditation, or for external control by organizations

with accreditation or inspection roles, for healthcare insurers or the public. Guidelines may also be used in disciplinary or judicial proceedings.
- *Basis for teaching and education*. A generally accepted and up-to-date clinical guideline offers a sound basis for training and continuing professional education on a specific topic. In contrast, textbooks often contain material that is general or out of date, whereas a clinical guideline provides specific recommendations based on recent research findings.
- *Basis for interdisciplinary collaboration and coordination of care*. Many clinical guidelines cover topics that involve different disciplines, for instance low back pain (primary care physicians, neurologists, orthopedic surgeons, rheumatologists, rehabilitation physicians, and professions allied to health such as physiotherapists and psychologists). In this context, a guideline can serve as a basis for interdisciplinary agreements about the management of a condition or disease.
- *Setting research and healthcare priorities*. Clinical guidelines can call attention to under-recognized health problems. If a systematic review of the available evidence fails to identify evidence on an important clinical area, this failure can be flagged for research funders as a research priority.

6.3.2 Possible Limitations

Clinical guidelines may also have limitations, such as:

- *Perception as "cookbook medicine."* A clinical guideline usually takes a hypothetical "average" patient as a point of reference and may not specifically address individual, unique patients with their own co-morbidities, circumstances, wishes, or preferences. Thus, guidelines may oversimplify clinical practice and neglect its complex reality (Shaneyfelt and Centor 2009; Greenhalgh et al. 2014), thereby encouraging users to apply recommendations rigidly or unthinkingly, even in situations for which departure from the clinical guideline may be desirable (Hurwitz 1999; Burgers 2015).

- *Unrealistic expectations and limited applicability.* Clinical guidelines formulate the way in which optimal healthcare should be provided. Adequate application of guidelines is expected to result in health gain. However, it is not clear to what extent this can be achieved in routine practice (Worrall et al. 1997; Grol and van Weel 2009). Many clinical guidelines are produced on the basis of results of clinical studies of selected patient populations with single diseases in standardized settings (Knottnerus and Dinant 1997; Starfield 1998). Results achieved in clinical trials are often not achieved in daily practice. Patients with co-morbidity are often excluded in clinical studies and therefore insufficiently taken into account by clinical guidelines (Boyd et al. 2005; Lugtenberg et al. 2011). The effect of interventions recommended in the guideline cannot be predicted with certainty.
- *Professional resistance and concern for legal consequences.* In general, healthcare professionals strive for professional autonomy. If clinical practice guidelines are interpreted in a rigorous way, this may threaten this autonomy (Tunis et al. 1994). Similarly, some professionals fear that guidelines will increase their medico-legal exposure (Hurwitz 1999), in part because clinical situations in which departure from the guideline might be appropriate are often unclear (Koerselman and Korzec 2008).
- *Unintended consequences of use by governmental authorities and the health insurance industry.* Clinical guidelines may also be used to develop performance indicators for assessing and monitoring healthcare performance. Benchmarking of healthcare organizations or individual healthcare providers can, however, lead to undesired competition and unreasonable requirements in healthcare contracts. Introducing guidelines together with financial sanctions might harm the image of clinical guidelines and

increase professional resistance (Durieux et al. 2000).
- *Uncertainty about cost-effectiveness.* The development of clinical guidelines makes large demands on resources. The cost of developing an evidence-based guideline varies from US$100 000 to more than $250 000, depending on the scope of the guideline and the number of stakeholders involved. There are also costs for dissemination and implementation of the guidelines (Haycox et al. 1999). Whether guidelines can improve the cost-effectiveness of healthcare has not been demonstrated, but there are examples where this is the case (Mason et al. 2001; Eddy et al. 2011).
- *Strategic motives and conflicts of interests.* Professional groups may produce clinical guidelines to strengthen their position in healthcare, at the cost of other professional groups. This might hamper professional collaboration to improve the coordination and quality of care.

6.4 Development of Effective Guidelines

Guidelines are preferably developed within a structured and coordinated program with methodological support from an organization or research institute experienced in guideline development (Wollersheim et al. 2005). Guidelines developed within such a program have higher quality than guidelines produced without any support (Burgers et al. 2003a). In view of acceptance and implementation, it is important that the organization that coordinates the guideline development process follows a clear procedure. Developing evidence-based guidelines involves several steps (Table 6.1), each of which needs to consider implementation.

6.4.1 Topic Selection

It is likely that the more relevant and appropriate a topic is for resolving problems encountered in practice, the more the guideline will

Table 6.1 Steps and activities in guideline development in the context of implementation.

Step	Aim related to implementation	Activities to promote implementation
Topic selection	Relevance	Definition of topic Definition of aims and target groups
Composition of guideline development group	Create conditions for a good and widely accepted product	Appointment of chair and working group members/clinical experts Declaration of potential conflicts of interest Patient involvement Methodological support Managerial and administrative support
Drafting the scope	Address specific problems perceived by professionals and patients in practice	Analysis of actual needs and problems Definition of health questions Patient involvement
Development of draft guideline	Credibility, scientific basis	Use of existing guidelines and reviews Collection and analysis of scientific literature Contribution from experts and practitioners/target user Formulation of recommendations
Consultation and authorization	Applicability Broad support and general acceptance among target groups and patient population	Consensus meeting, invitational conference, written survey among random sample of future guideline users Patient participation Pilot test Formal approval by professional societies and other organizations involved Accreditation or certification
Design and products	Accessibility and attractiveness	Publication in journals Accessible and attractive summaries Electronic versions on internet, tablets, or integrated in electronic patient records Patient versions/leaflets, decision aids Quality indicators
Evaluation	Monitoring guideline use	Evaluation of experiences from practice Evaluation with quality indicators
Revision and update	Keeping up to date	Determining ownership and procedure for updating Regular monitoring of literature Modification of recommendations if necessary

Source: Data from Grol (1993).

be accepted and used; thus, one should start with an analysis of problems that need to be addressed. Healthcare professionals as well as patients are able to define problems perceived in practice. Implementation will be facilitated if they have the opportunity to suggest topics, questions, and problems for guideline development. Prioritization and final selection of topics are mostly performed by professional societies and/or governmental agencies. Note that some problems are important or urgent, but cannot be resolved by developing and introducing guidelines, for example problems due to shortage or incorrect use of staff, beds, or resources; or malpractice resulting from inefficient procedures (Woolf et al. 1999).

In deciding whether a topic is appropriate for guideline development, the following questions could be answered:

- Which aspects of care are especially complicated; for which questions or problems in practice could guidelines provide an answer?
- What do we know about the actual care and what are the shortcomings; how often does the problem occur and who is involved; if care is inadequate, are there new methods or better techniques available that require a change in clinical practice?
- What barriers can be expected in developing guidelines for the topic suggested; is there a divergence of opinions between various groups of professionals, patient organizations, or other stakeholders involved; what can be done to overcome the barriers?

Once potential topics have been identified, there is a process of deciding whether they are really suitable for guideline development, especially from the perspective of implementation. To this end various criteria can be used (Box 6.3):

- The condition or disease occurs frequently and clinical guidelines have the potential to produce significant health benefits for a large group of patients. Examples are diabetes mellitus, cardiovascular risk management, asthma/chronic obstructive pulmonary disorder (COPD), depression, and breast cancer. In most countries, guidelines on these topics have been available for many years, including several updates.
- There are new insights about the topic and there is a need for an update of scientific knowledge and expertise. This particularly applies to problems or conditions for which many new drugs are developed, such as heart disease and various cancers.
- There is uncertainty or a difference of opinion about optimal care and there is sufficient scientific evidence available as input for useful discussions and to draw firm conclusions. In addition, there should be a real opportunity to achieve consensus about the final recommendations to reach agreement, and opinions and interest should not vary too much. For example, the development of a guideline on chronic fatigue syndrome in the UK was made difficult by the divergence in opinions between professionals and patient organizations. The final guideline was not widely accepted among patient advocates (Dyer 2009).
- The topic concerns an issue with significant social or macro-economic impact. It may concern disorders that are uncommon but with a high burden on resources, such as AIDS and multiple sclerosis. Other examples are whiplash and chronic fatigue syndrome, which can have major social impact through absenteeism and disability.
- The topic should allow feasible guidelines, which include recommendations that can be applied in practice without large

---

Box 6.3 Criteria for Topic Selection

- The topic concerns a prevalent problem and guideline development allows improvement in quality of care.
- There are new insights and there is a need for an up-to-date knowledge synthesis.
- There is uncertainty about optimal care, there is sufficient scientific information available, and there is a real opportunity to achieve consensus.
- There is social relevance or macro-economic impact.
- There are no substantial barriers for implementation in practice.

organizational, financial, or legal barriers to overcome. If the guideline reflects actual care and is compatible with existing norms and values, it is more likely to be accepted. An example of this phenomenon are guidelines on pregnant women at risk for herpes neonatorum in which vaginal birth was no longer considered malpractice, confirming the common sense and experience of many gynecologists and other healthcare professionals.

6.4.2 Composition of the Guideline Development Group

Most guidelines are developed by a guideline working group or team of experts. The composition of the group is important for the validity of the recommendations and acceptance of the guideline among target users (Pagliari and Grimshaw 2002; Raine et al. 2004). A balanced composition will contribute to the credibility and ownership of the guideline among the target users.

A crucial step is the selection of the *chair*, who should be as neutral as possible, sensitive to group dynamics, and may not necessarily be a clinical expert. The success of guideline development is often related to the status and performance of the chair. The chair should stimulate discussion, should make sure that all group members are involved, and should not dominate the discussions. In each group meeting, tasks, deadlines, and timelines for document submission and meeting schedule should be clear.

The working group includes *representatives* from all relevant professional groups. For most topics, at least three different disciplines

will be represented. A broad representation increases the future acceptance of the guideline; beyond physicians, nurses, allied health professionals, and patient representatives should be involved (G-I-N Public Working Group 2015). All group members sign a declaration of interests, concerning commercial, intellectual, and institutional activities that could result in a conflict of interest with the guideline content (Institute of Medicine 2011a,b; Schünemann et al. 2015).

The guideline development group should be representative of the target audience to increase the feeling of ownership among the guideline users. Group members can be well-known academic experts on the clinical topic, but non-academic clinicians working in daily practice can be valuable as well, contributing critical views on relevance for and feasibility in daily practice (Gøtzsche and Ioannidis 2012).

Methodological and group support is needed to ensure high-quality guidelines (Box 6.4; Shekelle et al. 1999). Specific methodological expertise is needed for literature searching and analysis, and for formulating specific recommendations (Hirsch and Guyatt 2009). Support of the chair can be helpful in moderating group discussions to prevent bias in outcomes by the possible dominance of certain group members.

Increasingly, *health economists* are involved in cost-effectiveness and budget impact issues, particularly when the guideline holds major implications for national or local healthcare budgets. An example is the impact of screening on cardiovascular risk factors, which potentially concerns large patient populations.

Box 6.4 Required Expertise for Guideline Development

- Literature searching and critical appraisal
- Epidemiology and biostatistics
- Health services research and health economics
- Clinical expertise
- Patients or patient representatives with experiential knowledge
- Group dynamics
- Writing and editing

Finally, *managerial and administrative support* of the guideline development process is necessary. These include the organization of the group meetings, invitational conferences, reimbursement of travel costs and attendance fees, and document production. These tasks are ideally performed by an organization experienced in developing and implementing guidelines.

6.4.3 Patient and Public Involvement

The experience and knowledge of patients are equally important in clinical decision making to scientific evidence and clinical expertise (Sackett et al. 1996). Therefore, it has been recommended that patients or patient representatives are involved in guideline development (Krahn and Naglie 2008; Boivin et al. 2009) and guideline implementation (van der Weijden et al. 2013). Investigating the experiences and preferences of patients is expected to contribute to the quality of the guideline and its implementation in practice. It is not known what the best ways are for effective patient and public involvement in guideline development (Schünemann et al. 2006), and there are several examples of failures (van de Bovenkamp and Trappenburg 2009).

A review of 71 studies revealed that patient and public involvement in guideline development is rarely evaluated with respect to its impacts (Légaré et al. 2011). Some organizations reported that the impact of patients' involvement is felt to be small (e.g. patients help choose the words used to formulate recommendations). Others reported that it may change the key questions for guideline development or key outcomes considered in the analysis of research. There is consensus that patient and patient representatives should at least be consulted in the scoping phase of the guideline, and when the draft guideline is ready for comments. In addition, the search for evidence could include specific empirical studies describing patients' preferences and concerns (Utens et al. 2016; Wessels et al. 2016).

The patient's opinion on relevant key questions in the scoping phase can be explored by organizing focus groups under skilled leadership or by conducting individual interviews (van Wersch and Eccles 2001; Légaré et al. 2011). Prioritizing the most relevant key questions can be done by means of written surveys. Patient involvement may not only lead to other or additional key questions, but may also lead to debate on the most desired outcomes of specific treatments. Outcomes that are relevant for patients, such as health-related quality of life, can be identified from patients through completion of a questionnaire (de Wit et al. 2013). An example from rheumatology shows that patient involvement has led to the insight that fatigue is an important outcome variable in this field, next to pain and swelling of joints (Kirwan et al. 2007).

The patient's opinion on the draft guideline can be explored by means of interviews and surveys. The benefit of surveys is that a larger number of patients or patient representatives can be invited to participate, thus increasing representativeness. Patient representatives can also be invited to national meetings or invitational conferences organized prior to authorizing the guideline. Patient support groups can have an important mediating role in these consulting activities. The possible existence of more than one patient support group (a society, association, or action group) in some clinical areas should be considered.

The most intensive and potentially fruitful method of participation is to invite patients or patient representatives to the guideline working group (Box 6.5). In this method, patients may participate in discussion in all phases of guideline development, and are directly involved in the consensus process. These patients are expected to have some basic medical and methodological knowledge on top of experiential knowledge to ensure effective participation in the discussions. For this purpose, specific guides and training programs have been developed (Dickersin et al. 2001). A preparation meeting could be organized to

---

Box 6.5   Ways of Facilitating Optimal Patient Involvement in the Working Group

- Patients need to be trained and prepared before the committee meetings start.
- The chair of the committee should be specifically instructed in ways that most effectively elicit helpful patient input.
- Patients need to be coached during the process by one of the staff members of the guideline development organization.

- At least two patients should have a formal position in the committee. They can support each other in their task and replace each other in case of inability to attend a meeting.
- The patients should be supported in a manner similar to all group members in terms of reimbursement for travel costs and working hours.

Source: Data from G-I-N Public Working Group (2015).

---

allow patient representatives to ask questions for clarification in a non-threatening environment and to build their confidence (Boivin et al. 2014).

Active participation of some patient representatives in the committee can be combined with consulting strategies to facilitate the representativeness of the patients' voice. A recent experiment with patient participation in guideline development by sharing draft texts in a wiki-web environment showed that social media may provide a low threshold to groups of patients to actively contribute to consultations for guideline development (see Box 6.6).

Box 6.6   Example of an Innovative Strategy for Patient and Public Involvement in Guideline Development

Patient and public involvement was organized in an innovative way in the development of the multidisciplinary guideline on subfertility in the Netherlands. In-depth interviews were held with couples suffering from subfertility in various stages of treatment. The analysis of the interviews was translated into a core set of key recommendations for the guideline. These recommendations were made available to members of the subfertility patient support group ("Freya") on their association's website. Associated patients and their partners were free to adapt or add recommendations by means of a Wikipedia-type method ("FreyaWIKI"). Over 250 recommendations were generated. This extensive set of recommendations was then made accessible to the same website with the purpose of ranking the top five of the most important recommendations. The final set of the top five recommendations generated by patients (n = 21) was directly integrated within the professional's guideline. Both the in-depth interviews with the couples and the website FreyaWIKI led to unexpected new insights on patient expectations and preferences with regard to patient education, communication, and their coaching needs in subfertility treatment. For instance, patients want their doctor to practice empathy instead of only working on the technical part of the treatment. Another particular preference that emerged from the study was to have separate waiting rooms for pregnant women and couples being treated for infertility. This was of high value for defining the final guideline.

Source: Data from den Breejen et al. (2012).

For guidelines in public health on screening, prevention, and health promotion, healthy consumers should participate. The UK National Institute for Health and Clinical Excellence (NICE) has a so-called Citizens Council for this purpose. The council gives advice on relevant expectations and preferences of the general public (Rawlins and Culyer 2004). It is possible that ethical issues, such as the role of age or gender, are discussed by the Citizens Council.

Since it is also important to evaluate whether the guideline recommendations have a sufficient fit with the needs and preferences of patients, there is another important role for patient representatives once the guideline is developed. They can be asked for their needs toward implementation of the guideline, and for the type of information they would like to receive about the guideline. They should be involved in the development of a patient version of the guideline or patient decision aids related to specific preference-sensitive recommendations within the guideline (Raats et al. 2008; van der Weijden et al. 2013).

6.4.4 Drafting the Scope

The next step is defining the scope of the guideline, which includes formulating key questions (Qaseem et al. 2012). Unlike a textbook, it is not useful to discuss all aspects of a topic in a guideline, such as screening, detection, diagnosis, treatment, and follow-up. Since limited time and resources are available for guideline development, the guideline should focus on the most vital issues. For determining these issues, an analysis of actual needs and problems among the target group (professionals and patients) is recommended. Involvement of the target group at an early stage raises awareness of the guideline and facilitates its implementation.

Various methods can be used for the analysis of actual needs and problems and defining the scope, such as written surveys, literature reviews, brainstorming sessions or focus groups, and interviews with professionals and patient representatives. An efficient method for this is to start with a list of actual needs and problems following a brainstorming session within a small working group (including the chair), followed by a written survey among a sample of healthcare professionals for prioritization of the needs and problems. Additional problems can also be suggested.

Based on the final selection of actual needs and problems, key questions are formulated, which are the basis for the literature research. The questions may cover all dimensions of quality of care relevant for the objectives (effectiveness, efficiency, safety, patient-centeredness, equity, accessibility) and should be formulated as specifically as possible, defining the patient population, the intervention, and the outcome measures (Table 6.2). This is also a prerequisite for efficient literature searching and for selection of evidence. As the literature

Table 6.2 Examples of non-specific and specific questions.

Non-specific questions	Specific questions
Is a screening program for prevention of prostate cancer useful?	Is screening for prostate cancer in men between 55 and 70 years cost-effective?
What is the best available treatment for influenza?	In which risk groups is treatment with antiviral agents in influenza useful to reduce hospital admissions and death?
What is the risk of malignancy in patients with thrombosis?	What is the risk of malignancy in a woman with leg vein thrombosis without apparent cause or risk factors?
What is the preferred care model in treatment of stroke?	What model for multidisciplinary team work and division of tasks is most cost-effective in the acute phase of stroke?

review is often resource intensive, and many healthcare professionals are confronted – on top of the overload of original research findings – with an overload of guidelines, the number of clinical questions needs to be limited. Depending on the expected amount of available literature, the number of key questions should not exceed 15. Consensus or ranking techniques such as the nominal group technique can be used to prioritize the key questions. To guarantee patient involvement, some guideline committees decide beforehand that at least one or two of the key questions should be derived from the patient's perspective.

6.4.5 Development of Draft Guideline

In developing a draft guideline, it is important to provide a proper scientific basis for the guideline, use clinical expertise optimally where scientific data are lacking or unclear, and translate the available knowledge from the different sources (scientific evidence, clinical expertise, experiential knowledge, economic modeling, and budget impact analysis) into concrete recommendations for practice (Wieringa et al. 2018).

Important steps in this process are:

- Identifying and reviewing existing guidelines and systematic literature reviews.
- Searching for scientific evidence and assessing its quality and relevance.
- Contribution of all relevant experts and experience.
- Formulating recommendations for practice.

Each of these steps will be discussed briefly in this section. For more details, guideline development manuals could be consulted (e.g. National Institute for Health and Care Excellence 2009; Institute of Medicine 2011a).

6.4.6 Identifying and Reviewing Available Guidelines and Reviews

The first step in compiling scientific evidence supporting specific recommendations is to determine whether national or international clinical practice guidelines on the same topic have already been published and whether systematic reviews are available or are under way. Existing clinical guidelines can be retrieved by searching guideline databases (Box 6.7), such as the library of the G-I-N, and websites of large guideline programs such as NICE in England and Wales, or the Scottish Intercollegiate Guidelines Network (SIGN). For optimal use of existing guidelines, the ADAPTE Manual and Resource Toolkit is recommended (Fervers et al. 2011). Guideline organizations can be consulted for more detailed information and to exchange literature and evidence tables. If the adoption of recommendations from other guidelines is considered, the healthcare context and healthcare system in which the guidelines have been developed should be taken into account. Some variation in guideline recommendations on the same topic based on the same evidence is acceptable, and can be explained by differences in the healthcare system and cultural and geographical factors (Fervers et al. 2006). A useful source of evidence is the Cochrane Library to identify existing systematic reviews

---

Box 6.7 Examples of Useful Guideline Websites

- G-I-N: www.g-i-n.net
- National Institute for Health and Care Excellence (England/Wales): www.nice.org.uk
- SIGN: www.sign.ac.uk

- National Health and Medical Research Council (NHMRC, Australia): www.nhmrc.gov.au/health-advice/guidelines
- Cochrane Library: www.cochranelibrary.com

and reviews under development. Cochrane Reviews Groups can be consulted for literature and more information on specific topics.

6.4.7 Collection and Evaluation of Scientific Evidence

Studies are best identified by systematic review using a range of electronic databases such as Medline, CINAHL, Embase, and the Cochrane Library (Institute of Medicine 2011b). Reviewing the reference lists of identified articles may identify further studies (the "snowball" method), as may consulting expert members of the guideline development group. This step minimizes the risk of missing important information. Relevant journals can be searched by hand, and the "gray" literature (not published in scientific journals) can be studied. The degree to which all of these are carried out depends on the time and resources available.

Relevant articles are usually selected on the basis of title and abstract. Subsequently, the selected articles are studied in full text and the quality of the studies described evaluated, including ratings of the level of evidence. Beyond the risk of bias (which is mainly related to study design and methods), other factors need to be considered in the assessment of research findings, such as the directness (or generalizability) of the results, and the consistency, precision, and size of the effects (Balshem et al. 2011). The GRADE approach specifies considerations for making the step from consolidated research evidence to recommendations. In this approach, the quality of research is only one component. Other considerations are the balance between benefits and harms, societal values and patient preferences, feasibility, resource use, and equity. The GRADE approach is currently the most frequently used approach to grade evidence (Table 6.3) and to support the process from

Table 6.3 GRADE rating system of the quality of evidence.

Study design	Quality of evidence	Lower if	Higher if
Randomized trial	High	Study limitations −1 Serious −2 Very serious	Large effect +1 Large +2 Very large
	Moderate	Inconsistency −1 Serious −2 Very serious	Dose response +1 Evidence of a gradient
Observational study	Low	Indirectness −1 Serious −2 Very serious	All plausible confounding +1 Would reduce a demonstrated effect, or +1 Would suggest a spurious effect when results show no effect
		Imprecision −1 Serious −2 Very serious	
	Very low	Publication bias −1 Likely −2 Very likely	

Source: Guyatt et al. (2011). Reprinted with permission from Elsevier.

evidence to recommendations or decisions (Guyatt et al. 2008, Guyatt et al. 2011; Andrews et al. 2013; Alonso-Coello et al. 2016). It has also been adopted by the Cochrane Collaboration and is implemented in Cochrane Reviews. Extensive information, including educational videos and support, is available online (www.gradeworkinggroup.org).

6.4.8 Contribution of All Relevant Expertise and Experience

Guideline development cannot succeed without the contribution of experts in the field concerned, primarily because for some questions or choices no or only conflicting evidence exists. It is estimated that less than half of the decisions in most disciplines are supported by good empirical studies (Buchan 2004). In the development of a clinical guideline for the management of patients with angina pectoris in England, for example, only 21% of the recommendations could be directly based on randomized studies or meta-analyses (Eccles et al. 1996). A study of 53 American guidelines showed that only 11% of the recommendations were based on the highest level of evidence (Tricoci et al. 2009). Even when there is internally valid and consistent evidence for a given clinical practice, the optimal method of proceeding is seldom immediately clear (Naylor 1995). Hence, it is always necessary to call upon the collective expertise and experience of the working group (Zuiderent-Jerak et al. 2012). Even if evidence is found for certain healthcare interventions, it may be valid only for specific subgroups of the patient population, and it will be necessary to determine whether the results can be extrapolated to those populations seen in routine care. For example, much of the evidence for practice in primary care is derived from more or less select groups of patients recruited from secondary care settings and with different prior probabilities of disease. Finally, the available evidence must still be interpreted in the light of the key questions and problems to which the guideline tries to provide an answer.

In the phase of the interpretation of scientific evidence, its translation to clinical practice guidelines, and the use of opinions of experts, various problems can arise, such as:

- Research findings may be used selectively, so that personal preferences or politics may tip the balance in the end (Kraemer and Gostin 2009).
- Consensus may be forced when the working group is under time or other pressures.
- Some working group members or the chair may dominate the discussion with their own opinions.
- Discussions may be dominated by considerations of feasibility to such an extent that research findings or new information are ignored.

By formalizing and structuring the discussions as much as possible, an attempt can be made to avoid such problems. Formal consensus methods are useful for this, allowing all group members to make their contributions, for example using nominal group methods (Raine et al. 2005) or Delphi methods. For acceptance of the guideline by the target group, it is important to be able to trust that the development process has proceeded very carefully and that all information and opinions have been considered (Sudlow and Thomson 1997).

6.4.9 Formulation of Recommendations

In formulating recommendations for practice, the scientific evidence and clinical and other relevant expertise (e.g. from patients, health economists, or implementation experts) are compiled. Here, in the formulation of appropriate or suitable care, considerations relevant to implementation need to be discussed (Box 6.8). In formulating recommendations, the following issues should be weighed:

- The nature and strength of the scientific evidence.

Box 6.8   Development of a Clinical Practice Guideline on Cardiovascular Risk Management

This study described the development of a guideline on cardiovascular risk management, including complex considerations. Randomized trials showed that treatment with cholesterol-lowering drugs was effective for many patient categories, including the elderly, patients with diabetes mellitus, and patients at increased risk of cardiovascular disease and only slightly elevated cholesterol values. The European guideline on the same subject recommended that large groups of patients should be offered drug treatment. A Norwegian study found that strict compliance with this guideline would imply that 22% of Norwegian women and 86% of Norwegian men over 40 years of age should be treated; and at the age of 55, 48.6% of women and 91.4% of men would need treatment. Implementation of the guideline would be impossible because of the limited capacity of healthcare providers. Moreover, the impact on the healthcare budget would be huge. Finally, there was the danger of undesired medicalization, as a large group of relatively healthy people with no symptoms would need medical treatment. Therefore, the guideline working group decided to increase the threshold of treatment. The guideline emphasizes that cardiovascular risk management needs to take into account individual circumstances and patient preferences.

Source: Data from Getz et al. (2005).

- The perceptions of professionals and patients of the balance of benefits of a given intervention and treatment burden and risks.
- The generalizability and applicability of the evidence to the population concerned.
- The medical and societal costs associated with the proposed care intervention, ideally derived from data on cost-effectiveness.
- The feasibility of the proposed intervention in terms of required skills, resources, available staff, and limitations of the healthcare system (e.g. legal regulations).
- Professional norms and values, patient views and preferences, and ethical considerations.

In the interpretation of the evidence and the use of expertise, normative and cultural values about the desired health benefit and the acceptable risks may play an important role (Eisinger et al. 1999; Burgers et al. 2002; de Kort et al. 2009). Considering these views is not inappropriate as long as the views are made explicit and care is taken to ensure that the recommendations are in agreement with the norms and values within the target group (see Box 6.9).

The effectiveness of the guideline may increase if the recommendations are formulated to be as specific as possible (Grol et al. 1998; Shekelle et al. 2000; Gupta et al. 2016). It should be clear what action is needed for which groups of patients and what the conditions are. The strength of the recommendation could be reflected in the wording, using words such as "must" and "should" or "strongly recommend" and "recommend" (Lomatan et al. 2010). In case of uncertainty "can" or "consider" can be used, but at the cost of the specificity of the recommendation. An alternative is to formulate options for management, including information on benefits and harms.

To enhance the "implementability" of recommendations, the Guideline Implementability Decision Excellence Model (GUIDE-M) can be used (Brouwers et al. 2015). This model comprises 7 domains, 19 subdomains, and 44 attributes, which can be applied to individual recommendations in the guideline. It can be used by guideline developers to help foster the creation of high-quality, unbiased, and usable recommendations.

Box 6.9   Guidelines for the Management of an Elevated Risk of Breast Cancer

An analysis of American and French clinical guidelines for the management of an elevated risk of breast cancer revealed interesting differences with regard to interpretation of the scientific evidence about the desired results and the norms and values of the guideline developers and the target group. American guidelines advise regular breast self-examination, while French guidelines point to the anxiety and insecurity that this can evoke in women. American guidelines also advise an active approach by physicians with regard to the preventive removal of associated lymph nodes, while French guidelines are more conservative in this area: they advise a "wait and see" approach to this intervention, suggesting delaying this step for a few months before a definitive decision is made. The authors point to the cultural differences underlying such divergent recommendations, such as the greater emphasis on autonomy for patients in the USA.

Source: Data from Eisinger et al. (1999).

6.4.10   Consultation and Authorization

To enhance the acceptance and ultimate use of the guideline, the guideline should be distributed for comments and approval to all relevant stakeholders and target groups. It also helps when the applicability of the guideline is pilot tested in practice.

6.4.11   Consultation

To promote wide support for the clinical guideline and to identify possible problems in its acceptance, it is recommended to ask the target users, others involved, and experts for their comments about the guideline. This can be done in various ways:

- *Survey*: a sample of users, experts, and other individuals (e.g. patients, insurers, policy makers, managers) receive a structured questionnaire, including questions on the guideline and specific recommendations. The aim is to provide feedback on the acceptability and applicability of the guideline and barriers to its implementation.
- *Website*: the draft guideline is published online and accessible for comments using a structured format following the content of the guideline. This method is often used by professional societies, providing useful information about acceptance of the guideline and feasibility in practice.
- *Face-to-face meetings*: the clinical guideline is presented at an open meeting for comment and approval. An organized discussion is held, based on the guideline recommendations which are explained by the working group. This can include soliciting participants' views on the most important conclusions and recommendations, allowing the audience to express their comments, criticisms, and suggestions, verbally or in writing. Such a meeting can be organized at a national level, regionally, or within an institution, inviting as many of the involved disciplines as possible. A meeting enables participation, but since it has the potential disadvantage that those with strong opinions can dominate the discussion, allowing for written comments or using a voting system can reduce this bias.
- *Focus group*: a purposive sample of target users with varying backgrounds is invited to discuss key recommendations in the guideline. The group facilitator may ask questions, such as: Do you agree with the recommendations? Do they reflect current practice? Would you be willing to change your behavior to adhere to the recommendations? What would

you need to adopt the guideline? The aim is not to achieve consensus among the group members, but to identify all potential barriers and facilitators for implementation.

6.4.12   Pilot Testing

Useful information on the applicability of the clinical guideline can be collected from a pilot test in a few healthcare organizations, practices, or healthcare teams. Care providers are asked to follow the guideline as closely as possible. Performance is recorded and barriers perceived in applying the guideline are reported. Comments of patients may also be included. The findings from the pilot test could be included in the guideline to inform the target group about possible problems in applying the guideline and how to address these.

6.4.13   Authorization

The results of the consultation process and pilot testing of the guideline are incorporated in the final version of the guideline. The uptake of a clinical guideline can be promoted if it has the support or endorsement of a professional association or an independent institution. Authorization may include a number of ritual characteristics intended to close ranks and preserve unity, which can be decisive in acceptance of the guideline by the target users. Authorization (or endorsement) can take a variety of forms:

- Formal approval of the clinical guideline can be requested from involved professional organizations, patient organizations, or other relevant stakeholders.
- An independent scientific council or committee can be established to verify the procedure and its results.
- The clinical guideline can be submitted for approval to an agency established for this purpose. Examples are NICE in England and Wales and the NHMRC in Australia.

6.4.14   Design of the Guideline and Related Products

From the perspective of implementation, it is crucial that the guideline is published in an accessible, understandable, and attractive format. This concerns both the layout and the adaptation of the design to the specific situation in which the guideline will be applied. Different users, purposes, conditions, and implementation strategies may need different tools (Table 6.4; Liang et al. 2017).

Implementation is more successful when a guideline is available in different formats (Stone et al. 2005; Kastner et al. 2015). If a guideline is to be used for educational purposes, for example, comprehensive texts, syllabi, and other teaching tools that explain and support the recommendations are needed. In routine practice, clear summaries and flow charts are likely to be useful. As an example, updates of clinical practice guidelines for primary care physicians in the Netherlands are made available in the following formats:

- Publication of a summary in the scientific journal explaining the most relevant issues and modifications.
- Electronic version on the website of the Dutch College of General Practitioners (www.nhg.org), also accessible for tablets and smartphones.
- Information on a public website for patients (Thuisarts.nl), explaining the recommendations in the guideline in lay terms.
- Electronic decision support, integrated in the electronic medical record, in particular the recommendations on drug treatment and chronic diseases, such as diabetes, COPD, heart failure, and renal failure.

For the purpose of clinical audit and measuring professionals' performance, the key recommendations of the guideline should be translated to review criteria, ideally in the format of validated quality indicators (see Chapter 7). It may be helpful to develop formats of strict protocols based on the guideline in which actions of all

Table 6.4 Framework of types of tools for guideline implementation.

Category	Type	Description
Patient support	Information	Print or electronic information about the condition, management options, or additional sources of information
	Guideline summary	Short versions of guidelines designed for patients and care partners
	Self-management support	Resources such as charts, templates, and action plans that can be used by patients to better manage their disease and daily activities
Clinician support	Guideline summary	Short versions of guidelines for clinicians in print or electronic format including pocket cards, summaries, or applications
	Algorithm	Flow charts or clinical pathways that provide step-by-step guidance for patient management
	Form or checklist	Print or electronic documents to be completed by clinicians for documentation in patient medical records
Implementation support	Training material	Resources to support educational meetings or self-directed learning such as slides for presentations or study modules
	Resources	Human, infrastructure, or funding resources, or instructions or processes needed for guideline implementation
Evaluation support	Audit tools	Guidelines or manuals to support the evaluation of guideline-compliant practice before and after guideline implementation
	Measures	Quality indicators or performance measures by which to assess compliance with guideline recommendations

Source: Data from Liang et al. (2017).

different disciplines involved within one region or setting are clearly described. For the purpose of informing patients about the content of the guideline, an accessible patient version of the guideline may be developed. As a guideline may contain recommendations that are preference sensitive due to a trade-off between benefits and harms, or because more than one option exist that different individuals may value differently, decision aids can support patients and involve them in decision making. Investment in such guideline-related products, for example by involving designers, text writers, and information and communication technology experts, is important in order to consider the needs of different target groups.

6.4.15 Evaluation

A final and important step in the development of clinical guidelines is the evaluation of their feasibility and applicability in the daily routines of healthcare, on the basis of a pilot implementation. Relevant elements of such evaluations are:

- How well are the guidelines known and to what extent are they valued? Are they discussed with colleagues? Are they well understood and remembered? Are they accepted and used in local meetings and quality improvement activities?
- To what extent are the recommendations applied and followed? If not, what recommendations are not followed? What are the problems in their application?
- If time and resources permit, a full-blown implementation study may be part of the guideline development: to what extent are the recommendations effective? Does their application lead to achievement of the objectives which were envisioned, such as better

health, fewer complications, lower costs, better quality of life, greater efficiency, and patient satisfaction?

Information that arises out of such evaluations can contribute to further implementation of the guideline and a tailored implementation plan. The results of the evaluation can raise questions about the validity and applicability of the guideline and the recommendations. A working group can try to find answers on these questions through additional literature reviews, discussions, and retesting of the recommendations in practice. This information can also be used in the updating of the guideline.

6.4.16 Updating Guidelines

While there is increasing consensus about methods for developing evidence-based guidelines, less attention has been paid to the process of assessing when guidelines should be updated (Alonso-Coello et al. 2011). The most common advice is for guidelines to include a scheduled review date. Shekelle et al. (2001) propose a set of principles and a pragmatic model for assessing whether guidelines need to be updated. They suggest that clinical guidelines may require updating due to changes in any or all of the following:

- Evidence on the existing benefits and harms of interventions.
- Outcomes considered important.
- Available interventions.
- Evidence that current practice is suboptimal.
- Values placed on outcomes.
- Resources available for healthcare.

They suggest applying a two-stage method to identify significant new evidence, and to assess whether the new evidence warrants guideline updating. A multidisciplinary group of experts reviews recommendations within the guideline and considers new evidence or developments in the field relevant to the guideline recommendation and, if so, whether this evidence is sufficient to invalidate the guideline

recommendation. This process is supplemented by targeted literature searches.

Within a guideline there may be some recommendations that are invalid while others remain current. A clinical practice guideline needs updating if the majority of recommendations are out of date, with new evidence demonstrating that the recommended interventions are inappropriate, ineffective, or superseded by new interventions. In other cases, a single, outdated recommendation may not invalidate the document. As a general rule, guidelines should be reassessed for validity at least every three years (Shekelle et al. 2001). In slowly evolving fields, it may take longer.

6.5 Quality of Guidelines and Guideline Development Programs

High-quality guidelines can improve the quality and outcomes of healthcare (Grimshaw et al. 2004), but low-quality guidelines can harm patients (Shekelle et al. 2000). Worldwide, many thousands of guidelines, aiming to direct healthcare, have been published to date (Alonso-Coello et al. 2010). As physicians can be confronted with multiple guidelines on the same topics (Feder 1994; Littlejohns et al. 1999), there is a need to consistently identify well-developed guidelines that can contribute to optimal patient care.

In 2001, the AGREE instrument was published (AGREE Collaboration 2003). This is an internationally developed and validated assessment tool for clinical guidelines. Not only the methodology and scientific validity, but also the clarity and applicability of the guideline are assessed with this instrument. It enables us to make a distinction between high- and low-quality guidelines. Moreover, the instrument can be used by guideline developers to improve the quality of guidelines that still need to be developed. A second version of the AGREE instrument – AGREE II (Box 6.10) – was

---

Box 6.10 Criteria of AGREE II

I Scope and purpose

1) The overall objective(s) of the guideline is (are) specifically described.
2) The health question(s) covered by the guideline is (are) specifically described.
3) The population (patients, public, etc.) to whom the guideline is meant to apply is specifically described.

II Stakeholder involvement

4) The guideline development group includes individuals from all relevant professional groups.
5) The views and preferences of the target population (patients, public, etc.) have been sought.
6) The target users of the guideline are clearly defined.

Rigor of development

7) Systematic methods were used to search for evidence.
8) The criteria for selecting the evidence are clearly described.
9) The strengths and limitations of the body of evidence are clearly described.
10) The methods for formulating the recommendations are clearly described.
11) The health benefits, side effects, and risks have been considered in formulating the recommendations.
12) There is an explicit link between the recommendations and the supporting evidence.

13) The guideline has been externally reviewed by experts prior to its publication.
14) A procedure for updating the guideline is provided.

Clarity and presentation

15) The recommendations are specific and unambiguous.
16) The different options for management of the condition or health issue are clearly presented.
17) Key recommendations are easily identifiable.

Applicability

18) The guideline describes facilitators and barriers to its application.
19) The guideline provides advice and/or tools on how the recommendations can be put into practice.
20) The potential resource implications of applying the recommendations have been considered.
21) The guideline presents monitoring and/or auditing criteria.

Editorial independence

22) The views of the funding body have not influenced the content of the guideline.
23) Competing interests of guideline development group members have been recorded and addressed.

---

developed after a new validation round led by researchers from McMaster University in Canada (Brouwers et al. 2010). The wording of some items has been modified and the manual has been expanded to the point where the instrument can be regarded as the international standard for reporting of guidelines (Brouwers et al. 2016).

The AGREE instrument has been translated into more than 20 languages and is used throughout the world. The results of research in which the quality of guidelines has been compared using the AGREE instrument are published regularly (see Box 6.1; Alonso-Coello et al. 2010). An overall conclusion is that there remains room for improving the quality of

---

Box 6.11   Characteristics of Effective Guideline Programs

Stakeholders involved in guideline development
- A reliable and independent guideline organization
- Target group of professionals from different disciplines
- Patient (or client) representatives

Methodology
- Defining scope and purpose by all relevant stakeholders
- Systematic literature reviews (including existing guidelines)
- Formulation of recommendations based on evidence and consensus among experts

- Consultation of external experts and potential guideline users
- Formal updating procedure
- Use of quality criteria for guidelines

Dissemination and implementation strategy
- Pilot implementation study
- Use of different guideline formats tailored to the target group, including patient versions
- Optimal use of electronic resources (including internet)
- Multiple interventions for implementation

---

guidelines and that more attention should be paid to describing the methods and the procedures followed. This conclusion also demonstrates a limitation of the AGREE instrument; that is, that a reliable judgment needs sufficient information. This information may also be included in accompanying documents or technical reports. If these documents are not studied, the quality score of the guideline may be underestimated. The AGREE instrument has proven to be a valid framework for guideline developers: many guideline organizations dealing with evidence-based guideline development use the AGREE criteria to raise the quality of their guidelines.

Guidelines developed within a coordinated guideline program are generally of better quality than those developed separately from such a program (Burgers et al. 2003b). As more groups in a country are involved in guideline setting and interests diverge, the process of guideline development and outcomes becomes more complex. Coordination by a center or program that combines knowledge and expertise on guideline development may guarantee both the quality and independence of guidelines. Acceptance of the infrastructure by the

stakeholders and sufficient involvement in the guideline development process are essential requirements for implementing the guidelines in daily practice. Box 6.11 summarizes the characteristics of effective guideline programs.

6.6 International Collaboration in Guideline Development

The production of evidence-based guidelines requires substantial resources. Existing guidelines can be used and adapted to the local context to reduce duplication of efforts (Fervers et al. 2011). Using guidelines from other countries raises the question of whether guidelines could be developed at an international level. The guidelines of the World Health Organization (WHO), in particular those on the prevention and treatment of infectious diseases, and the guidelines of the European Society of Cardiology are examples of such international guidelines. Governmental agencies and public health institutions are the main target groups of these guidelines. These organizations are also responsible for implementation of the guidelines in practice, in which case there remains an important role for national organizations to translate these global guidelines and adapt them to the national practice setting. An international guideline can provide a scientific basis, just like a systematic review, but the specific practice recommendations often need to be formulated in countries separately, considering the professional, cultural, and healthcare context. This explains why studies comparing guidelines from different countries may lead to different conclusions. Depending on the topic, recommendations may be similar while the evidence differs, for example in type 2 diabetes mellitus (Burgers et al. 2002) and breast cancer (Wennekes et al. 2008), or the recommendations differ in cases where the evidence is similar (Eisinger et al. 1999).

Collaboration within the G-I-N on guideline development focuses mainly on exchanging knowledge and experiences and developing new methods and standards, for example on searching and summarizing the literature in terms of search filters and evidence tables (Mlika-Cabanne et al. 2011) and management of conflicts of interests (Schünemann et al. 2015). The challenge is to summarize the evidence unambiguously and clearly, but to respect the countries' and regions' autonomy with regard to guidelines and decisions on optimal care (Eisenberg 2002).

6.7 Conclusion

Guidelines summarize the current state of knowledge and serve as an important aid in the implementation of new evidence in daily healthcare. Guidelines are not implemented automatically in practice, but require careful implementation. Considerations about the implementation of a guideline begin at the stage of preparation for guideline development and should be incorporated in all stages of the development process (Box 6.12). An analysis of problems that need to be addressed by the clinical guideline and the formulation of specific questions reflecting the problems in practice should lead to a product that professionals are eager to use in daily practice. Further, involving all relevant disciplines and patients in the guideline development process creates broad support and encourages the use of the guideline. In addition, a systematic evaluation

---

Box 6.12 Characteristics of Effective Guidelines

- *Relevance*: guidelines should provide an answer to questions that stem from relevant concerns in daily practice.
- *Credibility*: systematic development and rigorous, transparent procedures within a structured program are needed with support from an experienced guideline organization, and with involvement of the target group in the development, including patient representatives.
- *Scientifically based*: a systematic literature review forms the basis of the guideline.
- *Applicability*: the recommendations are commented upon or tested in practice by the intended users of the guideline, taking into account guideline implementation in terms of consequences for patients, required knowledge, skills, resources, materials, and facilities.
- *Accessibility*: a neat, clear, and attractive design with possibilities for electronic and web-based use.
- *Integration in usual care processes*: efforts need to be made to incorporate the guidelines in local care protocols, electronic decision-support systems, and systems for monitoring care.

of the guideline in daily practice provides insight into both the use and the applicability of the guideline; these results can be taken into account in the revision process. Finally, guideline development cannot be considered as an isolated activity, but as part of an iterative, quality circle in which implementation and evaluation also play an important role.

References

AGREE Collaboration (2003). Development and validation of an international appraisal instrument for assessing the quality of clinical practice guidelines: the AGREE project. *Qual. Saf. Health Care* 12: 18–23.

Alonso-Coello, P., Irfan, A.B., Sola, I. et al. (2010). The quality of clinical practice guidelines over the last two decades: a systematic review of guideline appraisal studies. *Qual. Saf. Health Care* 19: e58.

Alonso-Coello, P., Martinez Garcia, L., Carrasco Gimeno, J.M. et al. (2011). The updating of clinical practice guidelines: insights from an international survey. *Implement. Sci.* 6: 107.

Alonso-Coello, P., Oxman, A.D., Moberg, J. et al. (2016). GRADE evidence to decision (EtD) frameworks: a systematic and transparent approach to making well informed healthcare choices. 2: clinical practice guidelines. *BMJ* 353: i2089.

Andrews, J.C., Schünemann, H.J., Oxman, A.D. et al. (2013). GRADE guidelines: 15. Going from evidence to recommendation— determinants of a recommendation's direction and strength. *J. Clin. Epidemiol.* 66: 726–735.

Balshem, H., Helfand, M., Schunemann, H.J. et al. (2011). GRADE guidelines: 3. Rating the quality of evidence. *J. Clin. Epidemiol.* 64: 401–406.

Boivin, A., Green, J., van der Meulen, J. et al. (2009). Why consider patients' preferences? A discourse analysis of clinical practice guideline developers. *Med. Care* 47: 908–915.

Boivin, A., Lehoux, P., Burgers, J., and Grol, R. (2014). What are the key ingredients for effective public involvement in health care improvement and policy decisions? A randomized trial process evaluation. *Milbank Q.* 92: 319–350.

van de Bovenkamp, H.M. and Trappenburg, M.J. (2009). Reconsidering patient participation in guideline development. *Health Care Anal.* 17: 198–216.

Boyd, C.M., Darer, J., Boult, C. et al. (2005). Clinical practice guidelines and quality of care for older patients with multiple comorbid diseases. Implications for pay for performance. *JAMA* 294: 716–724.

Brouwers, M.C., Kerkvliet, K., Spithoff, K., and AGREE Next Steps Consortium (2016). The AGREE reporting checklist: a tool to improve reporting of clinical practice guidelines. *BMJ* 352: i1152.

Brouwers, M.C., Kho, M.E., Browman, G.P. et al. (2010). AGREE II: advancing guideline development, reporting and evaluation in health care. *CMAJ* 182: E839–E842.

Brouwers, M.C., Makarski, J., Kastner, M. et al. (2015). The Guideline Implementability Decision Excellence Model (GUIDE-M): a mixed methods approach to create an international resource to advance the practice guideline field. *Implement. Sci.* 10: 36.

Buchan, H. (2004). Gaps between best evidence and practice: causes for concern. *Med. J. Aust.* 180: S48–S49.

Burgers, J.S. (2015). Opschudding over evidence-based medicine. Van reductionisme naar realisme in de toepassing van richtlijnen [Criticism of evidence-based medicine: from reductionism to realism in the application of guidelines]. *Ned. Tijdschr. Geneeskd.* 159: A8376.

Burgers, J.S., Bailey, J.V., Klazinga, N.S. et al. (2002). Inside guidelines: comparative analysis of recommendations and evidence in diabetes guidelines from 13 countries. *Diabetes Care* 25: 1933–1939.

Burgers, J.S., Cluzeau, F.A., Hanna, S.E. et al. (2003b). Characteristics of high quality guidelines: evaluation of 86 clinical guidelines developed in ten European countries and Canada. *Int. J. Technol. Assess. Health Care* 19: 148–157.

Burgers, J.S., Grol, R., Klazinga, N.S. et al. (2003a). Towards evidence-based clinical practice: an international survey of 18 clinical guideline programs. *Int. J. Qual. Health Care* 15: 31–45.

De Wit, M., Abma, T., Koelewijn-van Loon, M. et al. (2013). Involving patient research partners has a significant impact on outcomes research: a responsive evaluation of the international OMERACT conferences. *BMJ Open* 3: 5.

Den Breejen, E.M.E., Nelen, W.L.D.M., Knijnenburg, J.M.L. et al. (2012). Feasibility of a wiki as a participatory tool for patients in clinical guideline development. *J. Med. Internet Res.* 14: e138.

Dickersin, K., Braun, L., Mead, M. et al. (2001). Development and implementation of a science training course for breast cancer activists: project LEAD (Leadership, Education and Advocacy Development). *Health Expect.* 4: 213–220.

Durieux, P., Chaix-Couturier, C., Durand-Zaleski, I., and Ravaud, P. (2000). From clinical recommendations to mandatory practice. The introduction of regulatory guidelines in the French healthcare system. *Int. J. Technol. Assess. Health Care* 16: 969–975.

Dyer, C. (2009). High court rejects challenge to NICE guidelines on chronic fatigue syndrome. *BMJ* 338: b1110.

Eccles, M., Clapp, Z., Grimshaw, J. et al. (1996). Developing valid guidelines: methodological and procedural issues from the North of England evidence based guideline development project. *Qual. Health Care* 5: 44–50.

Eddy, D.M., Adler, J., Patterson, N. et al. (2011). Individualized guidelines: the potential for increasing quality and reducing costs. *Ann. Intern. Med.* 154: 627–634.

Eisenberg, J.M. (2002). Globalize the evidence, localize the decision: evidence-based medicine and international diversity. *Health Aff. (Millwood)* 21: 166–168.

Eisinger, F., Geller, G., Burke, W., and Holtzman, N. A. (1999). Cultural basis for differences between US and French clinical recommendations for women at increased risk of breast and ovarian cancer. *Lancet* 353: 919–920.

Feder, G. (1994). Management of mild hypertension: which guidelines to follow? *BMJ* 308: 470–471.

Fervers, B., Burgers, J.S., Haugh, M. et al. (2006). Adaptation of clinical guidelines: a review of methods and experiences. *Int. J. Qual. Health Care* 18: 167–176.

Fervers, B., Burgers, J.S., Voellinger, R. et al. (2011). Guideline adaptation: an approach to enhance efficiency in guideline development and improve utilisation. *Qual. Saf. Health Care* 20: 228–236.

Getz, L., Sigurdsson, J.A., Hetlevik, I. et al. (2005). Estimating the high risk group for cardiovascular disease in the Norwegian HUNT 2 population according to the 2003 European guidelines: modelling study. *BMJ* 331: 551.

G-I-N Public Working Group (2015). *Public Toolkit: Patient and Public Involvement in Guidelines*. Pitlochry: G-I-N.

Gøtzsche, P.C. and Ioannidis, J.P. (2012). Content area experts as authors: helpful or harmful for systematic reviews and meta-analyses? *BMJ* 345: e7031.

Greenhalgh, T., Howick, J., Maskrey, N., and Evidence Based Medicine Renaissance Group (2014). Evidence based medicine: a movement in crisis? *BMJ* 348: g3725.

Grimshaw, J. and Russell, I. (1993). Achieving health gain through clinical guidelines. I. Developing scientifically valid guidelines. *Qual. Health Care* 2: 243–248.

Grimshaw, J.M., Thomas, R.E., MacLennan, G. et al. (2004). Effectiveness and efficiency of guideline dissemination and implementation strategies. *Health Technol. Assess.* 8: 1–72.

Grol, R. (1993). Development of guidelines in general practice. *Br. J. Gen. Pract.* 43: 146–151.

Grol, R., Dalhuijsen, J., Thomas, S. et al. (1998). Attributes of clinical guidelines that influence use of guidelines in general practice: observational study. *BMJ* 317: 858–861.

Grol, R. and van Weel, C. (2009). Getting a grip on guidelines: how to make them more relevant for practice. *Br. J. Gen. Pract.* 59: e143–e144.

Gupta, S., Rai, N., Bhattacharrya, O. et al. (2016). Optimizing the language and format of guidelines to improve guideline uptake. *CMAJ* 188: E362–E368.

Guyatt, G.H., Oxman, A.D., Schünemann, H.J. et al. (2011). GRADE guidelines: a new series of articles in the Journal of Clinical Epidemiology. *J. Clin. Epidemiol.* 64: 380–382.

Guyatt, G.H., Oxman, A.D., Vist, G. et al. (2008). Rating quality of evidence and strength of recommendations. GRADE: an emerging consensus on rating quality of evidence and strength of recommendations. *BMJ* 336: 924–926.

Haycox, A., Bagust, A., and Walley, T. (1999). Clinical guidelines: the hidden costs. *BMJ* 318: 391–393.

Hirsch, J. and Guyatt, G. (2009). Clinical experts or methodologists to write clinical guidelines? *Lancet* 374: 273–274.

Hurwitz, B. (1999). Legal and political considerations of clinical practice guidelines. *BMJ* 318: 661–664.

Institute of Medicine (2011a). *Clinical Practice Guidelines We Can Trust*. Washington, DC: National Academies Press.

Institute of Medicine (2011b). *Finding What Works in Health Care: Standards for Systematic Reviews*. Washington, DC: National Academies Press.

Jacoby, I. (1985). The consensus development program of the National Institutes of Health: current practices and historical perspectiveness. *Int. J. Technol. Assess. Health Care* 1: 420–432.

Kastner, M., Bhattacharyya, O., Hayden, L. et al. (2015). Guideline uptake is influenced by six implementability domains for creating and communicating guidelines: a realist review. *Clin. Epidemiol.* 68: 498–509.

Kirwan, J.R., Minnock, P., Adebajo, A. et al. (2007). Patient perspective: fatigue as a recommended patient centered outcome measure in rheumatoid arthritis. *J. Rheumatol.* 34: 1174–1177.

Knottnerus, J. and Dinant, G.J. (1997). Medicine based evidence, a prerequisite for evidence based medicine. *BMJ* 315: 1109–1110.

Koerselman, G.F. and Korzec, A. (2008). Voorstel voor een checklist bij het afwijken van richtlijnen [Proposal to Develop a Checklist in Case of Deviation of Guidelines]. *Ned. Tijdschr. Geneeskd.* 152: 1757–1759.

de Kort, S., Burgers, J.S., Willemse, P., and Willems, D. (2009). Hidden values in formulating guidelines for palliative chemo-therapeutic cancer treatments. *Neth. J. Med.* 67: 62–68.

Kraemer, J.D. and Gostin, L.O. (2009). Science, politics, and values: the politicization of professional practice guidelines. *JAMA* 301: 665–667.

Krahn, M. and Naglie, G. (2008). The next step in guideline development: incorporating patient preferences. *JAMA* 300: 436–438.

Légaré, F., Boivin, A., van der Weijden, T. et al. (2011). Patient and public involvement in clinical practice guidelines: a knowledge synthesis of existing programs. *Med. Decis. Mak.* 31: E45–E74.

Liang, L., Abi Safi, J., Gagliardi, A.R., and members of the Guidelines International Network Implementation Working Group (2017). Number and type of guideline implementation tools varies by guideline, clinical condition, country of origin, and type of developer organization: content analysis of guidelines. *Implement. Sci.* 12: 136.

Littlejohns, P., Cluzeau, F., Bale, R. et al. (1999). The quantity and quality of clinical practice guidelines for the management of depression in primary care in the UK. *Br. J. Gen. Pract.* 49: 205–210.

Lomatan, E.A., Michel, G., Lin, Z., and Shiffman, R.N. (2010). How "should" we write guideline recommendations? Interpretation of deontic terminology in clinical practice guidelines: survey of the health services community. *Qual. Saf. Health Care* 19: 509–513.

Lugtenberg, M., Burgers, J.S., Clancy, C. et al. (2011). Current guidelines have limited applicability to patients with comorbid conditions. *PLoS One* 6: e25987.

Lugtenberg, M., Burgers, J.S., and Westert, G.P. (2009). Effects of evidence-based clinical practice guidelines on quality of care: a systematic review. *Qual. Saf. Health Care* 18: 385–392.

Mason, J., Freemantle, N., Nazareth, I. et al. (2001). When is it cost-effective to change the behavior of health professionals? *JAMA* 286: 2988–2992.

Mlika-Cabanne, N., Harbour, R., de Beer, H. et al. (2011). Sharing hard labour: developing a standard template for data summaries in guideline development. *BMJ Qual. Saf.* 20: 141–145.

National Institute for Health and Care Excellence (2009). *Developing NICE Guidelines: The Manual*. London: National Institute for Health and Care Excellence www.nice.org.uk.

Naylor, C.D. (1995). Grey zones of clinical practice: some limits to evidence-based medicine. *Lancet* 345: 940–942.

Ollenschläger, G., Marshall, C., Qureshi, S. et al. (2004). Improving the quality of health care: using international collaboration to inform guideline programmes – by founding the Guidelines International Network G-I-N. *Qual. Saf. Health Care* 13: 455–460.

Pagliari, C. and Grimshaw, J. (2002). Impact of group structure and multi-disciplinary evidence-based guideline development: observed study. *J. Eval. Clin. Pract.* 8: 145–153.

Qaseem, A., Forland, F., Macbeth, F. et al. (2012). Guidelines International Network: toward international standards for clinical practice guidelines. *Ann. Intern. Med.* 156: 525–531.

Raats, C.J., van Veenendaal, H., Versluijs, M.M., and Burgers, J.S. (2008). A generic tool for development of decision aids based on clinical practice guidelines. *Patient Educ. Couns.* 73: 413–417.

Raine, R., Sanderson, C., and Black, N. (2005). Developing clinical guidelines: a challenge to current methods. *BMJ* 331: 631–633.

Raine, R., Sanderson, C., Hutchings, A. et al. (2004). An experimental study of determinants of group judgments in clinical guideline development. *Lancet* 364: 429–437.

Rawlins, M.D. and Culyer, A.J. (2004). National Institute for Clinical Excellence and its value judgments. *BMJ* 329: 224–227.

Robinson, K.A., Saldanha, I.J., and McKoy, N.A. (2011). Identification of research gaps from evidence-based guidelines: a pilot study in cystic fibrosis. *Int. J. Technol. Assess. Health Care* 27: 247–252.

Sackett, D.L., Rosenberg, W.M., Gray, J.A. et al. (1996). Evidence based medicine: what it is and what it isn't. *BMJ* 312: 71–72.

Schünemann, H.J., Al-Ansary, L.A., Forland, F. et al. (2015). Guidelines International Network: principles for disclosure of interests and management of conflicts in guidelines. *Ann. Intern. Med.* 163: 548–553.

Schünemann, H.J., Fretheim, A., and Oxman, A. D. (2006). Improving the use of research evidence in guideline development: 10. Integrating values and consumer involvement. *Health Res. Policy Syst.* 4: 22.

Shaneyfelt, T.M. and Centor, R.M. (2009). Reassessment of clinical practice guidelines: go gently into that good night. *JAMA* 301: 868–869.

Shekelle, P., Eccles, M.P., Grimshaw, J.M., and Woolf, S.H. (2001). When should clinical guidelines be updated? *BMJ* 323: 155–157.

Shekelle, P.G., Kravitz, R.L., Beart, J. et al. (2000). Are nonspecific practice guidelines potentially harmful? A randomized comparison of the effect of nonspecific versus specific guidelines on physician decision making. *Health Serv. Res.* 34: 1429–1448.

Shekelle, P., Woolf, S., Eccles, M. et al. (1999). Developing guidelines. *BMJ* 318: 593–596.

Starfield, B. (1998). Quality of care research. Internal elegance and external relevance. *JAMA* 280: 1006–1008.

Stone, T.T., Schweikhart, S.B., Mantese, A., and Sonnad, S.S. (2005). Guideline attribute and implementation preferences among physicians in multiple health systems. *Qual. Manag. Health Care* 14: 177–187.

Sudlow, M. and Thomson, R. (1997). Clinical guidelines: quantity without quality. *Qual. Health Care* 6: 60–61.

Tricoci, P., Allen, J.M., Kramer, J.M. et al. (2009). Scientific evidence underlying the ACC/AHA clinical practice guidelines. *JAMA* 301: 831–841.

Tunis, S.R., Hayward, R.S.A., Wilson, M.C. et al. (1994). Internists' attitudes about clinical practice guidelines. *Ann. Intern. Med.* 120: 957–963.

Utens, C.M.A., Dirksen, C.D., van der Weijden, T. et al. (2016). How to integrate research evidence on patient preferences in healthcare policy decisions: a qualitative study among Dutch stakeholders. *Health Policy* 120: 120–128.

Van der Weijden, T., Boivin, A., Burgers, J. et al. (2012). Clinical practice guidelines and patient decision aids. An inevitable relationship. *J. Clin. Epidemiol.* 65: 584–589.

Van der Weijden, T., Pieterse, A.H., Koelewijn-van Loon, M.S. et al. (2013). How can clinical practice guidelines be adapted to facilitate shared decision making? A qualitative key-informant study. *BMJ Qual. Saf.* 22: 855–863.

Wennekes, L., Hermens, R.P., van Heumen, K. et al. (2008). Possibilities for transborder cooperation in breast cancer care in Europe: a comparative analysis regarding the content, quality and evidence use of breast cancer guidelines. *Breast* 17: 464–471.

van Wersch, A. and Eccles, M. (2001). Involvement of consumers in the development of evidence based clinical guidelines: practical experiences from the North of England evidence based guideline development programme. *Qual. Health Care* 10: 10–16.

Wessels, M., Hielkema, L., and van der Weijden, T. (2016). How to identify existing literature on patients' knowledge, views, and values: the development of a validated search filter. *J. Med. Libr. Assoc.* 104: 320–324.

Westert, G.P. and Faber, M. (2011). Commentary: the Dutch approach to unwarranted medical practice variation. *BMJ* 342: d1429.

Wieringa, S., Dreesens, D., Forland, F. et al. (2018). Different knowledge, different styles of reasoning: a challenge for guideline development. *BMJ Evid. Based Med.* 23: 87–91.

Wollersheim, H., Burgers, J., and Grol, R. (2005). Clinical guidelines to improve patient care. *Neth. J. Med.* 63: 188–192.

Woolf, S.H. (1990). Practice guidelines: a new reality in medicine. I. Recent developments. *Arch. Intern. Med.* 150: 1811–1818.

Woolf, S.H., Grol, R., Hutchinson, A. et al. (1999). Potential benefits, limitations, and harms of clinical guidelines. *BMJ* 318: 527–530.

Worrall, G., Chaulk, P., and Freake, D. (1997). The effects of clinical practice guidelines on patient outcomes in primary care: a systematic review. *CMAJ* 156: 1705–1712.

Zuiderent-Jerak, T., Forland, F., and Macbeth, F. (2012). Guidelines should reflect all knowledge, not just clinical trials. *BMJ* 345: e6702.

Part III

Assessment of Performance

7

Indicators for Quality and Safety of Care

Jozé Braspenning[1], Rosella Hermens[1], Hilly Calsbeek[1], Stephen Campbell[2],
Philip van der Wees[1], and Richard Grol[3,4]

[1] Department IQ healthcare, Radboud Institute for Health Sciences, Radboud University Medical Center, Nijmegen, The Netherlands
[2] School of Health Sciences and NIHR Greater Manchester Patient Safety Translational Research Centre, University of Manchester, Manchester, UK
[3] Radboud University, Nijmegen, The Netherlands
[4] Maastricht University, Maastricht, The Netherlands

SUMMARY

- How to measure performance depends on the purpose of the assessment. Three broad purposes can be distinguished: internal quality measurement; external quality measurement; and research on quality of care and implementation of innovations.
- A rigorous and systematic procedure is needed to develop and test valid and reliable measures, such as quality and safety indicators. The involvement of stakeholders, including patients, is crucial in this procedure.
- Ideally, performance measures involve a low burden for participants and are part of the day-to-day activity of healthcare providers and routine quality improvement and patient safety management.
- Indicators should remain flexible to minimize measure fixation and ossification. Timely rotation and even "retirement" of indicators are therefore required.

7.1 Introduction

Getting insight into the quality and safety of care based on the performance data of healthcare professionals is an initial step to stimulate improvements in healthcare delivery. The objectivity of the data is important, as many healthcare professionals overestimate the quality of their performance (Davis et al. 2006). A description of the actual care delivered is required to identify aspects that need to be improved and to raise awareness and motivation among stakeholders. Performance data can provoke a sense of urgency that stimulates the implementation of

recommended practices or the de-implementation of redundant procedures.

A Cochrane review showed that audit and feedback have mixed effects, which are on average small but potentially important (Ivers et al. 2012; see also Chapter 13). This effect can be enhanced, among many other things, by setting clear goals and providing realistic action plans. Moreover, performance data can be formative in prioritizing the pursued outcomes of improvement programs and their associated objectives of change. Also, it is helpful to know what room for improvement exists before starting and during an implementation

Improving Patient Care: The Implementation of Change in Health Care, Third Edition. Edited by Michel Wensing, Richard Grol, and Jeremy Grimshaw.
© 2020 John Wiley & Sons Ltd. Published 2020 by John Wiley & Sons Ltd.

Box 7.1   Quality Indicators for Head and Neck Cancer Care

Head and neck cancer and its treatment have a significant impact on a patient's well-being. Patients often experience problems with speech, swallowing, and physical disfiguration due to surgery, systemic therapy, radiation, or a combination of these treatments. For optimal results, it is crucial that medical specialists and allied health professionals (AHPs) deliver integrated care throughout the care process. A quality registration was set up to monitor the care process, the Dutch Head and Neck Audit (DHNA). Quality indicators (QIs) were extracted from (inter)national head and neck cancer guidelines, additional literature, and websites for both medical specialists', AHPs' and patients' organizations, and decided on in a systematic RAND-modified Delphi method, including an individual written rating and a face-to-face consensus meeting (Van Overveld et al. 2017). This resulted in 5 outcome indicators (survival, recurrence, complication rate, and patient-reported outcomes and experiences), 13 process indicators on medical specialists' performance (on diagnostics, treatment, and follow-up), 18 process indicators on AHPs' performance (e.g. malnutrition screening), and 3 structure indicators (e.g. availability of case managers). Furthermore, to take account of the context, 10 determinants at patient level (e.g. tumor stage) and 1 at hospital level (number of operations) were selected.

In the first round, QI scores were calculated with data from 1667 curatively treated patients in 8 hospitals. QIs with a sample size of >400 patients were included to calculate reliable QI scores. Table 7.1 shows the results. Current care varied from 29% for

Table 7.1   Clinimetrics of nine indicators for integrated head and neck cancer care from medical and allied health professionals' perspective in eight Dutch centers.

Indicator	Patients, n	Score, %	Range between hospitals, %	Missing data, %	Influencing patient and hospital characteristics
Multidisciplinary team meeting (MTM) takes place before treatment of the patient	877	95.4	88–98	14.1	None
Treatment plan available (if patient discussed in MTM before start of treatment)	836	100	0	18.1	Not applicable
Registration if patient is treated according to protocol	835	97.2	86–99	17.7	Hospital volume
Involvement of dental team before start of radiotherapy	713	83.7	67–100	25.1	Tumor stage
Referral to the hospital (within 7 calendar days)	975	79.6	53–100	4.5	Hospital volume
Finishing diagnostics (= MTM) (within 21 calendar days)	1010	82.6	63–100	1.1	Tumor site Hospital volume
Start first treatment (within 28 calendar days) from first consult	978	48.4	24–78	26.3	None
Malnutrition screening at intake or before start of treatment	619	49.9	2–100	39.4	Tumor stage Performance status
Presence of case manager/nurse practitioner at conversation to discuss treatment plan	1013	28.9%	0–90	0.8	Tumor site

(Continued)

Box 7.1 (Continued)

the indicator on a case manager being present to discuss the treatment plan to 100% for the indicator on the availability of a treatment plan. Variation between hospitals was small for the QI on patients discussed in multidisciplinary team meetings (MTMs; 95%, range 88–98%), but large for the QI on malnutrition screening (50%, range 2–100%). Higher QI scores were associated with lower performance status, advanced tumor stage, and tumor in the oral cavity or oropharynx at the patient level, and with more curatively treated patients at hospital level (hospital volume).

Although the quality registration was only recently launched, it already visualizes hospital variation in current care. Four determinants were found to be influential: tumor stage, performance status, tumor site, and volume. More data are needed to assure stable results for use in quality improvement.

program. *Continuous monitoring* enables responsiveness and adaption of the implementation strategy. Public reporting of indicator scores and reimbursement for performance achievements (pay for performance) can also be seen as extra stimuli for improvement. Finally, valid measures are required to examine the outcomes of implementation strategies.

All these functions depend on valid and reliable information on actual care (see Box 7.1). Thus, measurement is important to determine actual care to identify important gaps in performance, to monitor progression made by improvements, and to assess the outcomes of strategies for improving healthcare. In more detail (see Figure 7.1), it can help:

- To set goals for improvement: when targets are not easily achieved (unrealistically high) or too easily achieved (unrealistically low) they can be adapted.
- To further analyze problems in changing care: when targets are not met a further analysis of the barriers and facilitating factors may be needed to better focus the implementation strategies.
- To alter strategies and measures for change: when targets are not achieved other, potentially more effective, strategies may be selected.
- To alter the implementation plan: not achieving the aims of an implementation

may be caused by failures in the implementation process.
- To determine the effects of strategies for improving healthcare.
- To integrate the change in daily routine: falling back into old habits could mean that the embedding of the new method in existing fixed routines has not yet succeeded and needs attention.

7.1.1 Aim of the Assessment

The approach to measurement of quality and safety of care depends on its purpose. It makes a difference whether the assessment aims to support the internal quality policy of healthcare professionals or is used to provide information to patients. For instance, a hallmark or smiley for children's hospitals to distinguish themselves positively in child-oriented facilities is mostly based on the environment and organization of care, which gives hardly any direction for pediatricians to take clinical action. Furthermore, the bundle of measures (indicators) will mostly vary between a one-off measurement or continuous measurement. In order to properly map out the actual care and monitor the improvement, it is necessary (see Figure 7.1, block 2):

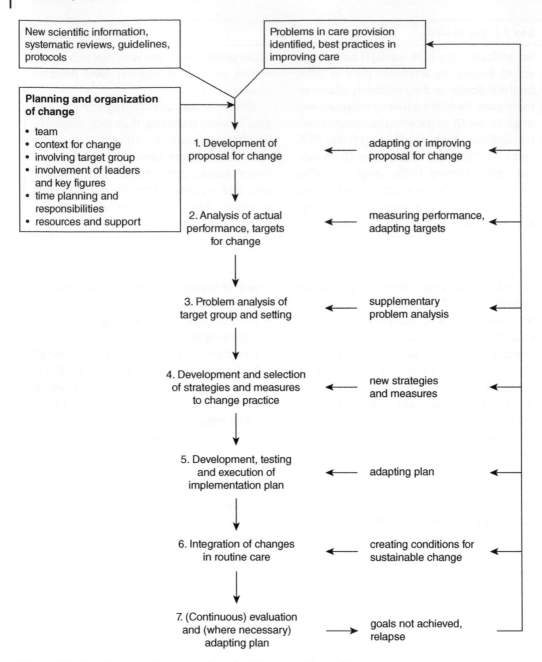

Figure 7.1 The Grol and Wensing implementation of change model.

- To develop or select valid and reliable indicators that express the correspondence between the actual and optimal care; the development and selection of these indicators preferably follows a systematic, careful procedure including a test in real practice.

- To develop clear and acceptable methods for calculating indicator scores, providing feedback that includes meaningful benchmarks.
- To formulate and prioritize specific improvement goals based on the measurements.

In the next few paragraphs these subjects will be discussed, but first we will define the concept of a Quality Indicator (QI) and relate it to the aims of the assessment, the various domains of quality, and the diverse perspectives of the target users as well as the different types of indicators. The chapter will conclude with some examples of the use and effectiveness of indicator sets and a wrap-up in the conclusion.

7.2 Indicators for Quality and Safety of Care

A QI is "a measurable element of practice performance for which there is evidence or consensus that it can be used to assess the quality, and hence change the quality of care provided" (Lawrence and Olesen 1997). As an example, Box 7.2 describes a QI on the influenza vaccination rate that showed that the Dutch influenza vaccination rate of the overall at-risk group decreased significantly in the period 2008–2013, from 71.5 to 59.6% (Tacken et al. 2015).

7.2.1 Aims of Measurement

The elaboration of the indicators is first of all related to the aim of the assessment. Solberg et al. (1997) therefore made a distinction in aims between quality improvement, accountability, and knowledge (see Table 7.2). The restrictions on data collection and how to handle confounders as well as the characteristics of the description (approximate or exact), the type of measurement (structure, process, or outcome indicators), and the time frame (short versus long term) vary between these three

Box 7.2 Quality Indicator on the Influenza Vaccination Rate

This indicator was defined as the number of vaccinated persons in the overall group at risk divided by the number of persons in the overall group at risk, multiplied by 100%. The group at risk was defined as persons of 60 years or older and persons who have certain chronic conditions (e.g. diabetes mellitus, chronic obstructive pulmonary disorder or COPD, some heart conditions). Data collected in general practices in the year 2013 showed an overall score of 59.6% (Tacken et al. 2015).

Table 7.2 Measurement characteristics according to their aim.

Aim	Quality improvement	Accountability	Implementation research
Data collection	Few measures	Very few measures	Many measures
Accuracy of measurement	Approximate	Very exact and valid	Exact and valid
Focus	Healthcare delivery	Patient safety and patient outcomes	Uptake of recommended practices
Time frame	Short term, prospective	Long term, retrospective looking	Long term, both retrospective and prospective
Confounders	Rarely measured	Described or measured and used for adjustments	Measured and used for adjustments
Confidentiality care provider	High	Low	High

Source: Data from Solberg et al. (1997).

Table 7.3 Framework of quality domains.

Safe	Avoiding harm to patients from the care that is intended to help them
Effective	Providing services based on scientific knowledge to all who could benefit and refraining from providing services to those not likely to benefit (avoiding underuse and misuse, respectively)
Patient centered	Providing care that is respectful of and responsive to individual patient preferences, needs, and values and ensuring that patient values guide all clinical decisions
Timely	Reducing waits and sometimes harmful delays for both those who receive and those who give care
Efficient	Avoiding waste, including waste of equipment, supplies, ideas, and energy
Equitable	Providing care that does not vary in quality because of personal characteristics such as gender, ethnicity, geographical location, and socio-economic status

Source: Data from IOM (2001).

types of evaluation and subsequent measurement. As a rule of thumb, 30% of the available budget for quality measurement should, according to Meyer et al. (2012), be spent on accountability and 70% on internal quality improvement.

7.2.2 Domains and Perspectives

Quality of care is an abstract concept, which needs to be operationalized in specific domains and aspects for measurement. The Quality and Outcomes Framework (QOF) in the UK (qof.ic. nhs.uk), for example, makes a distinction between clinical care, organization of care, and patient centeredness. The broadly used framework of the Institute of Medicine (IOM 2001) distinguishes six domains of quality of care. The IOM argued that care should become more (i) safe, (ii) effective, (iii) patient centered, (iv) timely, (v) efficient, and (vi) equitable (see Table 7.3).

Further elaboration of aspects within these domains relies strongly on the perspective of the stakeholder (Markhorst et al. 2012; Martirosyan et al. 2008). Both studies show that the different stakeholders (patients, healthcare providers, payers, inspectorate) varied in their description of these domains and their suggestion of appropriate QIs.

7.2.3 Categories of Indicators

Three categories of indicators are distinguished based on Donabedian's early classification of healthcare: the structure, process, and outcome of care (Donabedian 1980). Structure indicators focus on organizational aspects of service provision, such as the availability of diabetes or asthma clinics, appointment or recall systems, equipment, or the skills of staff. Process indicators focus on the actual care delivered to and negotiated with patients as well as communication with patients. Outcome indicators specify the ultimate goal of the care given and can relate either to health status or to patient evaluations of care (Table 7.4).

Structure indicators are mostly expressed in a number per 1000 patients, or as a numeric variable (yes/no). Process and outcome indicators can be expressed most simply as a numerator and a denominator. The denominator usually describes the target group in absolute numbers and the numerator represents the actual performance within the eligible target group; see for instance the description of the influenza vaccination rate in Box 7.2. By defining an indicator and expressing it with a precise numerator and denominator, the quality of care can be described explicitly as a percentage between 0 and 100. The expression of patient-reported measures is defined by the

Table 7.4 Examples of indicators.

Structure indicators	Number of professionals (full-time equivalents) per 1000 patients Presence of multidisciplinary deliberation for cancer patients
Process indicators	Diagnosis management Referral management Prescription management Vaccination rates
Outcome indicators	Hospital readmission rates Post-operative wound infection rates Patient-reported experience measure (PREM) Patient-reported outcome measure (PROM)

validated questionnaire in use. For instance, the mean and standard deviation for each subject (concept) of the questionnaire may be calculated.

There has been considerable debate about whether the focus in quality assessment should be on processes or outcome measures. There are advantages and disadvantages to measuring each and the choice rests with the aims of the research, assessment, or improvement

process (Eddy 1998; Davies 2005; Bilimoria 2015). Internal quality improvement usually focuses more on process indicators and external quality measurement on outcome indicators.

The use of patient-related outcome measures (PROMs) as an outcome indicator "is part of a shift in thinking about how to measure quality and a general movement towards the idea that the patient, properly queried, is the best source of information about how he or she feels" (Bren 2006). Many available PROMs have their origin in quality-of-life measures such as the Oxford knees score or the generic EQ-5D (Appleby 2012). The use of PROMs as outcome indicators was further stimulated by the movement of value-based healthcare, which tries to balance the cost of care and the value for patients (Porter 2010). Porter speaks of an overarching goal: achieving high value for patients in terms of high health outcomes, which should be reached for the lowest possible cost. In achieving this goal, Porter proposes a hierarchic framework of outcomes. Box 7.3 describes this framework and applies it to quality of care in breast cancer.

Box 7.3 Outcome Hierarchy for Breast Cancer

	Tier	Dimension	Breast cancer
1	Health status achieved or retained	Survival Degree of health or recovery	Survival rate Remission, functional status, breast preservation, breast-conservation surgery outcomes
2	Process of recovery	Time to recovery and time to return to normal activities Disutility of care or treatment process	Time to remission, time to achievement of functional and cosmetic status Nosocomial infection, nausea or vomiting, febrile neutropenia, limitation of motion, breast reconstruction discomfort or complications, depression
3	Sustainability of health	Sustainability of health or recovery and nature of recurrences Long-term consequences of therapy	Cancer recurrence, consequences of recurrence, sustainability of functional status Incidence of second primary cancers, brachial plexopathy, premature osteoporosis

Source: Data from Porter (2010).

Porter argues that measurement of the quality of care should cover at least one outcome at each tier, and ideally one at each level. In this way, trade-offs between different categories of outcomes can be made explicit. According to Porter, the performance measurement systems underlying pay for performance should cover the full care pathway of a patient through the healthcare system. The International Consortium for Health Outcome Measurement (www.ichom.org) aims at establishing international agreement on PROMs in order to facilitate international comparisons.

7.3 Methods to Develop a Set of Indicators

QIs can be developed in systematic or non-systematic ways (Campbell et al. 2002; Mainz 2003; Davies et al. 2011). Non-systematic approaches may be pragmatically applied while looking at available data. Nevertheless, systematic approaches are preferable, as they help to maximize the accuracy and validity of measurement. A systematic approach can be described in five steps: (i) define the aim of the measurement; (ii) select or develop a preliminary set of indicators; (iii) find consensus among target users; (iv) test the indicators empirically; and (v) create a feedback report. Possible aims of measurement (Step 1) were described in Section 7.2. The remaining steps will be elaborated in the subsequent sections.

7.4 Selecting or Developing a Preliminary Set of Indicators

While it is possible, and sometimes necessary, to develop indicators de novo, it is also possible to make use of indicators that are already available. There are many published sets of indicators for a wide variety of clinical problems or aspects of healthcare delivery (see Box 7.4 for examples). An advantage of using existing indicators is that reference data may

---

Box 7.4 Sources of Available Quality Indicators

qualitymeasures.ahrq.gov	USA
rand.org/health/projects/acove	USA
nice.org.uk/aboutnice/qof/indicators.jsp	UK
cihi.ca/en/health-indicators	Canada
health.gov.au	Australia
iqtig.org	Germany
ichom.org	International

---

be available. The disadvantage is that the original purpose of these indicators may not match the current need. For example, searching for prescribing indicators in diabetes care can be done from a safety or effectiveness perspective. A safety indicator might lead to an indicator of care such as "the percentage of type 2 diabetics with hypertension prescribed α blockers in mono-therapy," whereas an example of an indicator on effectiveness related to undertreatment might be "the percentage of type 2 diabetics with a systolic blood pressure over 140 mmHg and prescribed any antihypertensive drug" (Martirosyan et al. 2008). It is also not necessarily appropriate or feasible to use indicators developed in one country in other jurisdictions without testing their validity and relevance first (Marshall et al. 2003; Campbell et al. 2010).

A search of indicators on websites from agencies (Box 7.4) and in the scientific literature can result in a number of indicators that have to be judged on their appropriateness for inclusion based on the precise purpose of the evaluation. Once the goal or intended use of the indicator has been determined, several issues need to be considered (NHS 2008; Pencheon 2008):

- Does the indicator possess the desirable attributes as outlined by the concepts of importance, scientific soundness, and feasibility of an indicator?
- How many indicators will be used?

- What data sources are available? What are the feasibility and expense of collecting additional data?
- What are the possible unintended consequences of data collection and quality measurement?
- Do the indicators apply to the desired setting of care and to the providers who give the care to be assessed?
- Does the indicator belong to a domain of measurement that will produce relevant data?
- Have considerations been made about possible comparisons?

7.4.1 Indicator Attributes

Regarding the first issue, the attributes of indicators, the National Quality Measures Clearinghouse (qualitymeasures.ahrq.gov) provides the following criteria for the concept of importance: (i) relevance to stakeholders; (ii) health importance; (iii) applicability to measuring the equitable distribution of healthcare (for healthcare delivery measures) or of health (for population health measures); (iv) potential for improvement; and (v) susceptibility to being influenced by the healthcare system. We will elaborate on the criteria for scientific soundness and feasibility in Section 7.6.

7.4.2 Number of Indicators

A big issue is how may indicators should be selected. In general, the more indicators available, the better we can describe the quality of care delivered. However, the amount of time spent on data collection as well as the interpretation of a large amount of data ask for a limited set. As we also know that improvement activities should be prioritized to become successful (Chapter 3), the use of small sets of indicators is strongly recommended. Based on the IOM criteria (Table 7.3) and the triple aim domains (process, outcome, experience, cost), Meyer et al. (2012) suggested reviewing

the completeness of a set of QIs along the following topics for hospitals:

- Adverse event rate
- Safe practices implementation
- Healthcare acquired condition rate
- Functional health outcome score
- Hospital 30-day readmission rate
- Evidence-based care score
- Patient experience score
- Care transition measure score
- Health risk status score
- Rate of same-day access
- Hospital days per decedent last six months of life
- Healthcare costs per capita
- Equity: stratify measurement results by relevant subgroups.

7.5 Finding Consensus among Target Users

Whenever possible, indicators should be based directly upon published scientific evidence, such as well-conducted randomized trials (Hearnshaw et al. 2001). The stronger the evidence that specific care processes are linked to patient outcomes, the greater the potential for the indicators to reflect true reductions in morbidity and mortality or improvements in the health status of patients. However, many areas of healthcare have a weak, conflicting, or non-existent evidence base. Therefore, methods for indicator selection have been developed, which combine evidence and expert opinion, using consensus-building techniques (Murphy et al. 1998; Campbell et al. 2002). Because experts often disagree on the interpretation of evidence, systematic methods are needed to assess the level of agreement. Consensus methods include group facilitation techniques designed to quantify the level of consensus among a group of experts by synthesizing and clarifying individual expert opinion, thus pooling individual opinions into a refined aggregated opinion.

Consensus methods can be used to generate topics for indicator development. Consensus methods can also be employed when indicators are available from agencies or scientific literature to create broad agreement among target users. The members of the consensus panels can be health professionals, patients, or policy makers. Since their views on important quality aspects differ, it is necessary to decide beforehand which perspectives should be included in any given evaluation and any given consensus panel. Where views are diverse, separate groups are recommended (Krueger 1988). So consensus methods do not generate new knowledge, but help to interpret and aggregate evidence and opinion.

Consensus techniques are characterized by three aspects: the ratings or judgments of experts are anonymous; they comprise iterative processes with feedback; and individual responses are synthesized and aggregated into a group judgment (Normand et al. 1998). Group judgments are preferred to individual judgments, because they are more consistent and less prone to personal bias or lack of reproducibility. We will describe two of the most commonly used consensus techniques, which may be used separately or in combination (Kötter et al. 2012).

7.5.1 Delphi Technique

The Delphi technique is a structured, interactive method involving the repeated administration of confidential postal or online questionnaires, usually over two or three rounds (Campbell et al. 2002); panels rarely meet face to face. The main stages include:

- Identifying a (research) problem.
- Developing questionnaire statements to rate.
- Selecting appropriate panelists.
- Conducting anonymous iterative postal questionnaire rounds.
- Feeding back results (analyzed statistically, qualitatively, or both) between rounds.
- Summarizing and feeding back the findings.

The absence of any face-to-face meetings prevents panel discussion of potentially different viewpoints, but this remote method is less costly than face-to-face meetings and enables a larger panel of experts from a more geographically diverse population to be involved. The Delphi technique has been used to generate indicators for clinical care and service delivery. For example, to develop indicators on surgical management of irritable bowel disease (Morar et al. 2017), antibiotic use (Monnier et al. 2018), older adults with diabetes and co-morbid conditions (Petrosyan et al. 2018), management of adult potential donor after brain death (Hoste et al. 2018), and maternal health outcomes (Sauvegrain et al. 2019).

7.5.2 RAND/UCLA Appropriateness Method

The Agency for Healthcare Research and Quality (AHRQ, formerly AHCPR) used the RAND/UCLA Appropriateness Method to develop guidelines and QIs. The method has been developed on an ongoing basis and has been used extensively (Brook 1986; Shekelle et al. 1998). This approach combines systematic literature reviews and expert panels. Preliminary indicators are extracted from the literature. In the first round, panelists are sent the literature review and indicator rating forms by post. They are asked to read the review and then rate the indicators according to how necessary they are for high-quality care. The second round involves a face-to-face meeting in which the ratings from the first round are fed back; panel members discuss all the indicators and then re-rate them. Only second-round ratings are used to derive indicators.

The RAND/UCLA method has been used to develop QIs or appropriateness scenarios in primary and secondary care for many conditions, for example asthma (To et al. 2010), cardiology (Shekelle 2009), and safe prescribing (Avery et al. 2011). In contrast to the Delphi technique, the RAND/UCLA method is focused on combining scientific evidence, summarized in a review document, with the collective judgment of experts by deriving a consensus opinion from a group with individual opinions aggregated into a refined aggregated opinion following face-to-face discussions. There has been criticism of the definition of appropriate care used in this method and the lack of user/patient involvement (Hicks 1994; Ayanian et al. 1998). While the reliability of the rating procedure is weak, it has higher reliability than many widely accepted clinical procedures (e.g. reading of mammograms). The reliability of the method increases when using a higher cut-off point for determining consensus within a panel (e.g. an overall panel median rating of 8 out of 9; see Shekelle et al. 1996, 1998). While there are practical reasons for restricting the number of panelists to about 12, a review of studies using consensus methods suggested that including more participants seldomly changed the overall ratings (Murphy et al. 1998). Table 7.5 summarizes the key determinants of the quality of indicators, and Box 7.5 presents methods used in consensus panels.

Box 7.5   Consensus Panels to Develop Indicator Sets: Members, Procedure, and Decision Rules

A balanced group of panel members (experts, stakeholders) is invited. The selection of panel members depends on the purpose of the QIs (e.g. internal quality improvement or consumer's choice information). An expert can be a caregiver or a patient, but also someone who has contributed to the development of guidelines or relevant publications. The content validity of the indicators depends on the expertise of the panel members. Input from stakeholders also creates support among the future users of the quality information. The number of participants that will be approached for participation in the consensus process is approximately 15 people, of which often two-thirds will actually join the face-to-face meetings. The minimum number for a consensus procedure is 7 (Fitch et al. 2003), although no justification for this figure has been given.

Most indicator development procedures take at least two rounds. In the first round a draft of the indicators is evaluated by the panel, mostly by written methods. Suggestions can be given for new indicators. The second round is focused on the discussion points (more easily face to face) and the development of new or modified indicators. The evaluation of draft indicators requires clear criteria such as the indicator's relevance for patients health benefits or care efficiency. The judgment is mostly given on a 9-point rating scale. A common decision rule is that an indicator is selected for the second round in case of a median score of 7 or higher, unless there is disagreement (at least 30% of the scores in both the lowest tertile – score 1, 2, or 3 – and in the highest tertile – score 7, 8, or 9). Indicators with a median score of 1–3 or 4–6, respectively, are not selected or introduced in the second round for discussion (Campbell et al. 2000). If a strong selection is needed due to applicability, panelists can be asked to make a top 5 as well (Hermens et al. 2006).

There is a range of consensus methods for developing indicators systematically: evidence based, evidence combined with consensus, and guideline based (Campbell et al. 2002; Mainz 2003). The approach chosen should be appropriate to the topic and the panel. Irrespective of the method used, the result will largely depend on the panel's composition.

Table 7.5 Possible factors influencing the quality of indicators.

Subjects	Factors influencing the result
Indicator definition	Available evidence, precision of indicator wording
Panel members	Knowledge, coherence of panel view, dominant individuals, focusing on different aspects of quality, number of panel members
Rating procedure	Rating scale, selection criteria, possibility of adding free-text information
Consensus procedure	Method of feedback, cut-off point, face-to-face meeting or postal survey

7.6 Testing the Indicators Empirically

QI data can be gathered by using routinely available data sources or, if necessary, by developing new information systems. The feasibility of the data-collection method contributes to the reliability of the data collection. Considering feasibility, routine data to test the indicators and assess the quality of care are preferred, particularly data from electronic medical records. These case-based information systems based on clinical performance (including diagnostics, medication prescription, referrals, etc.) are increasingly being used for quality information. While such information offers much promise for accurate data collection, some caveats require consideration (Powell et al. 2003). Quality measurement needs accurate, complete, and consistent information systems. However, it is unusual that all aspects of clinical performance needed for the test are registered in the electronic medical record, and the available data are not always valid and reliable. One of the reasons is that they have been collected for a different goal. Thus, routinely collected data are often available, but their value can be constrained because they may be inconsistent, incomplete, and unreliable, both at micro (electronic medical records) and at macro levels (health insurance claims data; Pawson et al. 2007).

The data in these systems can combine different data-collection methods, such as prospective recording questionnaires, interviews, and/or observations, for example by using cameras. A combination of both routinely collected and other data is possible as well. Patient report questionnaires, for instance, may be most feasible, if they are integrated into routine healthcare delivery and in patient records. To assess the most convenient data collection method, both validity and feasibility have to be considered. Feasible methods (e.g. sampling of patients in a waiting room) may not be valid and vice versa (e.g. linkage of patient survey data to patient records).

Quality measures need to be valid and reliable, as well as acceptable and feasible. These attributes are facilitated by a clear definition and purpose, and can be tested by evaluating the psycho- or clinimetric properties of indicators and assessing their feasibility in daily practice. As such, quality measures should be subjected to a testing protocol, and be piloted, before being used in practice in order to evaluate if they meet key attributes of good quality measures.

7.6.1 Validity and Reliability

The validity of QIs is usually described in terms of content and construct validity. The content validity of an indicator is strongly related to the method for developing QIs. The more the indicator is grounded within evidence-based data on best practice, the stronger the content validity. In addition, consensus among relevant stakeholders can contribute to the content validity. Construct validity can be established by relating the measurement to the actual quality of healthcare. The measurement should be able to discriminate between different aspects of quality and different target groups with different levels of quality. Furthermore, construct validity can be supported by confirmation of expected associations with other measures and expected differences between individuals and organizations.

The reliability expresses the extent to which measurement results are a true reflection of the variables that have to be measured; it reflects the error, both random and systematic, inherent in any measurement (Streiner and Norman 1995). Inclusion of sufficient cases is important for the reliability of the measurement, as is taking into account specific patient characteristics when comparing performance measures of hospitals or primary care practices (see Box 7.6). In quality measurement, the focus is usually on the reliability of estimates at the level of healthcare providers or other aggregates. To examine the influence of random factors, the reliability can be expressed, for example, by a test–retest procedure. There are also issues of technical reliability, when data are extracted from (electronically) medical records, such as the accuracy and completeness of the medical records. Piloting enables data extraction to be tested and for any errors to be identified and rectified (Campbell et al. 2011).

Furthermore, a QI should be sensitive to changes in the quality of care, because the purpose of measurement is quality improvement and therefore it should be able to capture changes in behavior or setting. Longitudinal analyses can be used to learn more about the sensitivity for change of indicators, if they can be related to an obvious event (e.g. the start of a quality improvement program). Obtaining baseline data and data at the end of a specific pilot period will enable tracking of performance (Campbell et al. 2011).

Box 7.6 Development and Measurement of Indicators for Patients with Non-Hodgkin Lymphoma

Care providers often argue that complex patients defined in terms of poor health status, co-morbidities, old age, or refusing recommended care may account for suboptimal guideline adherence. To test this for non-Hodgkin lymphoma (NHL), a study was performed with a set of guideline-based QIs aimed at measuring important processes and structures in current NHL care and at examining the need for improvement, considering relevant arguments for non-adherence. The measurement was done in a random sample of patients with NHL (N = 431) diagnosed in 2006–2007 in 22 hospitals in the Netherlands, with data derived from medical records. Multilevel logistic regression analyses were used to estimate the relationship between indicator scores and complexity characteristics such as co-morbidity index (combined with age), disease stage, patients' own choices, and lymphoma type. Of the 20 indicators developed, 16 had improvement potential (score less than 90%). Half of these indicator scores were affected by the complexity characteristics. Table 7.6 describes five indicators with a particularly low score. The difference in indicator scores over 20 different indicators between the complex and less complex groups were not very large. The authors would therefore prefer a simple comparison between hospitals, unless a hospital definitely sees substantially larger numbers of more or less complex patients.

(Continued)

Box 7.6 (Continued)

Table 7.6 Adherence to quality indicators for non-Hodgkin lymphoma (NHL) care in 22 Dutch hospitals among 431 patients.

	Adherence		
Quality indicator	Total group	Complex group	Less complex group
• Staging techniques include computed tomography (CT) scans of neck, thorax, and abdomen; bone marrow aspirate; and bone biopsy	23%	15%	30%
• Assessment of International Prognostic Index for patients with aggressive NHL	21%	15%	25%
• Re-evaluation after chemotherapy with CT scans (or positron emission tomography); bone marrow aspirate; and bone biopsy (in stage IV cases)	37%	21%	44%
• Pathology report in which five items were reported (documentation of origin of tissue, tissue characteristics, biopsy method, receipt of material, whether tissue was frozen)	11%	n.a.	n.a.
• Patients discussed in multidisciplinary consultations	21%	n.a.	n.a.

n.a. = complexity characteristics did not contribute significantly to the indicator score.
Source: Wennekes et al. (2011).

Finally, risk adjustment of scores on QIs needs to be considered. In general, random variation should be accounted for to avoid overinterpretation in rankability (Van Dishoeck et al. 2011). Factors that are eligible for risk adjustment or case-mix correction are demographic characteristics of patients (age, gender, socio-economic status) or related to the disease itself, such as complications or co-morbidity. Which factors need to be considered varies across indicators. A systematic review of the correction factors needed for selected indicators of diabetes care – HBa1c, blood pressure, and cholesterol levels – showed that only body mass index (BMI) and marital status/housing situation influenced these indicators (Calsbeek et al. 2016).

Risk adjustment is commonly applied in the calculation of mortality rates, for instance in the Hospital Standardized Mortality Ratio (HSMR; Jarman et al. 2010). In this approach, the expected mortality rate based on the population under study is related to the actual mortality rate. However, applying risk adjustment on QIs can mask variation in the quality of care (Mant and Hicks 1995) or lead to the wrong conclusions (Nicoll 2007). Iezzoni (2003) warns about methodological restrictions and encourages proper use. Mortality figures based on administrative data and generic risk models can be useful for longitudinal monitoring, but not for comparison of healthcare providers. According to Iezzoni, four questions should be answered: (i) risk of what outcome, (ii) over what time frame, (iii) for what population, and (iv) for what purpose. For instance, it may be desirable not to correct for risk adjustment when the aim is to improve quality of care. Suppose we are running a screening program on colon cancer, and data show that the uptake rate is lower for people in urbanized areas. From a population point of view, the uptake rate should be adjusted for the urbanization level in comparisons of the performance of different screening organizations. However, for a single screening organization in an urbanized area, this adjustment would mean that they feel no urgency to improve, because insight on their low uptake rate is lacking due to correction.

7.7 Create a Feedback Report

7.7.1 Calculating Indicators and Benchmarks

To interpret the collected data and to find aspects of care in need of improvement, indicator scores are usually calculated as an aggregated average score (means or medians). In addition, benchmarks or reference figures may be defined (e.g. the scores of the best-performing care providers). If scores on QIs are compared between healthcare providers or organizations, rankings can be based on the indicator scores. In this comparison a *relative standard* is defined with regard to the quality of care delivered. The highest scores (e.g. scores from the highest quartile) function as a benchmark for others. Based on such a ranking, a healthcare provider or organization can decide to start an improvement aiming to reach the upper quartile (the best 25%) in the next measurement. The idea is that the recipients of the feedback become aware of the fact that high scores can be reached in daily practice, because others succeed as well. Studies suggested that defining *best practices* and giving feedback can achieve more improvement than a comparison with a mean or minimal norm (Edgman-Levitan et al. 2003).

It is also possible to define an *absolute standard* or target for each QI; that is, the score to be met for a positive evaluation. For instance, in the English QOF for primary care practices, each QI is accompanied by an absolute standard. The extent to which general practices adhere to this standard indicates the quality of care delivered and determines the financial incentive received. For example, 80% of diabetes patients must have blood pressure lower than or equal to a specified target. Defining such performance standards is complex. A systematic approach is the Angoff procedure (Angoff 1971). This method originates from education, but can be applied to performance standards in healthcare as well (Jelovsek et al. 2010).

Graphs can be supportive in wrapping up the quality information. Most common representations are pie charts or bar, dot, or line graphs. Little scientific evidence is available, however, on differences in their effect on understanding the information by decision makers in healthcare, although there is a body of research outside healthcare. Assada et al. (2017) argued that dot charts are easier to decode than bar charts. A quality register on integrated head and neck cancer care studied the preferences in feedback reports for three different target groups: patients, healthcare professionals, and health insurers (Van Overveld et al. 2017). They concluded that all stakeholders got along well with bar charts, but patients preferred pie charts for PROMs and patient-reported experience measures (PREMs), and medical specialists Kaplan–Meier survival curves.

7.7.2 Formulating Aims of Improvement

After measuring indicators in actual practice and before formulating concrete goals for change, the calculated indicators should be presented to the caregivers as feedback, whether or not accompanied by benchmarks. The purpose of feedback is to allow professionals to make choices concerning necessary changes and encourage active participation in a process of change. Sometimes it is difficult to interpret the indicator scores, particularly

---

Box 7.7   SMART Goals for Change

- *Specific*: the improvement activities are described in concrete and unambiguous terms. It has to be clear who is involved, what must be achieved exactly, where it has to take place, which conditions are necessary, which barriers will be encountered, and which profit is yield by reaching the goal.
- *Measurable*: the progress of the activities will be measured in order to direct the care providers in the right direction and to motivate them to continue.
- *Acceptable*: enough support for the activities will be created. This is particularly important for consolidation of the improvement. Attitudes, capacities, skills, and resources do not impede the execution of the plans.
- *Realistic*: the planned activities are feasible. The care providers want it, are able to do it, and think that they can achieve the goals.
- *Time restricted*: the improvement plan describes clearly who does what at which moment, what are the measurement moments, and within which period are the goals reached.

---

when indicators consist of different items. Written explanations can support understanding and interpretation. Generally, when the complexity of indicators decreases, the applicability increases.

Preferably, feedback is given soon after the performed behavior (Bradley et al. 2004). The use of QIs is most effective when they are integrated into a system of continuous monitoring and a cycle of measuring–checking–improving–evaluating. Chapter 13 includes more information on the best way to present feedback, in order to be effective and usable for implementation of new procedures.

Insight into actual performance does not automatically lead to improvement. When different targets for improvement arise, prioritization is necessary to increase the chances of success. To formulate concrete goals for change, the SMART methodology can be used (see Box 7.7).

7.8   Use and Effect of Quality Indicators

Quality measures are widely used now to measure the quality of healthcare. They are developed as part of accreditation programs, for public reporting, for improvement programs, or for patient evaluations, but more and more the indicators are applied as part of a payment scheme. In reviews on pay for performance it was concluded that the effect on performance is overall inconclusive (van Herck et al. 2010; Scott et al. 2011). Other researchers have concluded that pay for performance creates short-term improvement (Petersen et al. 2006; Sutherland et al. 2008). Campbell et al. (2009) corroborated this conclusion with their analyses of the impact of the QOF on quality of clinical care in the UK (Box 7.8). Indicators should not be used in isolation within a single quality assessment/improvement scheme. Research suggests that indicators used as part of, for example, pay for performance (Sutherland et al. 2008), feedback on the basis of patient surveys (Vingerhoets et al. 2001), and accreditation on the basis of measured organizational performance (Goetz et al. 2012) show evidence of small and often short-term gains. Indicators should be used therefore within multiple strategies incorporating external assessment and intrinsic quality improvement (Grol et al. 2004).

7.8.1   Unintended Effects

Unintended effects of publishing performance data and pay for performance need to be

---

Box 7.8   Results of the Quality and Outcomes Framework

Indicators used within pay for performance tend to show high levels of performance (Rosenthal et al. 2006; Doran et al. 2008). For example, the QOF in the UK has led to improvements in quality standards and patient outcomes in a number of incentivized conditions. Campbell et al. (2009) demonstrated that accelerated quality improvement, over and above underlying trends in existing improvement, were evident for clinical care for diabetes and asthma in the short term after the introduction of the QOF in 2003, but that there was no additional change in the quality of heart disease. However, there is also evidence that performance dips once the incentives are taken away (Lester et al. 2010).

---

considered as well. Smith identifies eight unintended consequences of publishing performance data, including measure fixation, tunnel vision, misinterpretation, and gaming (Smith 1995). There is some evidence that health practitioners prioritize targets attached to indicators over personalized care and listening to patients' concerns (Maisey et al. 2008; Lester et al. 2011). This is due to "measure fixation," where a focus on isolated incentivized aspects of care conflicts with patient-centered care (Lester et al. 2011) or result in less attention to non-incentivized clinical areas (Doran et al. 2011).

In general, using patient data to improve patient care can be regarded as a logical procedure in quality of care management. Ivers et al. (2012) did indeed show the impact of audit and feedback, although the outcomes are mixed (see Chapter 13). However, some systematic reviews also show inconclusive results. For instance, a review on polypharmacy in the elderly concluded that it is yet unclear if reviewing patients' prescriptions improved appropriate prescribing, although it probably has potential in reducing prescribing omissions (Rankin et al. 2018). A Cochrane review of 12 relevant studies on the effect of publicly releasing healthcare data presented some evidence that public release of performance data has little impact on the behavior of disadvantaged populations. No (adverse) effect was seen on healthcare utilization decisions by purchasers (Metcalfe et al. 2018). The specific conditions under which the data are presented (feedback), as well as guidance in the improvement (prioritizing and accomplishment), seem crucial for the impact of QIs.

7.9   Conclusion

A key question in measuring the quality of care concerns the purpose of the evaluation: Is it aimed at quality improvement, at (public) accountability, or at scientific development on effective innovations or implementation strategies? The exact measurement approach undertaken should be in line with the aim. Indicators of quality of care are widely used in quality improvement and patient safety management, focusing on the structure, process, or outcome of healthcare. We prefer a measurement system with a mix of structure, process, and outcome indicators to create a more balanced picture of the quality of care provided. In assessing the quality of care in an appropriate way, this chapter conveyed several messages. First, indicators should be tested for their validity, reliability, acceptability, unintended consequences, feasibility, sensitivity to change, and how communicable or understandable they are. Second, indicators should not be used in isolation, but as part of multiple quality improvement initiatives. Third, indicators should be flexible to minimize measure fixation and ossification. Fourth, and most important, patients play a crucial role in measuring quality. Evaluation and measurement of quality are complex and require a mixture of internal and external, subjective and objective approaches (Greenhalgh and Heath 2010a,b). Fifth, QIs should not become paper tigers, but be an instrument to help healthcare providers in continuous improvement efforts. Finally, QIs should not be seen as the ultimate method to improve the quality and safety of healthcare.

References

Angoff, W.A. (1971). *Educational Measurement*. Washington, DC: American Council on Education.

Appleby, J. (2012). Patient reported outcome measures: how are we feeling today? *BMJ* 344: d8191.

Assada, Y., Abel, H., Skedgel, C., and Warner, G. (2017). On effective graphic communication of health inequality: considerations for health policy researchers. *Milbank Q.* 95: 801–835.

Avery, A.J., Dex, G., Mulvaney, G. et al. (2011). Development of prescribing safety indicators for general practitioners using RAND appropriateness method. *Br. J. Gen. Pract.* 61: e526–e536.

Ayanian, J.Z., Landrum, M.B., Normand, S.L.T. et al. (1998). Rating the appropriateness of coronary angiography – do practicing physicians agree with an expert panel and with each other? *N. Engl. J. Med.* 338: 1896–1904.

Bilimoria, K.Y. (2015). Facilitating quality improvement. Pushing the pendulum back toward process measures. *JAMA* 314: 1333–1334.

Bradley, E.H., Holmboe, E.S., Mattera, J.A. et al. (2004). Data feedback efforts in quality improvement: lessons learned from US hospitals. *Qual. Saf. Health Care* 13: 26–31.

Bren, L. (2006). The importance of patient-reported outcomes... it's all about the patients. *FDA Consum* 40: 26–32.

Brook, R.H. (1986). *The RAND/UCLA appropriateness method*. In: *Methodology Perspectives*. AHCPR Pub No 95-009 (eds. M.C. KA, S.R. Moore and R.A. Siegel), 59–70. Rockville, MD: Public Health Service, US Department of Health and Human Services.

Calsbeek, H., Markhorst, J., Voerman, G.E., and Braspenning, J. (2016). Case-mix adjustment of quality indicators for diabetes mellitus: a systematic review of risk factors and their importance. *Am. J. Manag. Care* 22: e45–e52.

Campbell, S.M., Braspenning, J., Hutchinson, A., and Marshall, M. (2002). Research methods used in developing and applying quality indicators in primary care. *Qual. Saf. Health Care* 11: 358–364.

Campbell, S.M., Cantrill, J.A., and Richards, D. (2000). Prescribing indicators for UK general practice: Delphi consultation study. *BMJ* 321: 1–5.

Campbell, S.M., Kontopantelis, E., Hannon, K. et al. (2011). Framework and indicator testing protocol for developing and piloting quality indicators for the UK Quality and Outcomes Framework. *BMC Fam. Pract.* 12: 85.

Campbell, S.M., Reeves, D., Kontopantelis, E. et al. (2009). Effects of pay-for-performance on quality of primary care in England. *N. Engl. J. Med.* 361: 368–378.

Campbell, S.M., Scott, A., Parker, R. et al. (2010). Implementing pay-for-performance in Australian primary care: lessons from the United Kingdom and the United States. *Med. J. Aust.* 193: 408–411.

Davies, H. (2005). *Measuring and Reporting the Quality of Health Care: Issues and Evidence from the International Research Literature*. Edinburgh: NHS Quality Improvement Scotland.

Davies, S., Romano, P.S., Schmidt, E.M. et al. (2011). Assessment of a novel hybrid Delphi and nominal groups technique to evaluate quality indicators. *Health Serv. Res.* 46: 2005–2018.

Davis, D.A., Mazmanian, P.E., Fordis, M. et al. (2006). Accuracy of physician self-assessment compared with observed measures of competence: a systematic review. *JAMA* 296: 1094–1102.

Donabedian, A. (1980). *Explorations in Quality Assessment and Monitoring. Volume 1: The Definition of Quality and Approaches to Its Assessment.* Ann Arbor, MI: Health Administration Press.

Doran, T., Fullwood, C., Kontopantelis, E., and Reeves, D. (2008). Effect of financial incentives on inequalities in the delivery of primary clinical care in England: analysis of clinical activity indicators for the quality and outcomes framework. *Lancet* 372: 728–736.

Doran, T., Kontopantelis, E., Valderas, J.M. et al. (2011). Effect of financial incentives on incentivised and non-incentivised clinical activities: longitudinal analysis of data from the UK Quality and Outcomes Framework. *BMJ* 342: d3590.

Eddy, D.M. (1998). Performance measurement: problems and solutions. *Health Aff.* 17: 7–26.

Edgman-Levitan, S., Dale Shaller, P.A., McInnes, K. et al. (2003). *The CAPHS® Improvement Guide Practical Strategies for Improving the Patient Care Experience.* Boston, MA: Department of Health Care Policy, Harvard Medical School.

Fitch, K., Bernstein, S.J., Aguilar, M. et al. (2003). *The RAND/UCLA Appropriateness Method User's Manual.* Santa Monica, CA: RAND Distribution Services.

Goetz, K., Campbell, S.M., Rosemann, T. et al. (2012). Importance of social support for patients with type 2 diabetes – a qualitative study with general practitioners, practice nurses and patients. *Scand. J. Caring Sci.* 9: Doc02.

Greenhalgh, T. and Heath, I. (2010a). Measuring quality in the therapeutic relationship – part 1: objective approaches. *Qual. Saf. Health Care* 19: 475–478.

Greenhalgh, T. and Heath, I. (2010b). Measuring quality in the therapeutic relationship – part 2: subjective approaches. *Qual. Saf. Health Care* 19: 479–483.

Grol, R., Marshall, M., and Campbell, S. (2004). *Quality assessment and improvement in primary care.* In: *Quality Management in Primary Care. European Practice Assessment* (eds. R. Grol, M. Dautzenberg and H. Brinkmann), 9–19. Gütersloh: Bertellsmann Stiftung.

Hearnshaw, H.M., Harker, R.M., Cheater, F.M. et al. (2001). Expert consensus on the desirable characteristics of review criteria for improvement of health quality. *Qual. Health Care* 10: 173–178.

Hermens, R.P.M.G., Ouwens, M.M.T.J., Vonk-Okhuijsen, S.Y. et al. (2006). Development of quality indicators for diagnosis and treatment of patients with non-small cell lung cancer: a first step toward implementing a multidisciplinary evidence-based guideline. *Lung Cancer* 54: 117–124.

Hicks, N.R. (1994). Some observations on attempts to measure appropriateness of care. *BMJ* 309: 730–733.

Hoste, P., Hoste, E., Ferdinande, P. et al. (2018). Development of key interventions and quality indicators for the management of an adult potential donor after brain death: a RAND modified Delphi approach. *BMC Health Serv. Res.* 18: 580.

Iezzoni, L.I. (2003). *Risk Adjustment for Measuring Health Care Outcomes.* Ann Arbor, MI: AcademyHealth/HAP.

Institute of Medicine (2001). *Crossing the Quality Chasm: A New Health System for the 21st Century.* Washington, DC: Institute of Medicine.

Ivers, N., Jamtvedt, G., Flottorp, S. et al. (2012). Audit and feedback: effects on professional practice and healthcare outcomes. *Cochrane Database Syst. Rev.* (6): CD000259. https://doi.org/10.1002/14651858.CD000259.pub3.

Jarman, B., Pieter, D., van der Veen, A.A. et al. (2010). The hospital standardised mortality ratio: a powerful tool for Dutch hospitals to assess their quality of care? *Qual. Saf. Health Care* 19: 9–13.

Jelovsek, J.E., Walters, M.D., Korn, A. et al. (2010). Establishing cutoff scores on assessments of surgical skills to determine surgical competence. *Am. J. Obstet. Gynecol.* 203: e1–e6.

Kötter, T., Blozik, E., and Scherer, M. (2012). Methods for the guideline-based development of quality indicators – a systematic review. *Implement. Sci.* 7: 21.

Krueger, R.A. (1988). *Focus Groups: A Practical Guide for Applied Research*. Thousand Oaks, CA: Sage.

Lawrence, M. and Olesen, F. (1997). Indicators of quality in health care. *Eur. J. Gen. Pract.* 3: 103–108.

Lester, H., Hannon, K., and Campbell, S. (2011). Identifying unintended consequences of quality indicators: a qualitative study. *BMJ Qual. Saf.* 20: 1057–1061.

Lester, H., Schmittdiel, S., Selby, J. et al. (2010). The impact of removing financially incentivised indicators on physician performance: longitudinal time series. *BMJ* 340: c1898.

Mainz, J. (2003). Developing evidence-based clinical indicators: a state of the art methods primer. *Int. J. Qual. Health Care* 15: i5–i11.

Maisey, S., Steel, N., Marsh, R. et al. (2008). Effects of payment for performance in primary care: qualitative interview study. *J. Health Serv. Res. Policy* 13: 133–139.

Mant, J. and Hicks, N. (1995). Detecting differences in quality of care: the sensitivity of measures of process and outcome in treating acute myocardial infarction. *BMJ* 311: 793–796.

Markhorst, J., Martirosyan, L., Calsbeek, H., and Braspenning, J. (2012). Different stakeholder preferences for public quality information on diabetes care: a qualitative study. *Qual. Prim. Care* 20: 253–261.

Marshall, M.N., Shekelle, P.G., McGlynn, E.A. et al. (2003). Can health care quality indicators be transferred between countries? *Qual. Saf. Health Care* 12: 8–12.

Martirosyan, L., Braspenning, J., Denig, P. et al. (2008). Prescribing quality indicators of type 2 diabetes mellitus ambulatory care. *Qual. Saf. Health Care* 17: 318–323.

Metcalfe, D., Rios Diaz, A.J., and Olufajo, O.A. (2018). Impact of public release of performance data on the behaviour of healthcare consumers and providers. *Cochrane Database Syst. Rev.* (9): CD004538. https://doi.org/10.1002/14651858. CD004538.pub3.

Meyer, G.S., Nelson, E.C., Pryor, D.B. et al. (2012). More quality measures versus measuring what matters: a call for balance and parsimony. *BMJ Qual. Saf.* 21: 964–968.

Monnier, A., Schouten, J., Le Maréchal, M. et al. (2018). Quality indicators for responsible antibiotic use in the inpatient setting: a systematic review followed by an international multidisciplinary consensus procedure. *J. Antimicrob. Chemother.* 73: vi30–vi39.

Morar, P.S., Hollingshead, J., Bemelman, W. et al. (2017). Establishing key performance indicators (KPIs) and their importance for the surgical management of inflammatory bowel disease—results from a pan-European, Delphi consensus study. *J. Crohns Colitis* 10: 1362–1368.

Murphy, M.K., Black, N.A., Lamping, D.L. et al. (1998). Consensus development methods and their use in clinical guideline development. *Health Technol. Assess.* 2 (i-iv): 1–88.

NHS Institute for Innovation and Improvement (2008). *Guidelines for Selecting and Using Indicators*. Coventry: NHS Institute for Innovation and Improvement.

Nicoll, J. (2007). Case-mix adjustment in non-randomised observational evaluations: the constant risk fallacy. *J. Epidemiol. Community Health* 61: 1010–1013.

Normand, S.-L.T., McNeil, B.J., Peterson, L.E. et al. (1998). Eliciting expert opinion using Delphi technique: identifying performance indicators for cardiovascular disease. *Int. J. Qual. Health Care* 10: 247–260.

Pawson, L.G., Scholle, S.H., and Powers, A. (2007). Comparison of administrative-only versus administrative plus chart review data for reporting HEDIS hybrid measures. *Am. J. Manag. Care* 3: 553–558.

Pencheon, D. (2008). *The Good Indicators Guide: Understanding How to Use and Choose Indicators*. Coventry: NHS Institute for Innovation and Improvement.

Petersen, L.A., Woodward, L.D., Urech, T. et al. (2006). Does pay-for-performance improve the quality of health care? *Ann. Intern. Med.* 145: 265–272.

Petrosyan, Y., Barnsley, J.M., Kuluski, K. et al. (2018). Quality indicators for ambulatory care for older adults with diabetes and comorbid conditions: a Delphi study. *PLoS One* 13: e0208888.

Porter, M.E. (2010). What is value in health care? *N. Engl. J. Med.* 363: 2477–2481.

Powell, A.E., Davies, H.T.O., and Thomson, R.G. (2003). Using routine comparative data to assess the quality of health care: understanding and avoiding common pitfalls. *Qual. Saf. Health Care* 12: 122–128.

Rankin, A., Cadogan, C.A., Patterson, S.M. et al. (2018). Interventions to improve the appropriate use of polypharmacy for older people. *Cochrane Database Syst. Rev.* 9: CD008165. https://doi.org/10.1002/14651858. CD008165.pub4.

Rosenthal, M.B., Landon, B.E., Normand, S.L. et al. (2006). Pay for performance in commercial HMOs. *N. Engl. J. Med.* 355: 1895–1902.

Sauvegrain, P., Chantry, A.A., Chies-Dubrille, C. et al. (2019). Monitoring quality of obstetric care from hospital discharge databases: a Delphi survey to propose a new set of indicators based on maternal health outcomes. *PLoS One* 14: e0211955.

Scott, A., Sivey, P., Ait Ouakrim, D. et al. (2011). The effect of financial incentives on the quality of health care provided by primary care physicians. *Cochrane Database Syst. Rev.* (9): CD008451. https://doi.org/10.1002/14651858. CD008451.pub2.

Shekelle, P.G., Kahan, J.P., Bernstein, S.J. et al. (1998). The reproducibility of a method to identify the overuse and underuse of procedures. *N. Engl. J. Med.* 338: 1888–1895.

Shekelle, P.G., Kahan, J.P., Park, R.E. et al. (1996). Assessing appropriateness by expert panels: how reliable? *J. Gen. Intern. Med.* 10: 81.

Shekelle, P.G., MacLean, C.H., Morton, S.C., and Wenger, N.S. (2001). Assessing care of vulnerable elders: methods for developing quality indicators. *Ann. Intern. Med.* 135: 647–652.

Smith, P. (1995). On the unintended consequences of publishing performance data in the public sector. *Int. J. Public Adm.* 18: 277–231.

Solberg, L.I., Moser, G., and McDonald, S. (1997). The three faces of performance measurement: improvement, accountability and research. *Jt. Comm. J. Qual. Improv.* 23: 135–147.

Streiner, D.L. and Norman, G.R. (1995). *Health Measurement Scales: A Practical Guide to Their Development and Use*. Oxford: Oxford Medical Publications.

Sutherland, K., Christianson, J.B., and Leatherman, S. (2008). Impact of targeted financial incentives on personal health behavior: a review of the literature. *Med. Care Res. Rev.* 65: S36–S78.

Tacken, M., Jansen, B., Mulder, J. et al. (2015). Dutch influenza vaccination rate drops for fifth consecutive year. *Vaccine* 33: 4886–4891.

To, T., Guttmann, A., Lougheed, M.D. et al. (2010). Evidence-based performance indicators of primary care for asthma: a modified RAND appropriateness method. *Int. J. Qual. Health Care* 22: 476–485.

Van Dishoeck, A.-M., Linsma, H.F., Mackenbach, J.P., and Steyerberg, E.W. (2011). Random variation and rankability of hospitals using outcome indicators. *BMJ Qual. Saf.* 20: 869.

Van Herck, P., De Smedt, S.D., Annemans, L. et al. (2010). Systematic review: effects, design choices, and context of pay-for performance in health care. *BMC Health Serv. Res.* 10: 247.

Van Overveld, L.F.J., Takes, R.P., Vijn, T.W. et al. (2017). Feedback preferences of patients, professionals and health insurers in integrated head and neck cancer care. *Health Expect.* 20: 1275–1288.

Vingerhoets, E., Wensing, M., and Grol, R. (2001). Feedback of patients' evaluations of general practice care: a randomised trial. *Qual. Health Care* 10: 224–228.

Wennekes, L., Ottevanger, P.B., Raemaekers, J.M. et al. (2011). Development and measurement of guideline-based indicators for patients with non-Hodgkin lymphoma. *J. Clin. Oncol.* 29: 1436–1444.

Part IV

Problem Analysis

8

Determinants of Implementation

Michel Wensing[1,2,3] and Richard Grol[4,5]

[1] *Faculty of Medicine, University of Heidelberg, Heidelberg, Germany*
[2] *Department of General Practice and Health Services Research, Heidelberg University Hospital, Heidelberg, Germany*
[3] *Department IQ healthcare, Radboud Institute for Health Sciences, Radboud University Medical Center, Nijmegen, The Netherlands*
[4] *Radboud University, Nijmegen, The Netherlands*
[5] *Maastricht University, Maastricht, The Netherlands*

SUMMARY

- A wide range of factors can influence the implementation of innovations in healthcare practice. These factors can strengthen or weaken the impact of implementation strategies and the effectiveness of the implemented innovations. A diagnostic analysis of "determinants of implementation" is therefore an important component of planned implementation.

- Determinants of implementation ("barriers and facilitators of change") can be related to the innovation that is implemented, the individuals who are expected to adopt it (e.g. their cognitions, motivations, habits), the social world in which they act (e.g. teams, networks), the healthcare organization (e.g. aspects of its structure, culture, resources), and healthcare systems (e.g. health professionals' organizations, financial incentives, regulations).

- Most studies report on perceptions of the determinants of implementation. Research evidence on the actual impact of specific determinants is limited. Therefore, it is important to interpret the relevance of factors emerging from a diagnostic analysis carefully.

8.1 Introduction

When actual performance has been documented and goals for improvement have been chosen, the next step in a planned approach to implementation is a diagnostic analysis of factors associated with change (Figure 8.1). A diagnostic analysis of the target group and setting is important for each implementation program, because it is plausible that implementation strategies are more effective if they address key determinants of change (Baker et al. 2015). Determinants of change are factors that might hinder or enable improvements (see Box 8.1 for an example). Such factors are sometimes referred to as barriers and enablers, barriers and facilitators, problems and incentives, or moderators and mediators. A diagnostic analysis considers the following:

- Relevant stakeholders and their goals and interests.
- Determinants related to specific goals or targets of improvement.
- Relevant subgroups among (potential) adopters of the innovation.

Improving Patient Care: The Implementation of Change in Health Care, Third Edition. Edited by Michel Wensing, Richard Grol, and Jeremy Grimshaw.
© 2020 John Wiley & Sons Ltd. Published 2020 by John Wiley & Sons Ltd.

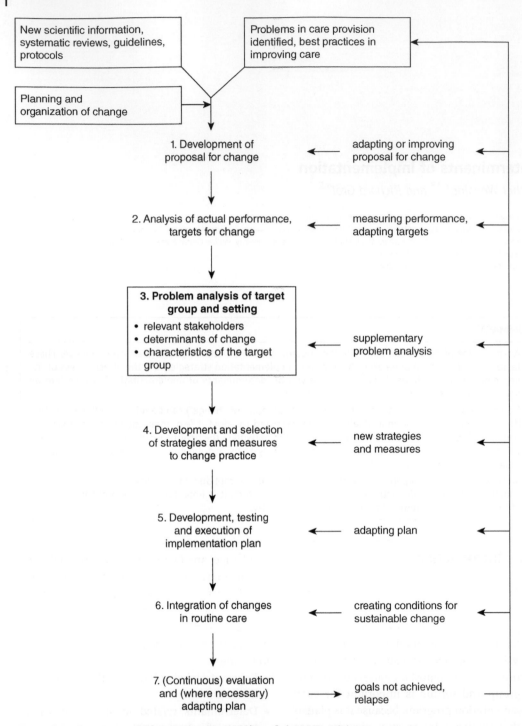

Figure 8.1 The Grol and Wensing implementation of change model.

Determinants of change can be explored in a pragmatic way, using for instance semi-structured interviews with health professionals. Alternatively, this exploration may be planned and performed as a scientific study, using systematic methods with a view on optimal validity and generalization to other settings than those studied. The study may be guided by a framework, which summarizes the types of factors identified in previous research. There are many frameworks and checklists of determinants of implementation, partly related to theories of change, which can guide such research (Strifler et al. 2018). Examples are the Consolidated Framework for Implementation Research (Damschroeder et al. 2009) and the Tailored Implementation for Chronic Diseases checklist (Flottorp et al. 2013). Many experts have argued for more systematic use of available theory, models, and frameworks in implementation research (Eccles et al. 2005; Grol and Buchan 2006).

Chapter 9 will elaborate on the methods for diagnostic analysis in the context of implementation. This chapter describes the types of factors to be considered in a diagnostic analysis preceding or during a program for improving healthcare. The chapter focuses on three aspects:

- Which parties are involved, and what are their goals and interests?
- Which factors may be associated with the start and process of change?
- What are the characteristics of the target group, which subgroups can be distinguished, and in which stage of change are they?

8.2 Analysis of Stakeholders

A comprehensive diagnostic analysis includes an analysis of individuals and organizations who are involved in a change process, or have an interest in it. Achieving the active participation of policy makers and organizational leaders requires specific activities (Lavis et al. 2003).

The role of scientific knowledge in decision making by policy makers and managers varies from minimal to reasonably large. It is influenced by a wide range of factors, such as the general degree of interest and understanding of knowledge and innovations among decision makers (Ouimet et al. 2006). Researchers and developers of innovations may influence these factors, for instance by initiatives to raise interest in research generally and the delivery of messages in formats that are attractive to decision makers (Lavis et al. 2008). They may actively disseminate research findings through various channels, so that different user groups are reached.

A first step is to map out stakeholders and identify their goals and interests, as far as relevant to the innovation of interest. For instance, organizational mission statements and performance in related cases in the past may be examined. In the example of cardiovascular risk management (Box 8.1), this analysis might look as follows:

- Most *patients* wish to reduce their cardiovascular risk, but patients vary in their willingness to change their lifestyle or use preventive medication. Some are reluctant to change their behavior or do not understand what is required due to limited (health) literacy.
- Most *primary care physicians* aim to provide recommended procedures, but some are reluctant to provide preventive procedures proactively. Maintaining a good long-term relationship with a patient is also important for most of them, which may reduce their inclination to persist with behavior change.
- *Cardiologists* and other medical specialists tend to treat cardiovascular risk factors more intensively than primary care physicians, but most do not have a comprehensive view of the patients and their context.
- *Other health professionals*, such as pharmacists, dieticians, and physiotherapists, have varying roles in the prevention of cardiovascular diseases. They tend to be dependent on

---

Box 8.1   Improving Cardiovascular Risk Management

A cluster randomized trial with 34 primary care practices tested an implementation program to improve cardiovascular risk management by introducing a risk table, information for patients, and training of physicians to use these tools (Van Steenkiste et al. 2007). The recommended procedure was to plan two consultations with each eligible patient to convey and discuss the information using motivating communication techniques. Six months after the start of the intervention, no differences were found on a range of outcomes. A survey among 239 participating patients showed that most patients had read and understood the information. The information had not induced worry, but also not led to behavior changes. In interviews the participating physicians mentioned a range of barriers for change, including shortage of knowledge on cardiovascular risk, suboptimal communication skills, inadequate skills to handle risk tables, high workload, and lack of time for shared decision making. The conclusion was that additional or different interventions were required to improve patients' health-related lifestyles. These barriers may have led to suboptimal implementation of the planned communication about cardiovascular risk. It may have been helpful to involve additional care providers, such as nurses, to provide counseling. In addition, the effectiveness of the approach for communication with the patient may have been strengthened by adding interventions that support behavior change, such as reminders and feedback.

---

referrals from physicians, but they may have independent initiatives in some settings.

- *Guideline-developing bodies* (related to health professions or to other stakeholders) use research evidence and possibly also considerations of financial cost to develop recommendations on cardiovascular risk management.
- *Health insurers* and other payers of healthcare aim to enhance quality while keeping cost at an acceptable level. A specific issue regarding preventive procedures is that cost saving (if any) may be realized in the future.
- *Companies* and organizations in the public sector may offer (cardiovascular) health checks or apps for mobile devices to employees or to the general public. These may be consistent with evidence-based recommendations, but this is not necessarily the case.

While the goals and interests of different stakeholders do not necessarily conflict, it is obvious that some do. Some conflicts are clear, such as the autonomy to choose any treatment versus the wish to contain the overall costs of healthcare. There are also subtler differences in the specific goals for different stakeholders. For instance, optimal outcomes of cardiovascular risk management are important for all stakeholders, but they have somewhat different meanings. The patient may want to avoid a major cardiovascular event, without changing lifestyle too much. The physician may want to reduce the cardiovascular risk by drug treatment of hypertension and hypercholesterolemia, leaving decisions on lifestyle to the patient, because of ethical considerations or to maintain a good relationship with the patient. On the other hand, national authorities may emphasize lifestyle changes, given the large number of individuals with an unhealthy lifestyle and its impact on population health. Finally, private companies focus on consumer demand in order to be financially viable. In the context of collectively funded healthcare, reimbursement is often conditional on the presence of reasonably convincing evidence on the safety and clinical effectiveness of interventions.

So, it is important to get an overview of relevant individuals and organizations involved in a specific implementation process. Their overall goals and interests cannot be influenced in most cases, at least not in the short run, but it is relevant to know these well before planning an implementation program. The goals and interests of different stakeholders are not necessarily different: they may also be well aligned. For instance, a large international study found few differences in ideas on barriers for change for improving chronic illness care between healthcare providers, managers and policy makers, and researchers (Wensing et al. 2014). A second important aim of knowing the stakeholders, obviously, is to get them on board and create a sense of ownership of the implementation process.

The involvement of stakeholders (e.g. patients, providers, payers) in the design and conduct of interventions to improve healthcare practice has been much emphasized in recent years. Involvement usually takes the form of consultation of stakeholders through interviews or surveys or participation of stakeholders in boards. Different concepts have been used to describe this idea, including "co-creation" and integrated knowledge translation. There is a need for better specification and validation of methods for the integration of stakeholders in the design and conduct of implementation projects, because a systematic review of studies found that the outcomes of stakeholder involvement are anecdotal and overall unclear (Gagliardi et al. 2016).

8.3 Determinants of Change

In this section we describe a number of specific determinants of practice which influence the implementation of innovations. After goals for improvement have been set and stakeholders have been involved, the next logical step is to identify determinants that need to be addressed (Wensing et al. 2010; Flottorp et al. 2013). Some of these factors are generic (they influence many implementation processes), while others are related to a specific innovation, target group, or healthcare setting. In many situations a wide range of different determinants needs to be considered.

In this chapter we do not consider features of the innovation itself, such as the strength of underlying research evidence and consistency with prevailing guidelines. These features have been considered in Chapter 5. The remaining factors have been categorized in this chapter as factors related to individual health professionals, patients, professional interactions, incentives and resources, capacity for organizational change, and societal, political, and legal aspects. The chapter does not provide a comprehensive overview of factors, but aims to provide an impression of the range of factors that may be relevant.

8.3.1 Individual Health Professional Factors

8.3.1.1 Cognitive Factors

This category includes many individual characteristics, such as intelligence, professional knowledge, information-seeking behaviors, decision-making patterns, and insight into current performance. The use of a guideline, technology, or new routine often requires specific knowledge and skills. Both identifying and learning about innovations by health professionals, managers, and patients are important for its implementation. This section focuses on healthcare professionals.

Health professionals' self-assessment of their professional performance is often inadequate. A systematic review (Davis et al. 2006) found 17 studies that mostly showed little association between self-assessment and external assessment of professional performance. Some studies found that the lowest agreement was in physicians with low competency and high self-confidence. The self-reported professional behavior of physicians showed low correlation with actual behavior, which was derived from patient records or surveys among patients; the latter two methods showed largely comparable methods (Montano and Phillips 1995).

It is crucial to identify and assess information on (potentially valuable) new treatments. In current times, access to information is less of a problem for many individuals. For instance, many clinical guidelines are available on platforms on the World Wide Web. Selection and prioritization of relevant pieces of knowledge from many items of information are often the main challenges. Information-seeking skills have thus become as crucial for healthcare professionals as for most highly educated professionals (Blumenthal 2002).

Research from before the era of evidence-based practice also suggests standardized patterns in clinical decision making. In a classic study from 1934, a panel of pediatricians assessed the need for tonsillectomy in children; they felt it was indicated in 45% of patients. The remaining 55% of children were reassessed by another panel of pediatricians; they felt tonsillectomy was indicated in 46% of these patients (Bakwin 1945). Similar results were found in a replication of this study several decades later (Ayanian and Berwick 1991). Physicians use implicit decision-making rules which can inhibit change of professional behaviors.

8.3.1.2 Motivational Factors

Motivational factors influence the intention to change behaviors (see Box 8.2). The impact of these factors may vary between innovations,

but it is nevertheless important to consider their potential role. The relationship between motivation and actual behavior is modest, yet relevant: 15–40% of variation in health professionals' behaviors was found to be influenced by motivation (Eccles et al. 2006). This is consistent with research in patients (Armitage and Conner 2001).

The psychology of behavior change has focused on behavioral intentions and related cognitions. Dissatisfaction with one's own performance can be the starting point of a change process (Geertsma et al. 1982). This dissatisfaction can be caused by a discrepancy between individual goals and current practice or by negative assessments of others. Individuals have varying tolerance for such discrepancies. The motivation to change may gradually increase as a result of experience or (repeated) information. Occasionally, a specific event, such as a patient safety incident, triggers a process of change (Armstrong and Reyburn 1996). For a sense of urgency of the need for change and the perception of responsibility for it, it is often crucial that credible information on professional performance is available.

The attitude regarding an innovation is another factor, which influences its implementation in practice. According to psychological theory, attitude is an important predictor of

---

Box 8.2   Motivations of Healthcare Providers to Change Behaviors

The motivations of healthcare providers, which drive their behaviors, are heterogeneous (Scott 1997) and may include:

- *Legal and ethical considerations*: risk of patient complaints and lawsuits, extent to which patients can actually be helped.
- *Job satisfaction*: satisfaction with their own professional performance, intellectual satisfaction of learning and applying knowledge, autonomy in decision making.
- *Income*: financial rewards, risks, and problems.

- *Social status*: esteem from colleagues, avoidance of negative publicity.
- *Work pressure*: number of contacts or procedures per hour, number of urgent contacts and house visits, volume of administrative work, unrealistic patient expectations.
- *Leisure time*: total hours per week, work during nights and weekends, burden of work on the family.
- *Societal engagement*: participation in activities outside direct patient care.

behavioral intention. Factors such as complexity, visibility, and the evidence base for the innovation influence attitudes of healthcare professionals regarding innovations (see Chapter 5). Healthcare professionals' attitudes regarding clinical practice guidelines, which are one important example of innovations in healthcare, have been widely studied. Many professionals hold generally positive views of guidelines, but some perceive that they may (inappropriately) reduce professional autonomy, may lack a strong evidence base, or may be misused for cost containment (Hayward et al. 1997). Some feel that clinical guidelines simplify the complexity of patient care too much, as clinical decisions need to be tailored to individual patients (Woolf et al. 1999; Grol and Weel 2009). Physicians who are members of professional organizations are more likely to have positive views of guidelines and other innovations (Grol and Wensing 1995).

8.3.1.3 Behavioral Factors (Routines)

Individual routines and institutionalized organizational processes often influence the likelihood of uptake of innovations. Routines seem related to professional training and to personality characteristics. For instance, internists appear to order a broader range of diagnostic tests in non-acute cardiological problems than do cardiologists (Glassman et al. 1997). A review of 56 studies showed that surgeons perform better if they treat more patients and have more years of experience, up to a specific point after which performance deteriorates (Muruthappu et al. 2015). Nurses who work

many hours or long shifts reported more problems in the quality and safety of healthcare (Griffiths et al. 2014). The tendency to order diagnostic tests seems to be related to the risk attitudes of physicians (Zaat and Van Eijk 1992).

8.3.2 Patient Factors

Patients' beliefs, knowledge, preferences, motivations, and behavior can also influence the uptake of innovations. These patient factors, such as beliefs about diseases and treatments, may differ from those held by physicians (see Box 8.3).

The effect of patients' views on the implementation of innovations is partly explained by the interpretation of these views by health professionals, who may adapt their behaviors to what (they think) patients think or want. A study found that the probability of a medication being prescribed was three times higher if the patient expected such a prescription. The probability was 10 times higher if the physician thought that the patient expected the prescription, regardless of whether this was accurate (Cockburn and Pit 1997). Another study showed that patients' preference influenced decisions on admission to an intensive care department for 71% of 402 Swiss intensive care physicians (Escher et al. 2004).

8.3.3 Professional Interactions

8.3.3.1 Team Processes

Patient care and prevention are often provided by teams or networks of healthcare providers. Formalized patient care teams meet regularly

---

Box 8.3 Patients Who Want Diagnostic Tests

A qualitative study with 22 patients (Van Bokhoven et al. 2006) focused on the question of why they wanted a laboratory test. The study showed that they had an overly positive view of the measurement quality of tests and that they interpreted positive test results as a sign of good health. Patients often perceived tests as a valid method for screening for major diseases. They felt supported in this belief by others in their environment and by the media. Most of these patients assumed that the physician would order laboratory tests for them.

(e.g. daily or weekly), but in ambulatory care the collaboration tends to be looser or based on intermittent interactions such as referrals of patients. Setting up or intensifying a patient care team or healthcare delivery network can be regarded as an implementation strategy (see Chapter 15). Here we elaborate on the impact of team processes on the uptake of innovations.

In social psychology many factors have been described as influencing team processes, including goal orientation, size of the team, psychological safety, leadership, and so on. Decision making in teams has been studied in cognitive psychology. Under specific conditions (e.g. little contact with the outside world, absence of procedures, strong cohesion), there is a risk that group decision making becomes coherent but is not optimal ("group think"). This is associated with a feeling of invulnerability, strong belief in group morality, shared rationalization of decisions, and illusion of unanimity (Park 2000).

Processes in patient care teams have been studied extensively, albeit not necessarily in relation to the uptake of innovations in healthcare. For instance, a study on intensive care departments showed that better (perceived) team functioning was associated with lowered mortality rates (Wheelan et al. 2003). An intensified team approach to patient care can improve patient outcomes (Bosch et al. 2009), but underlying mechanisms have not been completely clarified. Both improved coordination (such as use of a case manager for structured meetings) and broader clinical input (e.g. inclusion of a pharmacist or specialized nurse in the team) can improve team outcomes.

Another factor is "team climate," which includes aspects such as the vision of the team, psychological safety, task orientation, and attitude regarding innovations. A review of studies conducted in the UK's National Health Service found few associations of clinical processes or outcomes with team climate (Goh et al. 2009). Other studies have also found such a lack of associations (Bosch et al. 2008;

Goh et al. 2009). It is plausible that team processes influence outcomes, but it remains difficult to measure exactly which aspects are important.

8.3.4 Professional Networks

Health professionals and managers participate in a range of professional networks for information exchange and professional collaboration. Such networks may be purposefully created or emerge from multiple interactions. Several theories predict that network structures influence individual behaviors, and vice versa. For instance, the theory on diffusion of innovations predicts that network characteristics influence the uptake of innovations by individuals (Rogers 2003). The theory emphasizes the role of brokers (individuals who connect two networks) and opinion leaders (individuals who influence many others in the network). Although modern information technology facilitates access to others and to knowledge, network structures remain important because they influence the selection and prioritization of knowledge. These processes are influenced by fundamental behavioral mechanisms, such as social comparison and role modeling, which are structured by networks (West et al. 1999). For instance, networks with a high density (many connections) may spread innovations more quickly than networks with low density.

Research on local opinion leaders illustrates a specific social influence mechanism related to social networks (Lomas et al. 1991). Opinion leaders are individuals who are consulted by colleagues for advice and who set an example by their behaviors (Stross 1996). This requires that they are technically competent and dedicated members of the local community (Greer 1988). They are not necessarily the first users of an innovation. Studies in medical settings have shown that opinion leaders can be involved in the dissemination of knowledge, although the effects of this approach were modest (Flodgren et al. 2019).

While more research on networks is needed, studies have suggested that healthcare professionals are influenced by the opinion of peers in their immediate environment. In a classic study, several hundred physicians working in hospitals were interviewed (Greer 1988). The study showed that most physicians actively observed their colleagues and that most discussed new information and procedures with their colleagues. Professional performance tended to change only when local consensus was realized on the preferred approach. Scientific publications or marketing seemed relatively unimportant. Important conditions for uptake of an innovation were local communication about the benefit and risks of a new procedure, availability of local demonstration and education, and positive expectations among relevant individuals.

8.3.5 Organizational Factors

8.3.5.1 Capacity for Organizational Change

Most health professionals are based in organizations of various sizes, such as hospitals, hospital departments, primary care out-of-hours cooperatives, and office-based practices. Organizations restrain, facilitate, and direct the behaviors of individuals. Most health professionals behave under organizational constraints and opportunities, which relate to resources and power. Characteristics of organizations have indeed been found to correlate with performance empirically. Management of patients with a problematic use of alcohol was better in primary care practices which had defined this as one of their responsibilities and in practices with more staff available (Schutte et al. 2009). While small office-based primary care practices may provide high-quality chronic care, a study in seven European countries suggested that the quality of chronic care was more consistent and slightly better if practice nurses are actively involved in healthcare delivery (Nouwens et al. 2014).

A systematic review of 30 qualitative studies identified a range of characteristics of organizations struggling to improve the quality and safety of care (Vaughn et al. 2019). These related to organizational culture (limited ownership, not collaborative, hierarchic, with disconnected leadership), infrastructure (limited quality improvement, staffing, information technology, or resources), cohesive mission (mission conflicts with other missions, is externally motivated, poorly defined, or promotes mediocrity), system shocks (events such as leadership turnover, new electronic health record system, or organizational scandals), and dysfunctional external relations with other institutions and stakeholders. Another review of 11 studies, which involved interviews with 145 health professionals, identified a range of contextual determinants of the uptake of evidence-based practice (Squires et al. 2019). These included resource access, work structure, patient characteristics, professional role, culture, facility characteristics, system features, healthcare professional characteristics, financial, collaboration, leadership, evaluation, regulatory, or legislative standards, and societal influences.

8.3.6 Organizational Structure

Research from outside healthcare suggests that differentiation of functions, specialized workers, and spread of power in an organization are determinants of the uptake of innovations (see Chapter 2). Such factors may influence the willingness and capacity to develop and implement innovations. For instance, studies in healthcare have suggested that organizational size may influence the uptake of innovations (Halm and Teirstein 2002; Gandjour et al. 2003). More imaging tests were ordered for patients with low back pain in large practice organizations than in small practices (Pham et al. 2009). Underlying mechanisms are a selection effect (the best centers attract more patients), an efficiency effect (large centers can work efficiently due to the size of scale advantages), and a learning effect (a large volume of procedures induces a steep learning curve and the maintenance of skills at a high level). Organizational structure tends to have a broad yet indirect and non-specific impact on the uptake of a range of innovations.

8.3.7 Organizational Culture

Organizational culture comprises shared ideas and behaviors in an organization, which reflect fundamental values and beliefs. Open communication and appreciation of new ideas in an organization are expected to contribute to innovation in an organization. Signaling new technologies in the outside world and the needs of customers are other components of culture, which are expected to contribute to innovation in an organization. Organizational leaders can influence organizational culture, but culture also develops autonomously.

There is some empirical support for the role of organizational influence on the quality of care and knowledge implementation. A comparative case study examined three high-performing and three low-performing British hospitals (Mannion et al. 2005). In the high-performing hospitals, leadership tended to be transactional and stable rather than charismatic and frequently changing. They had strong middle management, transparency of performance, and incentives linked to good performance. In low-performing hospitals, information systems were underdeveloped and rewards linked to patronage. The director in a high-performing hospital was characterized as "Apollo" (because of the focus on rationality and harmony), while the director in a low-performing hospital was characterized as "Zeus" (because of many personal interventions and emphasis on patronage). This study generates many interesting hypotheses, which have to be examined in further research.

Quantitative research (using questionnaires to measure aspects of leadership or culture) is limited and has not consistently confirmed the proposed impact of leadership and culture on performance and outcomes (Øvretveit 2005). There is no convincing evidence that culture can be predictably changed (Parmelli et al. 2011). Nevertheless, it is plausible that leaders in healthcare organizations and professions have an important influence on the culture, and thus on the implementation of innovations.

8.3.8 Availability of Necessary Resources

Availability of the resources needed for a specific new procedure is obviously a crucial condition for the successful implementation of an innovation. For instance, practices that had facilities for imaging tests ordered four times as many tests as practices who had to refer for such tests (Hillman et al. 1990). In some settings, such as low-income countries and deprived healthcare sectors, resources are generally scarce. In other settings, the availability of resources is often the result of a political process to determine priorities. Organizational science studies have suggested that the availability of technical and financial resources is associated with organizational innovation (see Chapter 2). It is plausible that the availability of resources has an important impact, but the amount of empirical research on this is limited.

8.3.9 Societal Factors

8.3.9.1 Health Professions

Professions (such as physicians and nurses) are trained and socialized to have a number of characteristics, such as specialized skills, professional pride, an altruistic orientation, and high integrity (Van de Camp et al. 2004). As a consequence, individual professionals tend to have a strong orientation to their profession rather than to the organization in which they work. This orientation can be both a driver and a barrier for the uptake of innovations, depending on the position taken by the professional bodies regarding a specific innovation. For instance, in a study of 43 nursing organizations, only 10 actively promoted evidence-based practice (Achterberg et al. 2006). The hospitals and other healthcare organizations may serve the aims of the professions or provide counter-vailing power (Kitchener et al. 2005). In larger primary care organizations, specific physicians take a leading role and have a major impact on organizational policies (Sheaff et al. 2002). Their engagement with an implementation program is indispensable for its success.

8.3.9.2 Financial Incentives and Disincentives

Financial incentives, disincentives, and risks have a broad influence on the uptake of innovations. Some healthcare providers are highly aware of these and involve them in their decisions in patient care and practice management. Others are not aware of finan-cial aspects, as was shown in a study among physicians on the price of medication (Allen et al. 2007). Standard economic theory pre-dicts that a higher financial reward for a spe-cific service leads to more frequent delivery of that service (except if it does not cover the costs for providing it). This economic theory finds support from research evidence from healthcare settings. Reimbursement on the basis of volume of services results in higher numbers of those services compared to a fixed budget (Gosden and Torgerson 1997). Reim-bursement on the basis of a fixed budget per year seems associated to be with the implementation of specific practices, such as a lower rate of test ordering and more time for counseling of patients (Salisbury et al. 1998). Likewise, financial incentives for patients may influence the uptake of prac-tices (Sutherland et al. 2008). Chapter 17 describes the impact of financial incentives in some more detail.

8.3.9.3 Legislation

Laws and regulations provide the boundaries of performance for both healthcare providers and patients, and may also provide financial incentives. The contracts of healthcare provi-ders with health insurers or authorities also provide such boundaries and incentives. Research on the impact of laws, regulations, and contracts is limited. A study on the use of clopidogrel after heart surgery (percu-taneous transluminal coronary angioplasty or PTCA) in Canada showed that the use increased substantially when it was no longer necessary to ask permission for a prescription from a healthcare insurer. The same study also found a positive effect on cardiovas-cular outcomes at one year after surgery (Jackevicius et al. 2008). In some countries, laws and regulations are commonly used to change healthcare practice. For instance, Germany has laws and regulations with spe-cific requirements regarding the management of specific chronic diseases, primary care as the first point of access to healthcare, and hospital admission and discharge.

8.4 Subgroups in the Target Population

The target population of (teams of) health professionals, managers of healthcare organi-zations, and patients may consist of sub-groups in which different determinants are relevant. Individuals and organizations in dif-ferent subgroups are in different phases of a process of change (Table 8.1). The idea of sub-groups is supported by a number of theories and partly also by some empirical research. For instance, a study on physicians' adher-ence to guidelines for vaccination identified four subgroups (Pathman et al. 1996): physi-cians who had never heard of these guide-lines; physicians who knew the guidelines but did not accept them; physicians who knew and accepted the guidelines, but applied them only occasionally; and physi-cians who knew, accepted, and applied the guidelines in most patients. This cumulative model fitted with 90% of physicians. However, evidence from studies of stage models that individuals predictably move through sequen-tial stages is lacking.

Table 8.1 Phases in a process of change.

Steps	Examples of potential barriers for change
Orientation	
Awareness of the innovation	Not involved in continuing professional education
Interest and involvement	Little contact with colleagues
	No sense of urgency for innovation
	Limited insight into current shortcomings
Knowledge	
Understanding	Poor information-seeking skills
Insight into own routines	Lack of specific knowledge or forgetting details
	Denial of suboptimal performance
	Defensive attitude
Acceptance	
Positive attitude, motivation to change	Low utility: seeing more disadvantages than advantages
Positive intention or decision to change	Uncertainty about scientific evidence
	Little trust in developers of innovation
	No involvement in development process
	Anticipated problems for implementation
	Shortage of confidence regarding skills
Change	
Actual adoption in practice	Shortage of time and money
Confirmation of benefit or value of change	Lack of skills
	Small-scale testing not possible
	Negative first experiences
	Patients or colleagues do not cooperate or respond negatively Negative side effects
Maintenance	
Integration of new practice into routines	Relapse in old routines organization
Embedding of new practice in the organization	Forgetting new knowledge and skills
	Lack of facilities
	Lack of support from (higher) management

Source: Data from Grol and Wensing (2004).

8.5 Conclusions

A good diagnostic analysis can contribute to a tailored approach to the implementation of innovations. Theory and some research evidence suggest that tailored implementation is more effective than a standardized approach. This chapter provided a broad overview of the aspects which need to be considered in the diagnostic analysis. Prospectively identified factors proved to influence actual implementation processes, but new (not previously identified) factors can also be relevant (Wensing 2017). The following chapter will describe the methods for diagnostic analysis.

References

Achterberg, T. van, Holleman, G., Van de Ven, M. et al. (2006). Promoting evidence-based practice: the roles and activities of professional nurses' associations. *J. Adv. Nurs.* 53: 605–612.

Allen, G.M., Lexchin, J., and Wiebe, N. (2007). Physician awareness of drug costs: a systematic review. *PLoS Med.* 4: 1486–1496.

Armitage, C.J. and Conner, M. (2001). Efficacy of the theory of planned behaviour: a meta-analytic review. *Br. J. Soc. Psychol.* 40: 471–499.

Armstrong, D., Reyburn, H., and Jones, R. (1996). A study of general practitioners' reasons for changing their prescribing behaviour. *BMJ* 312: 949–952.

Ayanian, J.Z. and Berwick, D.M. (1991). Do physicians have a bias toward action? A classic study revisited. *Med. Decis. Making* 11: 154–158.

Baker, R., Camosso-Stefinovic, J., Gillies, C. et al. (2015). Tailored interventions to address determinants of practice. *Cochrane Database Syst. Rev.* (4): CD005470. https://doi.org/10.1002/14651858.

Bakwin, H. (1945). Pseudodoxia pediatrica. *N. Engl. J. Med.* 232: 691–697.

Blumenthal, D. (2002). Doctors in a wired world: can professionalism survive connectivity. *Milbank Q.* 80: 525–546.

van Bokhoven, M.A., Pleunis-van Empel, M.C.H., Koch, H. et al. (2006). Why do patients want their blood tested? A qualitative study of patient expectations in general practice. *BMC Fam. Pract.* 7: 75.

Bosch, M., Dijkstra, R., Wensing et al. (2008). Organizational culture, team climate and diabetes care in small office-based practices. *BMC Health Serv. Res.* 8: 180.

Bosch, M., Faber, M., Cruijsberg, J. et al. (2009). Effectiveness of patient care teams and the role of clinical expertise and coordination: a literature review. *Med. Care Res. Rev.* 66: S5–S35.

Cockburn, J. and Pit, S. (1997). Prescribing behaviour in clinical practice: patients' expectations and doctors' perceptions of patients' expectations – a questionnaire study. *BMJ* 315: 520–523.

Damschroder, L.J., Aron, D.C., Keith, R.E. et al. (2009). Fostering implementation of health services research findings into practice: a consolidated framework for advancing implementation science. *Implement. Sci.* 4: 50.

Davis, S.A., Mazmanian, P.E., Fordis, M. et al. (2006). Accuracy of physician self-assessment compared with observed measures of competence. A systematic review. *JAMA* 296: 1094–1102.

Eccles, M., Grimshaw, J., Walker, A. et al. (2005). Changing the behaviour of healthcare professionals: the use of theory in promoting the uptake of research findings. *J. Clin. Epidemiol.* 58: 107–112.

Eccles, M.P., Hrisos, S., Francis, J. et al. (2006). Do self-reported intentions predict clinicians' behaviour: a systematic review. *Implement. Sci.* 1: 28.

Escher, M., Perneger, T.V., and Chrevolet, J.C. (2004). National questionnaire survey on what influences doctors' decisions about admission to intensive care. *BMJ* 329: 425.

Flodgren, G., O'Brien, M.A., Parmelli, E., and Grimshaw, J.M. (2019). Local opinion leaders: effects on professional practice and health care outcomes. *Cochrane Database Syst Rev* 1: CD000125. https://doi.org/10.1002/14651858.CD000125.pub4.

Flottorp, S., Oxman, A.D., Krause, J. et al. (2013). A checklist for identifying determinants of practice: a systematic review and synthesis of frameworks and taxonomies of factors that prevent or enable improvements in healthcare professional practice. *Implement. Sci.* 8: 35.

Gagliardi, A.R., Berta, W., Kothari, A. et al. (2016). Integrated knowledge translation (IKT) in health care: a scoping review. *Implement. Sci.* 11: 38.

Gandjour, A., Bannenberg, A., and Lauterbach, K.W. (2003). Threshold volumes associated with higher survival in health care: a systematic review. *Med. Care* 41: 1129–1141.

Geertsma, R.H., Parker, R.C., and Krauss, S. (1982). How physicians view the process of change in their practice behaviour. *J. Med. Educ.* 57: 752–761.

Glassman, P.A., Kravitz, R.L., Petersen, L.P. et al. (1997). Differences in clinical decision making between internists and cardiologists. *Arch. Intern. Med.* 157: 506–512.

Goh, T., Eccles, M.P., and Steen, I.N. (2009). Factors predicting team climate, and its relationship with quality of care in general practice. *BMC Health Serv. Res.* 9: 138.

Gosden, T. and Torgerson, D.J. (1997). The effect of fundholding on prescribing and referral costs: a review of the evidence. *Health Policy* 40: 103–114.

Greer, A.L. (1988). The state of the art versus the state of the science. *Int. J. Technol. Assess. Health Care* 4: 5–26.

Griffiths, P., Dall 'Ora, C., Simon, M. et al. (2014). Nurses' shift length and overtime working in 12 European countries. The association with perceived quality of care and patient safety. *Med. Care* 52: 975–981.

Grol, R. and Buchan, H. (2006). Clinical guidelines: what can we do to increase their use? *MJA* 185: 301–302.

Grol, R. and Weel, C.v. (2009). Getting a grip on guidelines: how to make them more relevant for practice. *Br. J. Gen. Pract.* 59: e143–e144.

Grol, R. and Wensing, M. (1995). Implementation of quality assurance and medical audit: general practitioners' perceived obstacles and requirements. *Br. J. Gen. Pract.* 45: 548–552.

Grol, R. and Wensing, M. (2004). What drives change? Barriers to and incentives for achieving evidence-based practice. *Med. J. Aust.* 180: S57–S60.

Halm, E.A. and Teirstein, A.S. (2002). Clinical practice. Management of community-acquired pneumonia. *N. Engl. J. Med.* 347: 2039–2045.

Hayward, R.S., Guyatt, G.H., Moore, K.A. et al. (1997). Canadian physicians' attitudes about and preferences regarding clinical practice guidelines. *CMAJ* 156: 1715–1723.

Hillman, B.J., Joseph, C.A., Marry, M.R. et al. (1990). Frequency and costs of diagnostic imaging in office practice: a comparison of self-referring and radiologist-referring physicians. *N. Engl. J. Med.* 323: 1604–1608.

Jackevicius, C.A., Tu, J.V., Demers, V. et al. (2008). Cardiovascular outcomes after a change in prescription policy for clopidogrel. *N. Engl. J. Med.* 359: 1802–1810.

Kitchener, M., Caronna, C.A., and Shortell, S.M. (2005). From the doctor's workshop to the iron cage? Evolving modes of physician control in US health systems. *Soc. Sci. Med.* 60: 1311–1322.

Lavis, J.N., Oxman, A.D., Moynihan, R., and Paulsen, E.J. (2008). Evidence-informed health policy I – synthesis of findings from a multi-method study of organizations that support the use of research evidence. *Implement. Sci.* 3: 53.

Lavis, J.N., Robertson, D., Woodside, J.M. et al. (2003). How can research organizations more effectively transfer research knowledge to decision makers? *Milbank Q.* 81: 221–248.

Lomas, J., Enkin, M., Andersson, G.M. et al. (1991). Opinion leaders versus audit and feedback to implement practice guidelines. Delivery after previous cesarean arthritis. *JAMA* 265: 2202–2207.

Mannion, R., Davies, H.T.O., and Marshall, M.N. (2005). Cultural characteristics of "high" and "low" performing hospitals. *J. Health Organ. Manag.* 19: 431–439.

Montano, D.E. and Phillips, W.R. (1995). Cancer screening by primary care physicians: a comparison of rates obtained from physician self-report, patient survey, and chart audit. *Am. J. Public Health* 85: 795–800.

Muruthappu, M., Gilberg, B.J., El-Harasis, M.A. et al. (2015). The influence of volume and experience on individual surgical performance. A systematic review. *Ann. Surg.* 261: 642–647.

Nouwens, E., van Lieshout, J., van Hombergh, P. et al. (2014). Shifting cardiovascular care to nurses results in structured chronic care. *Am. J. Manag. Care* 20: e278–e284.

Ouimet, M., Landry, R., Amara, N., and Belkhodja, O. (2006). What factors induce health care decision-makers to use clinical guidelines? Evidence from provincial health ministries, regional authorities and hospitals in Canada. *Soc. Sci. Med.* 62: 964–976.

Øvretveit, J. (2005). Leading improvement. *J. Health Organ. Manag.* 19: 413–430.

Park, W. (2000). A comprehensive empirical investigation of the relationship among variables of the group-think model. *J. Organ. Behav.* 21: 873–887.

Parmelli, E., Flodgren, G., Beyer, F. et al. (2011). The effectiveness of strategies to change organisational culture to improve healthcare performance: a systematic review. *Implem Sci* 6: 33.

Pathman, D.E., Konrad, T.R., Freed, G.L. et al. (1996). The awareness-to-adherence model of the steps to clinical guideline compliance. The case of pediatric vaccine recommendations. *Med. Care* 34: 873–889.

Pham, H.H., Landon, B.E., Reschovsky, J.D. et al. (2009). Rapidity and modality of imaging for acute low back pain in elderly patients. *Arch. Intern. Med.* 169: 972–981.

Rogers, E.M. (2003). *Diffusion of Innovations*. Simon and Schuster: New York.

Salisbury, C., Bosanquet, N., Wilkinson, E. et al. (1998). The implementation of evidence-based medicine in general practice prescribing. *Br. J. Gen. Pract.* 48: 1849–1851.

Schutte, K., Yano, E.M., Kilbourne, A.M. et al. (2009). Organizational contexts of primary care approaches for managing problem drinking. *J. Subst. Abuse Treat.* 36: 435–445.

Scott, A. (1997). *Agency, Incentives and the Behaviour of General Practitioners: The Relevance of Principal Agent Theory in Designing Incentives for GPs in the UK*. Aberdeen: Aberdeen University.

Sheaff, R., Smith, K., and Dickson, M. (2002). Is GP restratification beginning in England? *Social Policy Adm.* 36: 765–779.

Squires, J.E., Aloisio, L.D., Grimshaw, J.M. et al. (2019). Attributes of context relevant to health professionals' use of research evidence in clinical practice: a multi-study analysis. *Implement. Sci.* 14: 52.

Strifler, L., Cardosa, R., McGowan, J. et al. (2018). Scoping review identifies significant number of knowledge translation theories, models, and frameworks with limited use. *J. Clin. Epidemiol.* 100: 92–102.

Stross, J.K. (1996). The educationally influential physician. *J. Contin. Educ. Health Prof.* 16: 167–172.

Sutherland, K., Christianson, J.B., and Leatherman, S. (2008). Impact of targeted financial incentives on personal health behaviour: a review of the literature. *Med. Care Res. Rev.* 65: S36–S78.

Van de Camp, K., Vernooij-Dassen, M.J.F.J., Grol, R.P.T.M., and Bottema, B.J.A.M. (2004). How to conceptualize professionalism: a qualitative study. *Med. Teach.* 26: 696–702.

Van Steenkiste, B.v., van der Weijden, T., Stoffers, H. et al. (2007). Improving cardiovascular risk management: a randomized, controlled trial on the effect of a decision support tool for patients and physicians. *Eur. J. Cardiovasc. Prev. Rehabil.* 14: 44–50.

Vaughn, V.M., Saint, S., Krein, S.L. et al. (2019). Characteristics of healthcare organisations struggling to improve quality: results from a systematic review of qualitative studies. *BMJ Qual. Saf.* 28: 74–84.

Wensing, M. (2017). Introduction to the article series on the tailored implementation in chronic diseases (TICD) project. *Implement. Sci.* 12: 5.

Wensing, M., Bosch, M., and Grol, R. (2010). The knowledge to action cycle: developing and selecting knowledge to action interventions. *CMAJ* 182: E85–E88.

Wensing, M., Huntink, E., Van Lieshout, J. et al. (2014). Tailored implementation of evidence-based practice for patients with chronic diseases. *PLoS One* 9: E101981.

West, E., Barron, D.N., Dowsett, J., and Newton, J.N. (1999). Hierarchies and cliques in the social networks of health care professionals: implications for the design of dissemination strategies. *Soc. Sci. Med.* 48: 633–646.

Wheelan, S.A., Burchill, C.N., and Tilin, F. (2003). The link between teamwork and patients' outcomes in intensive care units. *Am. J. Crit. Care* 12: 527–534.

Woolf, S.H., Grol, R., Hutchinson, A. et al. (1999). Potential benefits, limitations, and harms of clinical guidelines. *BMJ* 318: 527–530.

Zaat, J.O. and Van Eijk, J.T. (1992). General practitioners' uncertainty, risk preferences, and use of laboratory tests. *Med. Care* 30: 846–854.

9

Methods to Identify and Analyze Determinants of Implementation

Michel Wensing[1,2,3] and Richard Grol[4,5]

[1] *Faculty of Medicine, University of Heidelberg, Heidelberg, Germany*
[2] *Department of General Practice and Health Services Research, Heidelberg University Hospital, Heidelberg, Germany*
[3] *Department IQ healthcare, Radboud Institute for Health Sciences, Radboud University Medical Center, Nijmegen, The Netherlands*
[4] *Radboud University, Nijmegen, The Netherlands*
[5] *Maastricht University, Maastricht, The Netherlands*

SUMMARY

- A range of methods can be used to identify and analyze determinants of implementation. Theories and frameworks may be used as a guide and stakeholders may be involved to guide the study and interpret the results.

- For identifying determinants of implementation, we recommend starting with detailed exploration of a few cases, followed by a larger study to determine the relative importance of different determinants.

- Semi-structured interviews, group interviews, and observation are methods to collect data on a few cases. Questionnaires and large-scale observation (e.g. using routinely collected data) can be used to assess the relevance of determinants in a wider population.

- It is often necessary to select and prioritize factors from a large number of identified factors. Methods such as paretograms can be used to support this.

9.1 Introduction

As described in the previous chapter, a "diagnostic analysis" aims to provide insight into the determinants of implementation, which are also called barriers or enablers for improvement in patient care. This chapter presents a range of methods for conducting such analysis. Few of these methods have been validated in the context of improving patient care, but some validation research has been done (Box 9.1). Most methods were initially developed for use in scientific research, but can – in a simplified format – also be used in pragmatic improvement projects. It

can be challenging to identify determinants of implementation with a view to planning for implementation, before any actual change has actually happened. In many situations people have little experience of change and will report what determines their current performance. In this situation it is then up to the analyst to consider current performance and what might cause it to change. For ease of writing, within this chapter we consistently talk about determinants of implementation. The chapter will first describe a variety of methods to collect data and then methods for data analysis and prioritization (see Boxes 9.2 and 9.3 for examples).

Improving Patient Care: The Implementation of Change in Health Care, Third Edition. Edited by Michel Wensing, Richard Grol, and Jeremy Grimshaw.

Box 9.1   Tailored Implementation: Which Methods Are Useful?

Little is known about the usefulness of various methods for the identification of determinants of implementation (barriers and facilitators of change) and matching implementation strategies to those determinants. In practice and research, different methods are used. An international study compared different approaches and tested tailored implementation programs for depression in Norway, obesity in England, vascular disease in the Netherlands, multimorbidity in Germany, and chronic obstructive pulmonary disorder in Poland (Wensing et al. 2011). Important lessons included:

- Group interviews with healthcare providers provided many ideas about determinants of implementation and implementation strategies. Other stakeholders (such as quality management staff and health insurers) also provided ideas, but fewer and largely similar to those of healthcare providers.

- As the number of ideas was large, it was necessary to prioritize them, as improvement programs can only address a limited number of factors.
- The items mentioned in group interviews (preceding the implementation programs) were largely recognized by healthcare providers, who actually participated in the implementation program. However, new ideas about the determinants of implementation and implementation strategies also emerged after the start of the program. Monitoring and formative evaluation during the running of a program are therefore recommended.
- Not all interventions were actually used by all healthcare providers, although all were matched to previously identified determinants of implementation. This might have reduced the effectiveness of the programs.

Box 9.2   Barriers for the Management of Urinary Tract Infections and Sore Throat

This study aimed to identify barriers to implementing evidence-based guidelines for urinary tract infection and sore throat in primary care in Norway, and to tailor interventions to address these barriers (Flottorp and Oxman 2003). A pragmatic combination of qualitative research methods was used. Those who were involved in the process of developing the guidelines were specifically asked to comment upon factors that could influence implementation of the guidelines. An international group of implementation experts had a brainstorming session on possible barriers. Two focus group interviews with patients and one focus group interview with practice assistants were also conducted. A pilot study was performed in five practices to get feedback on factors influencing the implementation of guidelines. Physicians and assistants in an intervention study discussed barriers in small groups. Finally, the researchers had informal interviews throughout the project. A checklist of 12 barriers to change was developed during this process. Barriers were categorized according to practice environment (financial disincentives, organizational constraints, perception of liability, patient expectations); prevailing opinion (standards of practice, opinion leaders, medical training, advocacy); knowledge and attitudes (clinical uncertainty, sense of competency, compulsion to act, information overload). The implementation strategy was tailored to address these factors.

Box 9.3 Systematic Literature Analysis of Studies on Barriers to Adherence to Guidelines

This overview of studies focused on perceived barriers to the implementation of clinical guidelines (Cabana et al. 1999). After analysis of databases and other sources, 76 studies were found in which at least one barrier to the use of clinical guidelines was described; these comprised 5 qualitative studies and 120 surveys with structured questions, of which 58% only concerned one type of barrier. From these, 293 potential barriers were derived. The average percentages of respondents that perceived a barrier were as follows:

- 55% were not aware of the guideline.
- 57% were not aware of the exact content of the guideline.
- Between 6 and 68% reported little self-efficacy in applying the guideline.
- 13% reported no positive expectation of the result of using the guideline.
- 42% reported a lack of motivation to change.
- Between 5 and 17% reported external factors, such as time and resources.

9.2 Interviews

9.2.1 Individual Interviews

Face-to-face or telephone interviews with health professionals, managers of healthcare organizations, policy makers, and patients can provide insight into their views on the implementation of a specific innovation (such as a guideline or best practice) in healthcare (see Box 9.4 for an example). Conducting any significant number of interviews usually requires time and resources, but offers the opportunity to ask questions about ideas underlying perceived barriers and facilitators for change. In most cases the number of interviews is small and therefore the study does not necessarily provide a representative picture. Doing an informative interview requires preparation, training, and also talent. In small projects "conversations" rather than "interviews" are usually performed, which nonetheless can provide useful information. Ideally, these interviews are followed by structured methods that seek to categorize factors and explore the generalizability of the findings.

9.2.2 Group Interviews

The added value of group interviews is that the interactions between group members help to identify items that might not have been identified in individual interviews (see Box 9.5 for an example). Depending on practicalities, group interviews may also be more efficient than individual interviews in terms of time needed. However, they may be difficult to

---

Box 9.4 Barriers to Optimal Antibiotics Prescribing in Lower Respiratory Infections

In this qualitative study in three medium-sized hospitals in the Netherlands, semi-structured interviews were conducted to identify barriers to optimal antibiotics prescribing in lower respiratory infections (Schouten et al. 2007). Eighteen interviews were performed with medical residents and specialists at the departments for internal medicine, pulmonology, microbiology, and clinical pharmacology. A range of subjects was discussed, including the choice of recommended antibiotics, timely use of antibiotics, and dose adaptations because of renal failure. Perceived determinants of implementation were categorized according to a conceptual framework.

Box 9.5 Case Management for Patients with Chronic Heart Failure

Case management allocates the coordination of individual patients' care in the hands of a dedicated health professional, who may be a nurse or physician. It concerns an organizational innovation, which can contribute to better clinical performance and outcomes as well as lowered costs and higher patient satisfaction with care. In a German study of case management for patients with chronic heart failure, focus group interviews with 24 physicians were conducted to explore their perceptions of case management, subsequent changes in the practice team, and the potential future role (Peters-Klimm et al. 2009). Case management was provided in an ambulatory setting and comprised regular telephone monitoring, home visits, health counseling, diagnostic screening, and booklets for patients. Practice-based assistants (equivalent to nurses) adopted these new activities. Five group interviews were performed, using a semi-structured format. At the time the physicians had at least eight months' experience with case management.

All interviews were audiotaped, transcribed, and analyzed for themes using a software package for qualitative data analysis. Two researchers looked for similarities in the data and assigned the same code to data that had some common characteristics. The analysis proceeded via pattern and thematic coding and clustering the descriptive codes into groups of related conceptual subcategories or generic categories. Coding of aspects that did not fit into the conceptual framework created further concepts based on inductive concept analysis. The researchers met regularly to compare and to discuss coding schemes. The study showed that physicians found all components of case management feasible, except for geriatric assessment in patients not at high risk. The collaboration of physicians and assistants in teams showed substantial variation. Physicians mentioned a range of role changes in doctor's assistants, including more in-depth medical knowledge and higher responsibilities, yielding more recognition by patients and physicians.

---

organize with busy healthcare professionals or managers. Various methods for group interviews are available that differ from each other in the degree of interaction:

- *Brainstorming*: this method aims to generate ideas about a specified topic. The main rules are that as many different ideas as possible should be generated, including extreme or unfeasible ideas, and no criticism on these ideas is offered during the brainstorming session. After ideas are generated, they are then categorized and prioritized.
- *Focus group interviews*: this method includes four to twelve participants who exchange ideas on two to four topics, facilitated by a group moderator (Morgan 1988). This type of group interview is useful to explore a few topics in depth.
- *Nominal group technique*: this method uses a mix of individual tasks and group tasks to generate and categorize ideas. Individual tasks, usually individuals identifying ideas (when the group is "nominal"), are followed by interactive tasks.
- *Delphi technique*: this method aims to generate consensus on a defined topic, such as the main barriers to improvement. If consensus cannot be achieved, the method can be used to clarify opposing views. Participants complete two or more rounds of questionnaires, in which later rounds include feedback on group views expressed in an earlier round. Participants may meet physically, for instance at the last round, but in some cases they may never meet and may even remain anonymous to each other.

In the context of an international research project (see also Box 9.1), various methods were applied to identify the determinants of implementation (Krause et al. 2014). Brainstorming in groups of healthcare providers was compared with other methods. Ten brainstorming sessions, which involved about 40 participants, generated 194 plausible determinants of implementation. Subsequent structured focus group interviews added another 144 new items. Individual interviews, which had been performed with 50 other healthcare providers in parallel, generated 152 plausible determinants of implementation. Interviews with patients (in two of five countries) produced 63 items. Overall, brainstorming provided the largest number of unique items (items which were not generated by other methods). However, none of the interview methods offered a comprehensive or superior perspective on the determinants of implementation.

9.3 Surveys

Written postal and online surveys are a widely used method to gather insights into the determinants of implementation to be used in the implementation of an innovation, as perceived by health professionals, managers, or patients (see Box 9.6 for an example). Surveys can reach large numbers of individuals at relatively low costs, but achieving high response rates can be a challenge. It is crucial that the questionnaire is well designed: questions should be clear and straightforward and cover all relevant domains to be explored in a study. If questions are taken from questionnaires in a different language, a structured translation procedure should be applied. Pilot testing of a newly developed questionnaire is recommended.

Regardless of the quality of the questionnaire, individuals do not necessarily report about their behaviors in a way that is consistent with objective measures of those measures (e.g. based on patient records or administrative databases; Davis et al. 2006). Motivation or intentions for specific behaviors are moderately associated with actual behavior (Eccles et al. 2006; Godin et al. 2008). A disadvantage of questionnaires is that it is more difficult to explore underlying motivations for answers, but additional free-text response options can go some way toward rectifying this. The main advantage of surveys is that the relevance of a range of potential determinants of implementation can be explored among

---

Box 9.6 Post-operative Prophylaxis for Atrial Fibrillation

All 166 practicing cardiac surgeons in Canada were invited by email to participate in an online survey on prescribing medication for prevention of atrial fibrillation after coronary and cardiac valve surgery (Price et al. 2009). The effectiveness of beta-blockers, among other drugs, has been proven. Different sources were used to make a list of cardiac surgeons. Non-responders were mailed repeatedly and approached by fax and telephone. A total of 119 surgeons completed the online questionnaire (72%). The study found that 58% prescribed beta-blockers routinely, while 42% prescribed these drugs occasionally, rarely, or never (answered on a four-point scale). Among non-prescribers, 44% were not convinced of the efficacy, 12% preferred another therapy, and 7% mentioned side effects. Corticosteroids were never prescribed by 92% of cardiac surgeons, because they felt that the effectiveness was not convincingly shown (75%) and because they anticipated wound infection (39%) and hyperglycemia (30%). When asked about the estimated risk reduction resulting from corticosteroids, 43% said they did not know this and 42% estimated this to be 10% or lower. The remaining 15% mentioned a risk reduction of 20–30%, which is most consistent with clinical research evidence.

large numbers of healthcare professionals, patients, or managers. These factors may be derived from explorative research or theories on change of behaviors and organizations.

9.3.1 Questionnaires about Clinical Guidelines

A specific type of questionnaire focuses on health professionals' views on clinical guidelines. Clinical guidelines contain recommendations for healthcare practice, which are often not (completely) implemented and therefore require change of professional performance. Some questionnaires are about guidelines in general, while others focus on one specific guideline or specific recommendations within a guideline. Questions on guidelines in general provide a view on the overall attitude of a health professional regarding the relevance of scientific evidence underlying clinical decisions. Questions on specific recommendations provide insight into views that may be more closely linked to actual behaviors. Questions may cover a range of aspects, such as knowledge of recommendations, views, and attitudes, or perceived barriers and needs for the implementation of specific recommendations. See Box 9.7 and Table 9.1 for examples.

The validity of perceived barriers to and need for change in professional practice is probably higher if the questions in a questionnaire refer to specific situations in which the new activities have been performed. An interesting method therefore is interviewing care providers or patients shortly after a specific action or event. This is often time consuming, as experiences are collected prospectively over a period of time. An alternative may be to ask for experiences in the recent past (such as the previous month), but a disadvantage of this method is that the greater the time interval, the more the risk that the memory of the respondent may be unreliable. The case-specific questionnaire is most useful when relevant patients present, or events occur, frequently, so that a lot of data can be collected within a short period of time.

9.3.2 Questionnaires on Theory-Based Determinants of Implementation

Theories on (change of) behaviors or organizations suggest a range of potential determinants of performance and change, partly supported by scientific research (see Chapters 2 and 8). Examples are learning style, available resources, and team functioning. A potential advantage of

---

Box 9.7 **Questionnaire for Perceived Barriers to Change**

Comparison of the determinants of implementation across different innovations and settings requires a generic measurement instrument. A validated questionnaire was developed to identify perceived determinants of implementation, and next applied in 12 different implementation studies in the Netherlands (Peters et al. 2003). Literature analyses and focus groups with implementation experts were used to identify possible determinants of implementation. Validation studies were performed to test psychometric characteristics of the questionnaire. A study on the prevention of cardiovascular diseases in primary care practice (n = 329 primary care physicians) showed that perceived barriers, as measured with the questionnaire, explained 39% of the variance in self-reported clinical performance. The questionnaire includes questions on the characteristics of the innovation, the care provider, the patient, and the context. The questions on patients and context particularly focus on the implementation of preventive activities. The findings from three studies are presented in Table 9.1.

Table 9.1 Perceived barriers to change in three studies.

Percentage of professionals perceiving a barrier	Prevention of cardiovascular diseases (n = 190 physicians)	Management of lower urinary tract symptoms in men (n = 40 physicians)	Management of anemia in pregnant women (n = 160 midwives)
Innovation characteristics			
Compatibility	8	83	8
Time investment	52	75	7
Specificity/flexibility	12	70	15
Didactive benefit	11	53	2
Attractiveness	15	68	4
Care provider characteristics			
Attitude/role perception	15	78	6
Knowledge and motivation	13	80	9
Doubts about the innovation	27	80	17
Life style/working style	40	28	12
Education	15	—	—
Involvement	2	55	13
Patient characteristics			
Age	17	—	—
Ethnicity	68	—	—
Financial situation/socio-economic status	52	—	—
Number of patient contacts	62	—	—
Health status	58	—	—
Motivation to change	25	—	8
Context characteristics			
Group norms/socialization	18	58	24
Reimbursement/insurance system	61	68	4
Laws, regulations	34	—	10
Opening hours of practice	27	38	—
Supporting staff	70	—	—
Facilities	22	—	—
Practice building	38	—	—

Source: Data from Peters et al. (2003).

a theory-based approach is that relevant factors are identified (if the theory is valid), which may not have been found in pragmatic or qualitative research. Such a study may contribute to developing the theory as well. Scientific knowledge of the theoretical determinants of implementation in healthcare practice is limited, so that we do not recommend using an exclusively theory-based approach in quality improvement and implementation programs (Wensing et al. 2010).

Box 9.8   Diabetes Care in General Practice

A study with 335 physicians and nurses from 94 British general practices examined which factors were associated with six aspects of performance in patients with diabetes (Presseau et al. 2014). The prediction model included cognitive factors (intention, planning), routines (automated behavior), and individual characteristics (discipline, years of experience). All information was collected through surveys. The multivariate analyses showed that professional performance was influenced by both cognitive factors and routines. For the measurement, the researchers used validated questionnaires related to specific theories.

Questionnaires have been developed for measuring specific theory-based factors, such as factors derived from behavior change theory (see Box 9.8 for an example), including the Team Climate Inventory (for perceived team functioning) and Competing Values Framework (for organizational culture). The Theoretical Domains Framework offers a general theoretical framework for a diagnostic analysis from the perspective of individual behavior change (Michie et al. 2005). It is beyond the scope of this book to give a comprehensive overview of all available theory-based measures. The relevance of such questionnaires depends on the actual impact of measured factors on professional behaviors or aspects of healthcare delivery, and also on the validity of the questionnaire. Theory-based measures are probably most relevant for scientific studies of implementation in healthcare, but they may also be used in pragmatic improvement projects.

9.4   Observation

9.4.1   Routinely Collected Data

Large volumes of data are routinely collected in healthcare for clinical purposes (e.g. in patient records), financial administration, or healthcare development (e.g. clinical registers). The resulting databases have their strengths and weaknesses, which have been discussed in Chapter 7. Secondary analysis of routinely collected data can help to identify gaps in performance, and also to identify determinants of implementation (using multivariate data analysis). For instance, a study used administrative data to determine which factors were associated with the use of imaging tests in patients with acute low back pain in the USA (Pham et al. 2009). The study included 4500 physicians and 35 000 elderly patients with low back pain, of whom one-third had received an imaging test. Among other findings, multivariate analysis in the study showed that this was more frequently the case for physicians in large organizations. Box 9.9 provides another example of the analysis of routinely collected data.

9.4.2   Direct Observation

It is also possible to directly observe events and situations in clinical practice, or other settings, and thus collect data on the determinants of implementation. These determinants may be perceived by study subjects (e.g. observed statements) or be deduced from analysis of the observations (see Box 9.10 for an example). The observer may participate in the normal flow of activities, in that case the method is called "participatory observation," which may be part of a broader ethnographic study. The presence of an observer can influence normal working processes, which is common in training situations but raises the possibility of information bias. There is also the risk that an observer becomes too engaged with study subjects so that observations become biased.

Box 9.9 Organizational Determinants of Quality of Diabetes Care

Data on 11 751 diabetes patients in 354 general practices, which were originally collected for practice accreditation, were used to explore associations between practice organization and health outcomes in diabetes care (blood glucose, blood pressure, cholesterol; Van Doorn-Klomberg et al. 2014). Practice organization was measured on the basis of a questionnaire for participating practices, which documented aspects such as registration of diabetes patients, presence of patient leaflets, and training of practice nurses. An aggregated measure of quality of the practice organizations showed a positive association with blood glucose values (not on glucose or cholesterol values). This observational study confirmed the findings of controlled studies on the effectiveness of organizational changes on the outcomes of diabetes care.

Box 9.10 Participating Observation of Pediatric Cardiac Surgery

This study was based on prospective observations of 102 children who had cardiac surgery (Barach et al. 2008). The process was divided into seven phases: pre-operative care including transport to the operating theater; anesthetic; surgery before cardiac bypass; bypass surgery; transport to intensive care; handover to intensive care. Two researchers observed the whole process and made notes, which were elaborated later by the research team. The surgeon used a head camera, so that the surgical procedures could be followed. Outcomes were measured and the complexity of each patient was assessed. Adverse events were recorded and characterized in terms of type, impact, and mediating actions. The study found an average of 1.2 major adverse events per patient, which mainly occurred directly after bypass surgery. Minor adverse events (15.3 on average) occurred mainly during bypass surgery and were mainly related to coordination and communication. A linear regression analysis showed that higher patient complexity, longer duration of surgery, and more adverse events were all predictive of a higher risk of mortality.

Furthermore, direct observation is time consuming, so its feasibility may be limited. Nevertheless, it can provide data which cannot be easily obtained in any other way.

Table 9.2 provides an overview of methods to identify the determinants of implementation and their advantages and disadvantages.

9.5 Data Analysis

Research on the determinants of implementation does not always provide a clear result and firm guidance for an implementation strategy. In many cases, many factors are identified, of which not all can be addressed in an implementation strategy. The data thus have to be analyzed, categorized, and prioritized. Scientific methods of data analysis can be used, such as regression analysis for quantitative data and framework analysis for qualitative data. Quality management tools can be used to visualize descriptive results, for instance in relation to frequency (paretogram), causes (fishbone diagram), or the care delivery process (flow diagram). Group methods, which were described in previous sections (e.g. the Delphi procedure), can support priority setting.

Table 9.2 Methods to identify determinants of implementation in healthcare.

Method	Advantages	Disadvantages
Interviews	Possibly most useful to identify topic-specific factors Unanticipated factors may also emerge	Perceived determinants may not predict behaviors in reality Added value depends on rigorous data analysis, which is time consuming
Group interviews	Useful to identify a broader range of factors in a shorter time period than interviews with individuals	Group process may bias data Organization of sessions can be difficult if participants are busy
Surveys	Can provides more representative results than interviews Range of factors can be systematically explored	Less effective for identifying factors underlying motivations Getting acceptable response rates is often a challenge
Routinely collected data	Concerns actual behaviors rather than perceptions Impact of factors on behaviors can be quantified	Only a small number of factors can be examined in most cases Cross-sectional studies cannot identify causality
Direct observation	Observes actual behavior Unanticipated factors can be included	Observation may influence the observed reality Method is time consuming

9.5.1 Scientific Methods of Data Analysis

The actual impact of a factor on an outcome (like the process and results of an implementation strategy) cannot be directly observed, but has to be deduced from the analysis of data. The analysis of causal relationships is complex. Here only a few principles and methods are highlighted. Many methods for identification of the determinants of implementation (such as interviews and surveys) provide data on the perceived determinants of implementation. Analysis of such data is either qualitative (e.g. identification of themes in a series of interviews) or quantitatively descriptive (e.g. counting positive answers on a list of items). In some research, advanced methods for the categorization of views are applied (see Box 9.11 for an example). While perceptions do influence behaviors and organizational processes, it remains to be determined whether the factors resulting from interviews or surveys do indeed predict relevant outcomes. This is a particular issue when the proposed innovation is new to the participants (e.g. new information technology) and they lack practical experience with the proposed behavior.

Scientific research on the determinants of implementation often involves a comparison of observed individuals, organizations, or situations of successful implementation with the remaining observations. For this purpose, multivariate analysis techniques may be used, such as regression analysis and other quantitative modeling methods. The scientific validity of the conclusions from such analysis depends on a range of factors, such as the study design (e.g. experimental or observational), explanatory model (e.g. pre-defined or post-hoc developed), and other factors. Scientific training is required to use the methods and interpret findings appropriately.

For practical purposes, it is helpful to distinguish between factors that moderate the impact of an implementation strategy and factors that mediate the effects. Moderating factors are not influenced by the strategies, but specify effects for subgroups in the targeted

---

Box 9.11 Discrete-Choice Experiments to Examine Determinants of Implementation

This study concerned the potential of discrete-choice experiments as a method for identifying determinants of implementation (van Helvoort-Postulart et al. 2009). The study focused on the implementation of a guideline for day surgery for breast cancer. Participants were anesthetists, oncology surgeons, and breast cancer nurses. Twelve key recommendations were identified in the guidelines, and 17 potential determinants for adherence to these recommendations were identified after interviews with a few key informants. Then two methods were used to identify determinants of implementation: a survey among clinicians, which listed the potential determinants with a Likert answering scale to indicate their relevance for the targeted key recommendations; and a discrete-choice experiment, in which determinants (with two levels) were combined in different scenarios and the same participants were asked to rate the probability of implementation in the various scenarios. The participation rate among invited individuals was 10%. The methods resulted in different rankings of determinants, and thus the possibility of the different methods leading to a different choice of improvement intervention. About half of the participants (47%) felt that the discrete-choice experiment was complicated and time consuming.

---

population. For instance, the impact of feedback may differ between younger and older physicians, so "physician age" is a moderating factor. Knowledge of moderating factors helps to specify subgroups and potentially target these differently. Mediating factors are influenced by strategies, because they are part of a causal chain of changes. For instance, an education program enhances knowledge, which leads to behavior change; knowledge is a mediating factor. Knowledge of mediating factors helps to specify a "logic model" of the implementation program and to set short-term targets of an improvement program.

The best evidence for the impact of a factor on an outcome is provided by a well-designed and -conducted experimental study (see Chapter 20) accompanied by a (process) evaluation of working mechanisms (see Chapter 22). In research on quality improvement and implementation programs, the focus is often on comprehensive programs targeted at many goals and intermediate factors at the same time. This makes it difficult to attribute specific changes to specific interventions or contextual factors. Some researchers have suggested so-called modeling studies, in which the effects of

specific mediators and moderators may be explored in an experimental design, using an interim outcome measure (see Box 9.12 for an example).

9.5.2 Quality Improvement Methods

Quality improvement methods for analyzing data on the determinants of implementation describe and categorize determinants in a visual way, using descriptive graphs and figures. They have been developed for improvement projects in healthcare practice rather than for scientific research. Some methods involve statistical methods, which specify the uncertainty of the information. Here three important methods are briefly described: paretograms, fishbone diagrams, and flow charts.

9.5.3 Paretogram

The paretogram is a graph that is based on the idea that a few factors cause most of the problems in many situations. A rule of thumb is that 80% of problems are due to 20% of causes. Therefore, it would be efficient to focus on these main causes. In a paretogram, causes are placed on the x-axis in order of decreasing

---

Box 9.12   Modeling of an Intervention to Improve Antibiotics Prescribing

Using psychological theory, two implementation strategies were developed for improving prescribing of antibiotics by primary care physicians in patients with upper respiratory tract infections (URTIs; Hrisos et al. 2008). Both used a distance-learning approach. The first strategy targeted self-efficacy using the behavior change techniques of graded task, rehearsal, and action planning. The aim of this intervention was to increase the individual's belief in their capabilities to manage URTIs without prescribing antibiotics. The second strategy targeted the constructs of anticipated consequences and risk perception, using techniques from persuasive communication. In a randomized trial, educational packages and questionnaires were mailed to primary care physicians. The questionnaires included questions on behavioral intentions (using a structured format), psychological constructs, and patient scenarios,

with questions on (self-reported) behaviors. Completed questionnaires were returned by 397 (32.4%) physicians. Among these participants, completion of interventions was high. This study with simulated clinical behaviors found that both strategies (thus underlying psychological models) predicted behavior change, but with a differential role of the various psychological determinants. For instance, anticipated consequences had no role in the effect of the first intervention (which targeted self-efficacy), while in the second intervention (persuasive communication) many psychological factors played a role, including self-efficacy. The study provided a scientific rationale for understanding how and why the implementation strategies were effective, thus offering a sound basis for an implementation program in a "real-world" trial.

Box 9.13   Analysis of Determinants of Dissatisfaction in Patients Who Received Endoscopic Tests

A sample of 537 patients who had had an endoscopy or colonoscopy were invited to complete a seven-item questionnaire on their experiences. The responses were presented in a paretogram format (Figure 9.1). This illustrated which questions yielded most expressions of dissatisfaction. Waiting time before

the appointment (I) and not receiving information (II) contributed substantially to overall dissatisfaction (60% of the variation in an aggregated dissatisfaction score). Interventions to improve patient experiences could focus on these aspects of care. Figure 9.1 presents the results in a paretogram.

---

frequency. The *y*-axis presents the frequency of the causes, based on measurement or the perceptions of participants (see Box 9.13 and Figure 9.1; del Rio et al. 2007).

9.5.4   Fishbone Diagram

A fishbone diagram presents potential causes of problems in a number of pre-defined

categories. Problems are usually placed on the right in the diagram, for example suboptimal adherence to guidelines or other innovation. A common classification of causes separately identifies people, resources, materials, and methods (other classifications may also be used). The causes are placed on the left in the diagram (see Box 9.14 and Figure 9.2).

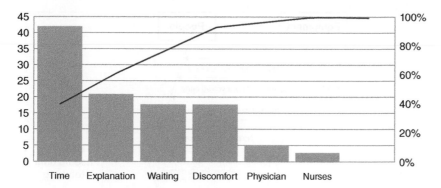

Figure 9.1 Paretogram on determinants of dissatisfaction (proportion of answers "poor" and "fair"). *Source:* Data from del Rio et al. (2007).

Box 9.14	Door-to-Needle Time in Acute Myocardial Infarction

This project aimed to assess and reduce delays in delivering coronary thrombolysis to patients with acute myocardial infarction (AMI; Bonetti et al. 2000). The prognosis of patients with AMI is significantly improved by early thrombolysis. The time interval between hospital admission and the initiation of thrombolytic therapy is referred to as the door-to-needle time (DTNT). A DTNT of 30 minutes was seen as acceptable. During 16 months, the DTNT was recorded of all consecutive patients with AMI receiving intravenous thrombolysis at the intensive care unit. First, DTNTs of 16 patients were documented and compared with the standard of 30 minutes. It showed that the average DTNT was 57 minutes. Then, in an interdisciplinary meeting, a formal process analysis was performed to detect factors that caused delays in in-hospital management. Every participant named the factors for delay that they had personally experienced and the factors were depicted in a fishbone diagram (Figure 9.2).

Factors causing delays were identified in the fields of "communications," "people," and "methods/rules/guidelines." An important finding was an apparent lack of communication – too many people showing up at the bedside, slow coordination, internal medicine staff not arriving on time, and wasting time by not focusing on essentials. The process analysis showed that, after the implementation of new guidelines, mean DTNT was significantly lower than before (now 32 minutes), with much less variability than before.

9.5.5 Flow Chart

A flow chart presents the order of activities of phases in a process visually. They have to be read from left to right or from top to bottom; blocks represent activities or events. The different steps may represent a cause–effect chain, but this is not necessarily so. In many applications, different phases in a process of healthcare delivery are specified. Some clinical guidelines and protocols include such flow charts. In a study of determinants of implementation, barriers and enablers are linked to one or more phases in the flow chart. Implementation strategies should address the determinants of phases in which adherence to recommended procedures is particularly low.

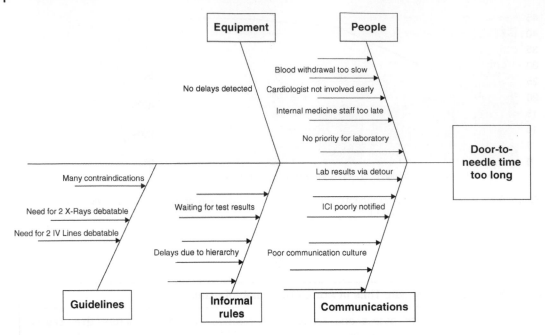

Figure 9.2 Fishbone diagram of figures identified as causing delays to treatment. *Source:* Data from Bonetti et al. (2000).

9.6 Prioritization and Goal Setting

After problems in current healthcare practice have been clearly identified, along with their most important determinants, goals need to be set for an improvement program. Several theories on change in behavior and organizations suggest that goal setting in itself contributes to the effectiveness of improvement programs. Goals should be limited in number, ambitious but not unrealistic, and defined in measurable terms. They should relate to the most relevant outcomes and determinants of implementation that can be influenced by an improvement program. Goals should be defined at two levels: (i) which specific aspects of healthcare practice need to be changed (and also how much change is aimed for); and (ii) which specific determinants of implementation are to be addressed to achieve this (and how much measurable change is aimed for). The linkage between the different goals

of a program should be clarified; for instance, some specific goals may contribute to other, broader goals. Ideally, a logic model is developed, which specifies the linkages between activities and the short- and long-term goals of the program. Participants can be involved in goal setting in similar ways as they can be involved in prioritizing the determinants of implementation, using structured group methods such as the Delphi procedure. Goals for improvement can be tailored to local settings, such as a specific hospital department, a geographical region, or individual physicians. In many cases, goals can be (somewhat) adapted while the program runs, ideally on the basis of intermediate evaluations.

9.7 Conclusions

This chapter has provided an overview of methods to identify and present determinants of the implementation of innovations. Ideally, both in-depth qualitative explorations and large-scale observational studies are used. Interviews and direct observations are particularly useful for in-depth exploration of situations. Surveys and routine data can be used to provide representative information. Both descriptive and visual methods and scientific methods for data

analysis may be useful. The validity and usefulness of methods are areas of ongoing research. For practical purposes, the analysis of the determinants of implementation should provide a clear set of goals for the improvement of healthcare practice, which guides the development of the implementation program.

References

Barach, P., Johnson, J.K., Ahmad, A. et al. (2008). A prospective observational study of human factors, adverse events, and patient outcomes in surgery for pediatric cardiac disease. *J. Thorac. Cardiovasc. Surg.* 136: 1422–1428.

Bonetti, P.O., Waeckerlin, A., Schuepfer, G. et al. (2000). Improving time-sensitive processes in the intensive care unit: the example of "door-to-needle time" in acute myocardial infarction. *Int. J. Qual. Health Care* 12: 311–317.

Cabana, M., Rand, C., Power, N. et al. (1999). Why don't physicians follow clinical practice guidelines. *JAMA* 282: 1458–1465.

Davis, S.A., Mazmanian, P.E., Fordis, M. et al. (2006). Accuracy of physician self-assessment compared with observed measures of competence. A systematic review. *JAMA* 296: 1094–1102.

Eccles, M.P., Hrisos, S., Francis, J. et al. (2006). Do self-reported intentions predict clinicians' behaviour: a systematic review. *Implement. Sci.* 1: 28.

Flottorp, S. and Oxman, A.D. (2003). Identifying barriers and tailoring interventions to improve the management of urinary tract infections and sore throat: a pragmatic study using qualitative methods. *BMC Health Serv. Res.* 3: 3.

Godin, G., Bélanger-Gravel, A., Eccles, M., and Grimshaw, J. (2008). Healthcare professionals' intentions and behaviours: a systematic review of studies based on social cognitive theories. *Implem Sci* 3: 36.

van Helvoort-Postulart, D., van der Weijden, T., Dellaert, B. et al. (2009). Investigating the complementary value of discrete choice experimentation for the evaluation of

barriers and facilitators in implementation research: a questionnaire survey. *Implement. Sci.* 4: 10.

Hrisos, S., Eccles, M., Johnston, M. et al. (2008). Developing the content of two behavioural interventions: using theory-based interventions to promote GP management of upper respiratory tract infection without prescribing antibiotics #1. *BMC Health Serv Res* 8: 11.

Krause, J., Van Lieshout, J., Klomp, R. et al. (2014). Identifying determinants of care for tailoring implementation in chronic diseases: an evaluation of different methods. *Implement. Sci.* 9: 102.

Michie, S., Johnston, M., Abraham, C. et al. (2005). Making psychological theory useful for implementing evidence based practice: a consensus approach. *Qual Saf Health Care* 14: 26–33.

Morgan, D.L. (1988). *Focus Groups as Qualitative Research*. Beverly Hills, CA: Sage.

Peters, M.A.J., Harmsen, M., Laurant, M.G.H., and Wensing, M. (2003). *Ruimte voor verandering? Knelpunten en mogelijkheden voor verbeteringen in de patiëntenzorg (Room for Change? Barriers and Facilitators for Improvements in Patient Care)*. Nijmegen: WOK.

Peters-Klimm, F., Olbort, R., Campbell, S. et al. (2009). Physicians' view of primary care-based case management for patients with heart failure: a qualitative study. *Int J Qual Health Care.* 21: 363–371.

Pham, H.H., Landon, B.E., Rechovsky, J.D. et al. (2009). Rapidity and modality of imaging for acute low back pain in elderly patients. *Arch. Intern. Med.* 169: 972–981.

Presseau, J., Johnston, M., Heponiemi, T. et al. (2014). Reflective and automatic processes in health care professional behaviour: a dual process model tested across multiple behaviours. *Ann. Behav. Med.* 48: 347–358.

Price, J., Tee, R., Lam, B.K. et al. (2009). Current use of prophylactic strategies for postoperative atrial fibrillation: a survey of Canadian cardiac surgeons. *Ann. Thorac. Surg.* 88: 106–111.

del Rio, A.S., Baudet, J.S., Fernandez, O.A. et al. (2007). Evaluation of patient satisfaction in gastrointestinal endoscopy. *Eur. J. Gastroenterol. Hepatol.* 19: 896–900.

Schouten, J.A., Hulscher, M.J.E.L., Natsch, S. et al. (2007). Barriers to optimal antibiotic use for community-acquired pneumonia at hospitals: a qualitative study. *Qual. Saf. Health Care* 16: 143–149.

Van Doorn-Klomberg, A., Braspenning, J., Wolters, R. et al. (2014). Organisational determinants of high-quality routine diabetes care. *Scand. J. Prim. Health Care* 32: 124–131.

Wensing, M., Bosch, M., and Grol, R. (2010). The knowledge to action cycle: developing and selecting knowledge to action interventions. *CMAJ* 182: E85–E88.

Wensing, M., Oxman, A., Baker, R. et al. (2011). Tailored implementation for chronic diseases (TICD): a project protocol. *Implement. Sci.* 6: 103.

Part V

Strategies for Change

10

Selection of Strategies for Improving Patient Care

Richard Grol[1,2] and Michel Wensing[3,4,5]

[1] *Radboud University, Nijmegen, The Netherlands*
[2] *Maastricht University, Maastricht, The Netherlands*
[3] *Faculty of Medicine, University of Heidelberg, Heidelberg, Germany*
[4] *Department of General Practice and Health Services Research, Heidelberg University Hospital, Heidelberg, Germany*
[5] *Department IQ healthcare, Radboud Institute for Health Sciences, Radboud University Medical Center, Nijmegen, The Netherlands*

SUMMARY

- There are numerous strategies (interventions and policies) for implementing innovations and improving healthcare, including professional-oriented strategies, patient-oriented strategies, financial measures, organizational changes, regulations, and laws.

- No strategy is superior or predictably effective. Which strategies are applied should be based on a rigorous analysis of barriers to and enablers of change, and a systematic use of the results of this analysis in the selection of implementation strategies.

- In selecting interventions, consideration must be given to:

  - Results of the "diagnostic analysis" of the target group and the setting of the implementation.
  - The full range of available implementation strategies, for which several classifications have been proposed.
  - Phases in the process of change and segments in the targeted population.
  - The available research evidence on the effectiveness of strategies.

10.1 Introduction

Ideally, implementation strategies which correspond as closely as possible to the results of a "diagnostic analysis" will be chosen and enacted. While this may seem logical, it is often not the case in practice (see Box 10.1). Individuals may become attached to a single, familiar intervention, such as educational refresher courses or financial incentives, which they apply in all situations. Underlying such a choice are implicit ideas concerning the most important bottlenecks in implementation (such as a

lack of knowledge or response to payment) that may not be uniformly true. However, tailoring interventions is not a straightforward process, since there is no unique match between barriers identified and possible strategies to overcome them. For instance, refresher courses can enhance knowledge but also change attitudes. Attitudes, however, may be changed more effectively by persuasive communication from a credible expert, offering an attractive perspective or providing compelling evidence.

A range of approaches and methods has been used to design interventions to change

---

Box 10.1   Tailored Implementation Interventions

A systematic review analyzed 20 studies of implementation strategies with respect to which methods were used to identify barriers and facilitators and to tailor interventions (Bosch et al. 2007). Methods used to identify barriers were mostly qualitative, such as focus groups and face-to-face interviews with healthcare providers. The fact that a prospective barriers analysis was performed did not necessarily imply that the intervention selected was based on the barriers identified. In many studies, it appeared that the choice of intervention had already been made. Further, methods for tailoring interventions were rarely described explicitly. The results also suggested there was often a mismatch between the type of barriers identified and the choice of interventions; for example, educational interventions were often selected for those studies indicating organizational barriers. In addition, half of the studies involving improvement interventions with at least one organizational component reported no organizational barriers to change. There were no obvious differences in methods used between studies selecting purely educational strategies and studies also incorporating organizational interventions.

Box 10.2   Designing Interventions

A systematic review conducted by Colquhoun et al. (2017), aimed at identifying published methods for designing interventions to change health professionals' behavior, screened 64 full-text papers to yield 15 papers. The papers were characterized, for example, with respect to the level of change (aimed at individuals or organizations), the context of development, and the methods used. Barrier identification was included 13 papers and explicit linking of barriers to intervention components in 13, but not the same 13. The use of theory and user engagement were included in 13 papers. The authors conclude that there is agreement about four tasks to be completed when designing individual-level improvement interventions: identifying barriers, selecting intervention components, using theory, and engaging end-users.

---

professional behavior in healthcare (see Box 10.2). As yet, evidence regarding the added value of tailoring interventions to barriers for implementation is limited (Baker et al. 2015; Wensing 2017). In a study among implementation researchers and health practitioners, few consistent associations were found between barriers for implementation and prioritized implementation strategies (Waltz et al. 2019). Nevertheless, it is highly plausible that tailored interventions are more likely effective. In any improvement program, the choice and design of strategies should be a comprehensive and balanced process, and ideally, strategies need to be piloted on a small scale before undertaking large-scale efforts. This chapter aims to provide guidance for selecting and developing strategies for change and ensuring they match the characteristics of the innovation, target groups, and setting to create the most effective intervention possible (Figure 10.1).

10.2   Methods to Select and Develop Implementation Strategies

Guidance for the development of complex interventions, such as implementation strategies, has

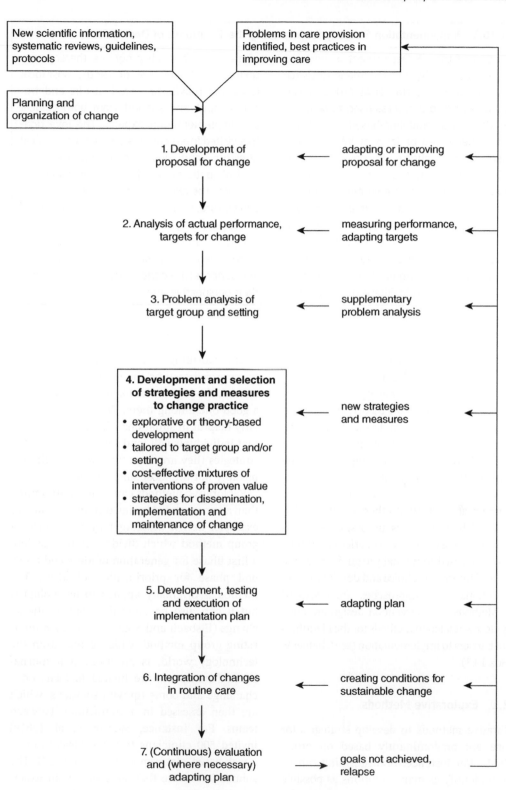

Figure 10.1 The Grol and Wensing implementation of change model.

Box 10.3   Implementation Strategy for Improving the Treatment of Depression

As a part of the US Department of Veterans Affairs (VA) Quality Enhancement Research Initiative (QUERI), Curran et al. (2008) developed and studied a process used to facilitate the adoption of guideline-based practices in treating depressed patients at VA substance abuse disorder clinics. In developing the implementation strategy, the investigators identified several pre-intervention conditions necessary for successful implementation. They included the presence of frameworks to guide intervention development and data collection, an evaluation strategy that would provide local, meaningful data, a partnership with clinical staff to facilitate the adaptation of materials for their programs, thereby contextualizing the intervention at the most local level and maximizing staff buy-in, and frequent input and support from both clinical and implementation experts. The investigators visited intervention sites, met with clinical directors, and posed questions regarding clinical policies. Additionally, investigators observed the existing organizational structure and culture, noting formal and informal structures, reporting relationships, staffing, social networks, and more. Also, the study team interviewed many program staff members and patients to see the barriers to change from their perspective and assess their readiness.

---

emphasized development as a dynamic iterative process, involving stakeholders, reviewing published research evidence, drawing on existing theories, articulating program theory, undertaking primary data collection, understanding context, paying attention to future implementation in the real world, and designing and refining an intervention using iterative cycles of development with stakeholder input throughout (O'Cathain et al. 2019). As there is little understanding of how strategies are best chosen, this process is often explorative. Theories and frameworks can be used additionally to guide the exploration and inform the choice and development of interventions. Both approaches are discussed here. Methods for intervention design are obviously closely related to methods for the identification of barriers to implementation (see Chapter 9; see Box 10.3).

10.2.1   Explorative Methods

Explorative methods to develop strategies for change are predominantly based on group methods. For instance, brainstorming can be used to identify as many solutions as possible to a certain problem. The underlying premise in brainstorming is that quantity of items leads to increased quality: the more suggestions are offered, the higher the likelihood that there is a good one among them. This can be particularly helpful in situations where there is a risk that individuals will tend simply to choose the strategies they are most familiar with, though possibly not the most suitable ones.

Explorative methods can be more structured than an open-ended brainstorming session. For example, *design thinking* may be applied: a group method which divides the process into a first phase for generation of ideas and a second phase for prioritization of ideas. The method is originally applied to technologies, but it can also be applied to organizational change (Elsbach and Stigliani 2018). An interesting group method, which comes from the technology world, is an innovation tournament. Participants are invited to focus on a challenge and come up with solutions, which are then assessed in a competition between teams. For instance, Stewart et al. (2019) invited 500 clinicians to share ideas through a web-based platform ("crowdsourcing"). The submissions were then assessed by an expert panel, involving behavioral scientists, system leaders, and payers. In a final event, six winning ideas were presented to an audience of clinicians and organizational leaders.

Another method is *intervention mapping*, which has its origins in the field of health education and promotion (see Box 10.4; Bartholomew et al. 1998, 2001), a process that has also been applied for the design of strategies to implement innovations (Van Bokhoven et al. 2003). The main benefits of structured approaches may be that more relevant aspects and steps are addressed, and they increase the transparency

---

Box 10.4   Intervention Mapping

An example of a structured, step-wise method to arrive at a selection of interventions, coupled to important factors, comes from the health promotion field – the "intervention mapping" method. It offers a process to turn the results from a diagnostic analysis into a concrete program for change. The process also appears to be suitable for the development or selection of interventions aimed at implementing changes in healthcare. The following steps are usually taken (Bartholomew et al. 1998, 2001):

- *Needs assessment*: the healthcare problem is phrased in terms of behaviors that need to be changed and targets that need to be reached.
- *Specifying determinants of (current) practice*: determinants that may influence practice are identified.
- *Developing matrices of proximal program objectives*: determinants and performance objectives are then mapped in a matrix. The cells of the matrix contain the behavioral elements that are needed to change a particular factor. This matrix is the intervention map and forms the basis of further work to develop the interventions.
- *Consider theoretical methods and practical strategies*: potentially suitable strategies to overcome the different barriers are then studied (for example, using an analysis of the literature or brainstorm technique).
- *Design the program*: various strategies are organized into a deliverable program with discrete components and mechanisms of delivery. The draft program is then

pre-tested in representatives of the target group that have not been involved in the development.

- *Monitoring and program evaluation*: to study if and how the targets are reached.

Schmid et al. (2010) used intervention mapping to develop an evidence-based secondary stroke program locally tailored to two healthcare facilities in a national organization. The process helped to support the implementation of existing stroke prevention tools into practice. The needs assessment included semi-structured interviews with the targeted users of the program: 44 clinical providers of stroke care, working in either facility. The structured interviews covered current provider practices in secondary stroke risk management, barriers, and needs to support risk factor management, and suggestions about how to enhance secondary risk stroke management throughout the continuum of care. Performance objectives were based on the secondary stroke guidelines, and included items such as the assessment of patient risk factors during hospitalization for stroke, and the ordering of investigations. Change objective statements were identified and added. Next, theory-based and practical strategies identified in the interviews were mapped. The previous steps were combined to design and organize the implementation program. The intervention was then tailored to meet local needs and interests. Subsequently it was decided how to track and monitor the delivery and use of the program, before the program was actually evaluated.

Box 10.5   Use of the Theory of Planned Behavior to Reduce Antibiotics Prescribing

Despite evidence demonstrating that antibiotics are ineffective in patients with an uncomplicated viral sore throat, and the fact that prescribing them in these cases contributes to antibiotic resistance at the population level, many primary care physicians continue to prescribe them. In this study (Walker et al. 2001), a search of the literature, as well as observations of and interviews with physicians, was conducted to design questionnaires that were sent to a random sample of 185 physicians in one region in the UK. The theory of planned behavior (TPB) was used to measure the strength of intention of physicians to prescribe antibiotics, as well as other variables described by the theory, such as attitudes regarding prescription,

perceived consequences, perceived behavioral control, and previous prescription behavior. The questionnaire was returned by two-thirds of the sample. The majority of physicians intended to prescribe fewer antibiotics in this patient group. TPB variables explained 48% of the variation in intention, while previous prescription behavior explained an additional 15%. The authors concluded that attitudes regarding prescribing and perceived behavioral control were important determinants of intention, and therefore strategies to reduce the prescription of antibiotics could be aimed at persuading physicians of the importance of reducing antibiotics and increasing their self-efficacy.

---

of the process. An obvious disadvantage is that they require more resources. Also, they do not provide guidance on which interventions may be used to address specific barriers and facilitators for change. In other words, they provide a structure and a method, but no guidance on the content.

10.2.2   Theory-Based Methods

Currently, hardly any fully systematic method exists for selecting and developing implementation strategies based on theories of change. An exception may be a framework for behavior change techniques, which links psychological interventions for individual behavior change to psychological determinants of behavior (Michie et al. 2013). While this has been primarily developed for change in health-related behaviors, it can also be used for behavior change in health professionals. It does not, however, well address the organizational constraints, which are typical for most healthcare professionals. Factors related to working in teams, to the organization in which the professionals practice, and to the health system may, in some cases, have

a larger impact on change processes (Ferlie and Shortell 2001; Grol 2010). A wide range of theories may be helpful in gaining insight into factors related to these higher levels, as discussed in Chapter 2 (Wensing et al. 2005; Grol et al. 2007). Most theories, however, provide only global ideas on the linkages between interventions and barriers. A "common-sense" approach to the use of such theories would be to use the theoretical concepts to guide the selection of strategies in a reflective process. If one knows which determinants may influence the change process, theory can then be used to hypothesize which strategies may influence changes in these determinants (Eccles et al. 2005). Boxes 10.5 and 10.6 provide examples of such a "theory-informed" approach.

10.3   Classification of Implementation Strategies

The literature provides a wide variety of strategies to implement change in professional behavior and healthcare delivery. Varying in

---

Box 10.6   Use of the Theory of Planned Behavior to Change Disclosure of Dementia

Foy et al. (2007) developed an intervention to promote appropriate disclosure of a diagnosis of dementia using a theoretical and empirical framework. To do so, they identified three key disclosure behaviors: finding out what the patient already knows or suspects about the diagnosis; using the words "dementia" or "Alzheimer's disease" when talking to the patient; and exploring what the diagnosis means to the patient. They subsequently conducted a survey of older people's mental health teams (MHTs) based upon theoretical constructs from the theory of planned behavior and social cognitive theory and used the findings to identify factors that

predicted mental health professionals' intentions to perform each behavior and selected behavior change strategies likely to alter these factors. The change strategies selected were persuasive communication to target subjective norms; behavioral modeling and graded tasks to target self-efficacy; persuasive communication to target the attitude to the use of explicit terminology when talking to the patient; and behavioral modeling by MHTs to target perceived behavioral control for finding out what the patient already knows or suspects, and exploring what the diagnosis means to the patient.

---

scope and complexity, they range from sending printed materials to care providers by mail to redesigning entire multidisciplinary care processes or providing financial incentives to stimulate the performance of desired behaviors. Different ways to categorize these methods exist. One is the taxonomy of the Effective Practice and Organization of Care Group (EPOC), used for Cochrane reviews. The first version was published in 1999 (Thorsen and Mäkelä 1999) and updated versions have been published since then. The 2015 version of the taxonomy (EPOC 2015) makes a distinction between four domains of strategies:

a) *Delivering arrangements*: changes in how, when, and where care is delivered and by whom.

b) *Financial arrangements*: changes in the way funds are collected, people are insured, healthcare services are paid, and financial incentives are used.

c) *Governance arrangements*: regulations or processes that influence authority and accountability in healthcare.

d) *Healthcare worker strategies*: interventions that target healthcare workers' performance, using information and communication strategies.

Note that category (d) is actually labeled implementation strategies, but strategies for implementation of change can be found across all four domains.

Other implementation scientists have undertaken complementary and alternative efforts to define and categorize interventions to improve healthcare practice (e.g. Mazza et al. 2013; Kastner et al. 2015). For instance, Michie et al. (2011) described a comprehensive framework for behavior change, which links policy categories (e.g. guidelines, legislation) to intervention functions (education, persuasion, incentivization, coercion, training, enablement, modeling, restructuring, restrictions) and sources of behavior (motivation, capability, opportunity). An international group compared and integrated four existing taxonomies, including the EPOC taxonomy (Colquhoun et al. 2014). The group developed a new framework, which consists of four components: strategies and techniques (active ingredients); how they work (causal mechanisms); how they are applied (mode of delivery); and at what targets they focus (Bragge et al. 2017). A similar exercise took place in the USA in the ERIC project (Powell et al. 2015). A panel of experts was involved in a Delphi procedure, in which a new list of discrete implementation interventions was developed. The process resulted in a list of 73 different interventions, including a number for the preparation of implementation programs. A final example is Leeman et al. (2017), who proposed a different classification of implementation strategies, making a distinction between five classes of strategies: dissemination strategies, implementation process strategies, integration strategies, capacity-building strategies, and scale-up strategies.

A different approach to the classification of implementation strategies is focused on the degree of facilitation (assuming internal motivation to change) and direction (assuming that external pressure is needed for change; Grol 1992). To a certain extent, it is possible to rank existing strategies on a scale that ranges from educational and facilitating methods to controlling and compulsory methods, as perceived by the targeted individuals (see Figure 10.2).

In summary, different frameworks for classification of strategies for the implementation of change exist and it seems likely that further proposals can be expected in the coming years. It is recommended to use one or more of the available frameworks to consider the full range of possibilities in strategies for improving healthcare.

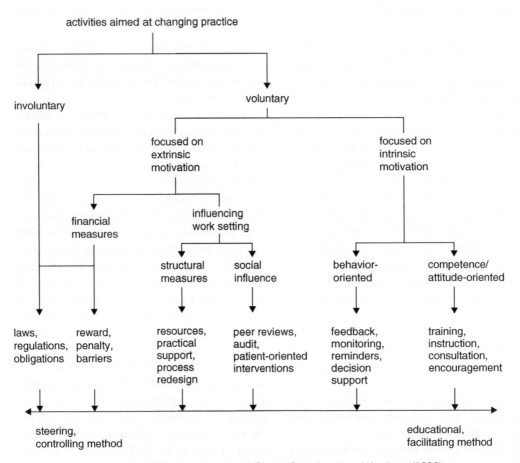

Figure 10.2 Methods for implementing change. *Source:* Data from van Woerkom (1990).

10.4 Implementation Strategies in the Different Phases of Change

Another way to arrange, plan, and describe strategies and interventions for the implementation of change is to use the perspective of the target group and link that to the different phases in the change process that individuals and groups have to go through (Grol and Wensing 2004; see Chapter 3). Those who are not familiar with, or are not interested in, the innovation require a different approach to those who are familiar with it, but do not believe that it can be accomplished successfully. If one is willing, but encounters problems in establishing the change in the normal care processes in one's own team or practice, other approaches may be needed. Since different subgroups are usually in different phases of the process of change, a combination of different strategies is often desirable. Examples of possible interventions are given in Table 10.1.

Table 10.1 Implementation strategies in different phases of the change process of the target group.

Steps and possible barriers to change	Possible strategies
1) Orientation	
• Not familiar (the provider does not read, has little relevant contact with colleagues) • No interest (the provider sees no need, does not think it is relevant)	Brief messages via all communication channels, approach key figures and networks Attention-catching brochure, personal approach and explanation, confrontation with own performance
2) Insight	
• No knowledge or understanding; information too complex or extensive • No insight or overestimation of own performance	Useful instruction materials, concise messages, information based on problems in practice, regular repetition Audit, peer review, and feedback
3) Acceptance	
• Negative attitude (sees disadvantages, doubts about developers or feasibility, not feeling involved) • Not prepared to change (doubts about success and own possibilities)	Adapt innovation to wishes of target group, local discussion and consensus, discuss resistance, good scientific arguments, involve key individuals and opinion leaders Demonstrate feasibility by colleagues, inventory of bottlenecks and seeking solutions, change plans with feasible objectives
4) Change	
• Has not started (provider lacks time, materials, ability; innovation does not fit in existing care procedures) • Insufficient success with attempts to change	Extra resources, support, training in skills, redevelopment of care processes, bringing in temporary support or consultants, information materials for patients, plan with feasible objectives
5) Maintenance	
• Innovation not integrated in routines (relapse, forgetting) • Innovation not embedded or supported in organization	Monitoring, feedback, and reminder systems, integration in care plans and protocols Providing resources, support from top management, organizational measures, rewards, payment for certain tasks

10.4.1 Orientation

- *Promote awareness of the innovation*: Care providers must first come into contact with an innovation and become aware that it is available. This step can fail simply because those concerned do not read the book, journal, or online platform in which the information is published, do not attend courses, or have little relevant contact with colleagues. Such individuals may read selectively and only take in information that confirms their own ideas, rather than being open to new ones if there is no immediate sense of urgency. In this situation, other ways are needed (via mass media, social media, or personal contacts, for example) to inform care providers not reached via the usual channels to trigger them to consider the innovation. In particular, a personal, attractively designed mailing and the involvement of colleagues and key figures from the individual's surroundings, who could make direct contact, would be appropriate strategies.
- *Stimulate interest and involvement*: the implementation must also generate interest among those in the target group, stimulating them to want to know more. This can be difficult if the subject is not seen as relevant and if the design of the information is not attractive or does not make it readily understood, so that the reader is not encouraged to explore it further. Equally problematic is a situation in which the information is not presented from the perspective or interests of the target group and is thus not recognized as being relevant for daily practice. The manner in which information is presented should address these issues. This can be accomplished by simple, quickly digested printed materials or computerized messages, or by discussion of the problems in care delivery during meetings of the care providers concerned. Engaging end-users in the design of the information may help to develop better materials. An enthusiastic report about the innovation by those who have already worked with it can also be helpful.

10.4.2 Insight and Understanding

- *Create understanding*: The target group must not only be interested in the new procedure or proposal for improvement, but must also understand what it involves and the arguments behind it. Care providers should know exactly what is expected from them and why it is important. This can be a problem if they do not have enough background knowledge or experience to understand the information. A presentation that is too technical, too abstract, or too detailed can also be a hindrance to understanding. Finally, what is learned can also quickly be forgotten. While it is important to provide good information and instructional materials or well-organized and short presentations on courses and deal with the translation of the central message to everyday practice, such messages must also be repeated in order to achieve full understanding and to prevent the information from being forgotten. This may need to happen many times and be offered in such a way (by printed, computerized messages and other means) that knowledge can be refreshed very quickly.
- *Develop insight into current practice*: to achieve change, it is often not sufficient for the individual to know exactly what must be done and how it must be done. Individuals must also examine their performance and see where improvement is needed. They should see where their routines differ from a proposal for change and accept that a change is necessary or desirable. Lacking objective performance data, many care providers overestimate their own performance or are unable to reflect critically on their own way of working. Manageable and acceptable methods are necessary to help them over this. Audit and feedback methods relating to the performance of the practice, self-assessment tools, peer review methods, and simple systems for continuous monitoring of care can be used to detect possible problems in care delivery and to offer practice benchmarks.

10.4.3 Acceptance

- *Develop a positive attitude to change*: at this stage, individuals in the target group need to carefully evaluate the advantages and disadvantages of the new way of working and decide their attitude to the innovation. This evaluation may be negative if individuals see more disadvantages than advantages (in terms of effectiveness, demands, or financial consequences), consider the change unfeasible in their own work setting, doubt the scientific basis of the proposed change, or question the credibility or expertise of those who developed the innovation. The change may also be disregarded if it is seen as having originated elsewhere and the target group does not feel that it has been sufficiently involved in the development. The type of attitudes that are relevant initially (e.g. evidence on clinical effectiveness and costs) may be different from those that influence whether to pursue implementation in a later phase (e.g. personal and patient experiences with the change). This process cannot be easily handled in writing; engaging participants in arguments for and against the innovation is a more effective method of addressing these issues. Resistance should be discussed seriously and openly, the arguments for changing must be adequately demonstrated, and the opportunity should be offered to adapt the process of changing to the situation and needs of the target group. For this, respected colleagues can be brought in who have already had a positive experience with the innovation and can describe its advantages as well as possible limitations.
- *Create positive intentions or decisions to change*: if an opinion about the change has been formed, the next step is a firm commitment to carry it through in practice. In organized settings, the initial decision to implement a change may be taken by a team leader or manager for a group of care providers. It is possible to be in favor of a change and yet be unable to see exactly how things can or should be other than the way they are, or to have little confidence in one's own ability to really begin doing otherwise. Specific resistance may also be anticipated from patients, colleagues, directors, or financiers. Further, problems may be foreseen in the organization or resources needed for the change that will make implementation difficult. The expected problems in introducing the change should therefore be carefully considered (see Chapter 8), and specific solutions for these problems sought. This might include a demonstration of others' experience with the innovation and insights into the costs, investments, and outcomes so that those who will have to use it can see that it is feasible. Finally, the change can be divided into simple, manageable steps that, taken in succession, offer the assurance that they are all feasible; a usable plan for the change with achievable objectives can be a useful aid.

10.4.4 Change

- *Try out the change in practice*: the next move is to the real change in performance. The essential step here is to actually try out the innovation, the pathway, or the new program and see whether its introduction is possible. Necessary skills may be lacking, and therefore specific training may be needed. Equally important, a trial period may reveal organizational problems that have yet to be resolved. Local organizations and the temporary help of experts can support individuals through this. What is important is that the change can be tried out without great risks and consequences before widespread implementation.
- *Confirm the benefit and value of change*: a formal evaluation can convince the target group that change is possible and that it brings the anticipated advantages. Failing this, there will be a quick return to the former ways of working. Collecting data and providing feedback about the achieved improvements,

as well as documenting any positive reactions from patients and providers, can support the motivation to continue during this phase. If this innovation requires partial adjustments, this may motivate individuals to embrace and implement it.

10.4.5 Maintenance

- *Integrate the new practice into routines*: if it is found to be useful, the new procedure will have to be integrated into existing care protocols or pathways, care plans, and work routines, since individuals can easily fall back into former ways of working. After a vacation, for example, one forgets how things were or precisely how they had to be done. Appropriate strategies may then be needed to assist the care provider, team, or care organization through such a period and to stabilize the change. One can consider regular monitoring and feedback on the desired method, reminders about its application, or rewards for achievement of agreed objectives. It may be particularly important to revise the entire care process of which the new procedure is now a part, to incorporate the change in the multidisciplinary care processes in a practice or hospital and to monitor its use.
- *Embed the new practice in the organization*: the last step is for the new procedure to be completely incorporated in, and supported by, the care organization so that its continuing application is possible. This might mean embedding the innovation in the reimbursement system, in budget agreements, in institutional policies, and possibly in regulations and laws. In general, the organizational, structural, and financial conditions must be such that they support the embedding of the new procedure in the organization or practice. This requires attention to the organizational culture, leadership involvement (administrators, managers, directors, and clinical leaders) in the innovation, and cooperation between disciplines and departments.

10.5 Subgroups within the Target Group

As noted in earlier chapters, *subgroups* within the target group can differ with regard to needs, characteristics, and barriers and incentives to change. Some groups may not understand or may oppose a specific change in routines, while other groups are struggling to master the new procedure. Different subgroups can thus need different approaches. In Chapter 3, for example, a distinction was made among "innovators," the "middle majority," and "laggards" (Rogers 2003). It has been suggested that different groups have different motives for changing and thus require a different approach (see Table 10.2).

Innovators may be adequately served by scientifically sound information obtained via

Table 10.2 Approach to different groups in the introduction of innovations.

	Innovators	Middle majority	Laggards
Motivation to change	Intrinsic, seeing the advantages	Belonging to a group, relation to others	Extrinsic, coercion, economic pressure
Effective influence	Aimed at cognition	Aimed at attitude	Aimed at behavior
Methods	Good information, credible sources, written methods	Personal sources, opinion leaders, activities with colleagues, feedback from colleagues	Regulations and agreements, rewards and sanctions, help with practical problems, clear leadership

Source: Data from Green et al. (1989); Grol (1992); Rogers (2003).

journals, online platforms, and qualified refresher courses. Those in the middle majority are more likely to respond to influences in their professional network, including the opinion of respected colleagues who introduce the new procedures or insights and translate them to their own local situation. The middle majority is also sensitive to the social pressure arising out of activities with colleagues (quality collaboratives, team discussion, mutual agreements, peer review, small-scale education in which opinion leaders introduce new guidelines or new working methods, local consensus meetings, etc.). Those in the third group, the "laggards," are relatively insensitive to these social influences, partly because they are inclined to go their own way. They have to be won over by an extra effort in the form of practical support or material reward, or if necessary by pressure, such as a statement of the official "standard," or by formal regulations or financial incentives from responsible managers or purchasers of healthcare.

10.6 The Effectiveness of Different Strategies and Interventions

There are many strategies that can be used for improving healthcare. The possibilities and research evidence for effectiveness will be elaborated in some detail in subsequent chapters. In short, the following lessons can be drawn:

- All strategies for implementation and improvement show variable effects and none is consistently effective in all target groups and settings.
- It seems plausible that multifaceted strategies are most effective – because they can address more barriers for change than single strategies – but research on this topic showed mixed findings.
- The effects of implementation strategies on professional behavior and healthcare delivery tend to be small to moderate, but such changes can still be relevant.

- A range of factors associated with the effects of implementation strategies have been identified, but further research is required to predict the effects more reliably.
- Given the current state of knowledge, it remains crucial to evaluate any implementation or improvement program, and to use the evaluation to optimize the approach.

The published body of scientific research on implementation strategies is large, which can be overwhelming. For instance, an estimated number of several thousand randomized trials of implementation and improvement strategies in healthcare has been published in the international scientific literature. Finding a way through this literature can be challenge for health professionals, managers, policy makers, as well as scientists, particularly if they have a primary focus on other domains (e.g. public health or a clinical discipline). It is generally recommended that decision makers focus on the full body of relevant research, rather than single studies, and this is no different for research on implementation and quality improvement. A good starting point is the systematic reviews of the EPOC Group in the Cochrane Collaboration; currently about 150 reviews have been published in the Cochrane Library. They focus on specific modes of intervention delivery (e.g. "educational material"), broad categories of professional behavior (e.g. "prescribing medication"), or settings (e.g. "low-income countries"). Many journals publish relevant systematic reviews as well, some of which are of good quality.

It can be challenging to assess the applicability of findings from a study in a specific setting, target group, and historical point in time to the setting, target group, and time that are relevant to a decision maker. Organizational context, history, and culture influence the adoption and outcomes of quality improvement and implementation strategies. For instance, research on pay-for-performance schemes for health providers or monitoring of patient-reported outcomes in a specific region or health system in the USA may not be generalizable to other regions or systems. Therefore, studies that focused on the target group and targeted setting are often considered to be most relevant. Decision makers must find a balance between such a legitimate focus on "local research" and the international body of evidence. This is straightforward if the two are consistent with each other, but challenging if there are major differences in results.

A further consideration is the cost and efficiency of the interventions; more expensive is not necessarily always better. For instance, it is reasonable to suppose that multifaceted interventions will cost more to deliver and, therefore, for a given effect will be less efficient. Changes in the reimbursement of care providers can be associated with substantial costs. When there is a limited budget for implementation, the choice of strategy will also be influenced by considerations of efficiency. There may be occasions where it is more cost-effective to use a less costly, but also less effective intervention rather than a costly, but marginally more effective one.

10.7 Conclusions

In this chapter, we focused on the selection of strategies for quality improvement and implementation of innovations. A wide variety of options is available, which have been classified in different ways. Most importantly, the need was emphasized to link the choice of strategies to a diagnostic analysis of barriers for implementation. In many cases, several interventions are required to address different phases of the change process and different segments of the target population. There is now a large body of research evidence, but its application to a given population and setting can be challenging. Besides the selection of strategies, it is equally important to design their components carefully (see Box 10.7). For instance, continuing professional education is highly variable with respect to its components. The design of implementation strategies and evidence on effectiveness will be elaborated for different types of strategies in Chapters 11–18.

Box 10.7 Improving Care in Nursing Homes

The challenge in improving healthcare is that while most improvers appreciate the importance of carefully designing an improvement intervention, they rarely do so. In a paper by Marshall et al. (2017), the authors described how they designed an intervention to improve the safety of people living in care homes and how the failure to design a better intervention from the start reduced the overall impact. The aim was to reduce the prevalence of falls, pressure ulcers, and urinary tract infections in 90 care homes and to reduce unnecessary attendances at the Emergency Department and admissions to the hospital. An improvement program included benchmarking, learning improvement skills, and awareness of the safety culture in the care homes. The program was based on theory, empirical evidence, and the experience of the developers. The evaluation found, however, that most of the intervention components were not completely implemented as planned and that changes measured were small. Reflection on this lack of success resulted in various ways in creating more effective improvement interventions, among them the use of theories to optimize the design, the fact that improvement efforts are usually evaluated too early in their development, and the need for a more active process of co-design of improvement initiatives, involving service users, practitioners, improvers, and academics.

References

Baker, R., Camosso-Stefinovic, J., Gillies, C. et al. (2015). Tailored interventions to address determinants of practice. *Cochrane Database Syst. Rev.* (4): CD005470. https://doi.org/10.1002/14651858.

Bartholomew, L.K., Parcel, G.S., and Kok, G. (1998). Intervention mapping: a process for developing theory- and evidence-based health education programs. *Health Educ. Behav.* 25: 543–563.

Bartholomew, L.K., Parcel, G.S., Kok, G., and Gottlieb, N.H. (2001). *Intervention Mapping: Designing Theory- and Evidence-Based Health Promotion Programs*. New York: McGraw-Hill.

Bosch, M., van der Weijden, T., Wensing, M., and Grol, R. (2007). Tailoring quality improvement interventions to identified barriers: a multiple case analysis. *J. Eval. Clin. Pract.* 13: 161–168.

Bragge, P., Grimshaw, J.M., Lokker, C., and Colquhoun, H. (2017). AIMD – a validated, simplified framework of interventions to promote and integrate evidence into health practices, systems and policies. *BMC Med. Res. Methodol.* 17: 38.

Colquhoun, H., Leeman, J., Michie, S. et al. (2014). Towards a common terminology: a simplified framework of interventions to promote and integrate evidence into health practices, systems and policies. *Implement. Sci.* 9: 51.

Colquhoun, H., Squires, J., Kolehmainen, N. et al. (2017). Methods for designing interventions to change healthcare professionals' behaviour: a systematic review. *Implement. Sci.* 12: 30.

Curran, G.M., Mukherjee, S., Allee, S., and Owen, R.R. (2008). A process for developing an implementation intervention: QUERI series. *Implement. Sci.* 3: 17.

Eccles, M., Grimshaw, J., Walker, A. et al. (2005). Changing the behavior of healthcare professionals: the use of theory in promoting the uptake of research findings. *J. Clin. Epidemiol.* 58: 107–112.

Effective Practice and Organisation of Care (EPOC) (2015). EPOC taxonomy. epoc.cochrane.org/epoc-taxonomy (accessed November 6, 2019).

Elsbach, K.D. and Stigliani, I. (2018). Design thinking and organizational culture; a review and framework for future research. *J. Manag.* 44: 2274–2306.

Ferlie, E.B. and Shortell, S.M. (2001). Improving the quality of health care in the United Kingdom and the United States: a framework for change. *Milbank Q.* 79: 281–315.

Foy, R., Francis, J.J., Johnston, M. et al. (2007). The development of a theory-based intervention to promote appropriate disclosure of a diagnosis of dementia. *BMC Health Serv. Res.* 7: 207.

Green, L., Gottlieb, N., and Parcell, G. (1989). Diffusion theory extended and applied. In: *Advances in Health Education and Promotion* (eds. W.B. Ward and F.M. Lewis), 3. Greenwich, CT: JAI Press.

Grol, R. (1992). Implementing guidelines in general practice care. *Qual. Health Care* 1: 184–191.

Grol, R. (2010). *Kwaliteit en veiligheid. Variaties op een complex thema [Quality and Safety. Variations on a Complex Theme]*. Nijmegen: Radboud Universiteit Nijmegen.

Grol, R., Bosch, M., Hulscher, M. et al. (2007). Planning and studying improvement in patient care: the use of theoretical perspectives. *Milbank Q.* 85: 93–138.

Grol, R. and Wensing, M. (2004). What drives change? Barriers to and incentives for achieving evidence-based practice. *Med. J. Aust.* 180: S57–S60.

Kastner, M., Bhattacharyya, O., Hayden, L. et al. (2015). Guideline uptake by six implementability domains for creating and communicating guidelines: a realistic view. *J. Clin. Epidemiol.* 68: 498–509.

Leeman, J., Birken, S., Powell, B. et al. (2017). Beyond "implementation strategies":

classifying the full range of strategies used in implementation science and practice. *Implement. Sci.* 12: 125.

Marshall, M., de Silva, D., Cruickshank, L. et al. (2017). What we know about designing an effective intervention (but too often fail to put into practice). *BMJ Qual. Saf.* 26: 578–582.

Mazza, D., Bairstow, P., Buchan, H. et al. (2013). Refining a taxonomy for guideline implementation: results of an exercise in abstract classification. *Implement. Sci.* 8: 32.

Michie, S., Richardson, M., Johnston, M. et al. (2013). The behavior change technique taxonomy of 93 hierarchically-clustered techniques: building an international consensus for the reporting of behavior change interventions. *Ann. Behav. Med.* 46: 81–95.

Michie, S., Van Stralen, M.M., and West, R. (2011). The behavior change wheel: a new method for characterizing and designing behavior change interventions. *Implement. Sci.* 6: 42.

O'Cathain, A., Groot, L., Duncan, E. et al. (2019). Guidance on how to develop complex interventions to improve health and healthcare. *BMJ Open* 9: e029954.

Powell, B., Waltz, T., Chinman, M. et al. (2015). A refined compilation of implementation strategies: results from the Expert Recommendations for Implementing Change (ERIC) project. *Implement. Sci.* 10: 21.

Rogers, E.M. (2003). *Diffusion of Innovations*. Simon and Schuster: New York.

Schmid, A.A., Andersen, J., Kent, T. et al. (2010). Using intervention mapping to develop and adapt a secondary stroke prevention program in Veterans Health Administration medical centres. *Implement. Sci.* 5: 97.

Stewart, R.E., Williams, N., Byeon, V. et al. (2019). The clinician crowdsourcing challenge: using participatory design to seed implementation strategies. *Implement. Sci.* 14: 63.

Thorsen, T. and Mäkelä, M. (eds.) (1999). *Theory and Practice of Clinical Guidelines Implementation*, DSI Rapport 99.05. Copenhagen: DSI Danish Institute for Health Services Research and Development.

Van Bokhoven, M.A., Kok, G., and van der Weijden, T. (2003). Designing a quality improvement intervention: a systematic approach. *Qual. Saf. Health Care* 12: 215–220.

Van Woerkom, C. (1990). *Voorlichting als beleidsinstrument: nieuw en krachtig? Inaugurale rede [Education as a Policy Tool: New and Powerful? Inaugural Lecture]*. Wageningen: Landbouw-universiteit Wageningen.

Walker, A.E., Grimshaw, J.M., and Armstrong, E.M. (2001). Salient beliefs and intentions to prescribe antibiotics for patients with a sore throat. *Br. J. Health Psychol.* 6: 347–360.

Waltz, T.J., Powel, B.J., Fernandez, M.E. et al. (2019). Choosing implementation strategies to address contextual barriers: diversity in recommendations and future directions. *Implement. Sci.* 14: 42.

Wensing, M. (2017). The Tailored Implementation in Chronic Diseases (TICD) project: introduction and main findings. *Implement. Sci.* 12: 5.

Wensing, M., Bosch, M., Foy, R. et al. (2005). *Factors in theories on behaviour change to guide implementation and quality improvement*. Nijmegen: Radboud University.

11

Dissemination of Innovations

Richard Grol[1,2] and Michel Wensing[3,4,5]

[1] *Radboud University, Nijmegen, The Netherlands*
[2] *Maastricht University, Maastricht, The Netherlands*
[3] *Faculty of Medicine, University of Heidelberg, Heidelberg, Germany*
[4] *Department of General Practice and Health Services Research, Heidelberg University Hospital, Heidelberg, Germany*
[5] *Department IQ healthcare, Radboud Institute for Health Sciences, Radboud University Medical Center, Nijmegen, The Netherlands*

SUMMARY

- Effective dissemination of innovations, such as guidelines and best practices, is often a necessary step toward uptake and use in practice.
- Dissemination strategies can use mass media and personalized approaches to reach target groups; a combination of the two may be most effective.
- Social media methods play an increasingly large role in the dissemination of innovations, but systematic research on their effectiveness is scarce.
- Effective dissemination of an innovation is an important prerequisite for uptake, but it usually does not result in actual use if applied as a single strategy.

11.1 Introduction

In order to adopt new insights or new procedures in existing routines, it is a necessary prerequisite that the target group is aware of their existence, takes notice of them, understands what they are about, is prepared to study them carefully, and actually does something with them, such as thoughtful reading and discussion with colleagues. Therefore, it is necessary to present individuals with information on the innovation, preferably in a stimulating manner (see Box 11.1 for an example). The importance of a systematic and well-planned dissemination is often underestimated. There are many examples of well-designed guidelines, program descriptions, and prototypes which never left

the shelf. Lomas (1997) distinguished five possible target groups: (i) policy makers and politicians; (ii) managers and administrators; (iii) care providers and healthcare policy makers; (iv) patient or consumer groups; (v) researchers and developers of support materials or instruments, and others. Depending on the aims, one or of more of these groups may be targeted in a structured approach to dissemination.

In a dissemination plan, consideration should be given to (NHMRC 2000):
- A clear definition of the target group.
- A description of segments of the target groups that have to be approached differently.
- The most suitable media or channels for distribution for each target group.

Improving Patient Care: The Implementation of Change in Health Care, Third Edition. Edited by Michel Wensing, Richard Grol, and Jeremy Grimshaw.
© 2020 John Wiley & Sons Ltd. Published 2020 by John Wiley & Sons Ltd.

Box 11.1   Dissemination of Guidelines among Physicians

To accelerate the adoption of national guidelines for primary care physicians, a special package was compiled containing 10 national guidelines and related self-evaluation methods (Grol et al. 1998; Grol 2001). In a controlled study, different methods for disseminating the package were compared:

- Mailing the package to all local coordinators of continuous medical education and to representatives of local physician groups in one district.
- Mailing it as above to physicians in another district, with the additional support of two colleague-physician outreach visitors, who sought contact with key figures, enquired whether they required any form of assistance with using the materials, and if necessary offered support at group meetings (one comparable district).
- The rest of the country served as control group: physicians were informed about the existence of the materials by publications in journals. If they were interested, they could request them.

All physicians in the first and second districts (527 and 504, respectively) and 500 from the rest of the country were asked to complete a questionnaire before and after the intervention period (1.5 years). A total of 762 physicians responded. The results included the following:

Situation after intervention	By post + outreach visitor (n = 269)	Only by post (n = 244)	Control group (n = 249)
Were aware of the existence of the package	66%	25%	20%
In possession of the materials	49%	14%	6%
Have read the materials	35%	9%	6%
Made use of the materials	25%	4%	2%

There was clearly more effect in the district that received the combined intervention – that is, with the input of so-called outreach visitors – than in the district that only received post or where advertisements had been made by the media. However, actual use of the materials was limited, even in the district where the target group had been reached most effectively.

- The allocation of responsibilities: which organization takes care of informing which target group and which media channels will be used.
- A plan for the development, production, and distribution of the various presentation forms for the different subgroups, including adequate measurements (e.g. are the aims being achieved? what are the financial costs?) and feedback.
- A budget itemizing components of the development, production, and distribution of the various forms of presentation of the innovation.

For dissemination of the innovation, a useful distinction can be made between (non-personalized) mass media and personalized communication channels (Table 11.1).

It seems plausible that a combination of approaches, including mass media and personalized methods, provides the highest likelihood for reaching the target group. Furthermore, a one-off presentation in a journal, a conference, or as a personalized message in an email is seldom sufficient to get the attention of the entire target group. Frequently, dissemination activities have to be repeated and continued for a considerable period of time in order for the

Table 11.1 Examples of mass media and personalized methods for dissemination.

Mass media	Personalized methods
Publication in scientific journals	Interactive types of continuing professional education
Publication in professional journals and newsletters	Local group meetings, e.g. quality circles
Direct mailing of paper-based texts, books, folders	Inter-collegial contacts with peers
Inclusion in databases, which can be consulted (e.g. Cochrane Library)	Communication with patients and stakeholders, e.g. payers of healthcare
Dissemination of information devices (DVDs, USB sticks)	Support by key figures and opinion leaders
Audiovisual communication (TV, radio)	Visits by trained outreach visitors
Non-personalized communication by internet, email, or social media	Personalized communication by social media, e.g. online discussion groups

target group – preoccupied by myriad other items of importance – to become aware of the message. In addition to the varying channels by which the "message" is relayed, the source and form of the message have to be considered. For instance, the message that antibiotics are better avoided in uncomplicated airway infections may be packaged as the message that they have no place in a healthy life style. Chapter 5 provides further detail on the presentation of innovations. The credibility of the source or the medium of information is another important factor in the success of implementation. Care providers are often more readily convinced by information from reputable journals, by guidelines from their own professional society (see Box 11.2), and by professional opinion leaders from their own social network.

Box 11.2 Dissemination of Guidelines among Medical Specialists in the Netherlands

Via a written survey among six groups of medical specialists (cardiologists, pediatricians, anesthetists, chest physicians, neurologists, and urologists), information was obtained about their knowledge of four nationally developed guidelines in their own field and the sources they had used to acquaint themselves with that knowledge (van Everdingen et al. 2003). The percentages of physicians who were aware of the guidelines ranged from 23% for the urologists to 73% for the chest physicians. Major sources (as percentages) were:

Sources used for information about guidelines	Cardio. (175)	Ped. (248)	Anes. (221)	Chest (225)	Neuro. (180)	Uro. (122)
Journal from own society	33	10	16	7	3	6
General professional journal	13	11	14	16	25	6
CME courses	22	14	11	25	25	7
Scientific meeting	17	9	10	26	16	9
Mailing from own society	10	9	15	12	21	6

This study demonstrated that an average of about half of the medical specialists were informed about the existence of specific national guidelines in their own field; also, various sources had been used, both written and personal. Rates varied between specialists, depending on the existence of adequate scientific journals in their own field or continuing medical education (CME courses).

In this chapter, we elaborate on the possible approaches and effects of using mass media and personalized methods to inform care providers and other agents about innovations. Patients and citizens can also be the target of dissemination activities. Here we focus on the impacts on awareness, knowledge, understanding, perceived usefulness, and interest with respect to innovations.

11.2 Mass Media Approach

The majority of innovations and new insights in health are reported in scientific and professional journals. Target groups are also often informed via paper-based mailings, digital newsletters (e.g. via email), and social media. The role of social media platforms, such as Twitter and Facebook, as well as Wikipedia, LinkedIn, chatrooms, discussion fora, and blogs, has been expanding quickly, but research on their impact in the uptake of innovations in healthcare is still limited. It is probably wise to make a distinction between segments in the target group on the basis of their information-seeking behavior. Also, people may use specific media privately, but not professionally. Various mass media can be used for the dissemination of information, as usually no single medium is able to reach everybody.

11.2.1 Written Materials

In most developed countries, new insights, guidelines, or best practices are first published in scientific or professional journals. However, many care providers do not read the information at all, or do not read it carefully, or only have time and interest to choose items that are in line with their preferences. Given the numbers of research papers in many fields and the high workload in healthcare practice, it seems unlikely that this will change. A classic study by Lomas et al. (1989) on the dissemination of a guideline on cesarean section among obstetricians showed, for instance, that 90% were aware of the existence of the guideline. However, only 3% could correctly repeat all eight central recommendations. Nearly two decades later, Wagnon et al. (2009) found similar findings when studying the impact of disseminated guidelines on awareness of osteoporosis in inflammatory bowel disease.

It seems likely that the situation in many countries today is better than in the past, as a result of the systematic development and active dissemination of clinical guidelines adopted by scientific societies of professionals in healthcare and other organizations. For instance, many written guidelines are now accompanied by implementation tools, such as summary cards and decision trees for clinicians (Liang et al. 2017). However, this may not apply to other types of innovations, such as recommended healthcare delivery models and new information technologies.

Another approach to informing target groups about innovations is through mass media campaigns. These tend to target both healthcare providers and the general public. For instance, Lecouturier et al. (2010) analyzed 10 studies to study the impact of such strategies to improve the detection, referral, and treatment of patients with stroke. The studies showed an overall improvement in the awareness of the problem and the symptoms. Box 11.3 (Morgenstern et al. 2002) gives an example of a mass media approach to detection and treatment of stroke.

11.2.2 Internet-Based Approaches

Internet-based approaches, such as email, online information platforms (e.g. Wikipedia), social media, and other communication tools (e.g. chatrooms, videoconferences, virtual patients) offer interesting possibilities for quickly spreading and sharing information (McKimm et al. 2003). Different media have different functions (Ventola 2014). They can facilitate:

Box 11.3   A Mass Media Approach to Early Detection and Treatment of Patients with Stroke

In a controlled study in east Texas, an extensive campaign was aimed at both health professionals and the general public to enable the early recognition, referral, and treatment (thrombolysis) of stroke patients. The program targeting the public included billboard advertising, radio and TV messages, news stories, brochures, and posters. Volunteers were trained in the early recognition of symptoms, who in turn trained new volunteers. In total 60 persons were trained who managed to bring the message to about 50 000 individuals in personal contacts. Over 60 000 brochures and 5000 posters were disseminated. The message was presented on TV 675 times and on radio more than 3300 times. To reach professionals in healthcare both mass media and brochures were used, while in hospitals care pathways for the management of stroke were introduced. In contrast, in a different control region no campaign was held. While time to treatment decreased in both regions, thrombolysis was significantly better in the intervention region. The authors concluded that the campaign had a significant impact on professionals and less on the general public.

- Mail, including alerts and newsletters (email programs).
- Communication and sharing in networks (e.g. LinkedIn, Myspace, Twitter).
- Sharing photos and videos (e.g. YouTube, Flickr, Instagram).
- Producing and sharing information (blogs such as Tumbler, Blogger, Twitter).
- Aggregation of knowledge from multiple contributors (e.g. Wikipedia).
- Virtual reality and gaming, e.g. skills training in surgery.

Advantages of this type of media include the speed of dissemination, the possibility of interactivity, and the ability to target specific individuals. They may also present disadvantages, such as a lack of control on the quality of the information, (non-disclosed) commercial and political interests, and suboptimal security of individual data. Also, communication within social media networks tends to exclude diverging views, so that these become "bubbles" of like-minded people. The privacy of users is often not well established and legal aspects of their use are not yet clear and are under debate, particularly in Europe (Ventola 2014; Dosemagen and Aase 2016).

The actual impact of these approaches on awareness and knowledge of innovations among professional groups is unclear (see Box 11.4). It should be considered that not all care providers are skilled users of information technology systems, despite their higher education degrees, although younger generations may on average be more skilled. A review of six studies on the use of electronic information systems found that training can actually

---

Box 11.4   Impact of Social Media on Dissemination of Guidelines

The American Academy of Neurology (AAN) developed a strategy for dissemination of its clinical practice guideline on "complementary and alternative medicine in multiple sclerosis," including social media methods. They evaluated the impact on awareness and knowledge of the recommendations (Narayanaswami et al. 2015). Outcomes were measured by four surveys among patients and clinicians. Both awareness and knowledge of the guideline increased after traditional dissemination, and did not further increase after the use of social media.

enhance the use of these systems by care providers (Fiander et al. 2015). However, in reality many physicians use trial and error and help from others to learn about computer systems, rather than manuals, online help functions, or courses (Wensing et al. 2019).

A review of 16 studies showed that internet-based information and education can be equally effective in terms of knowledge compared to traditional education (Wutoh et al. 2004). A meta-analysis of 201 studies was performed on the impact of internet learning compared to no intervention and to non-internet educational activity. On average, substantial effects were found for the internet intervention versus no intervention, and a small positive effect was found when compared to traditional education (Cook et al. 2008). Positive correlations with positive outcomes were noted for the duration of the activity and the degree of interactivity. Box 11.5 provides an example of mailing educational materials to physicians.

Because the field of social media has developed rapidly and the best strategies for dissemination of information through these media among healthcare providers and other professional agents are as yet unclear, more research is needed. In particular, the field deserves answers to questions about better ways to involve the target group in the adaptation of innovations and change proposals and to increase acceptance of the desired change (Greysen et al. 2010). The risks of the use of social media should be considered as well, because the information disseminated may be preliminary, superficial, or one-sided. Boxes 11.6 and 11.7 offer examples.

11.2.3 Factors Associated with the Impact of Mass Media Strategies

In order to increase the likelihood that a mass media approach will achieve its goal, a number of measures can be considered. The essence of the new information can be summarized into a concise, easy-to-grasp text, with an attractive presentation. For example, guidelines might be summarized on a plastic card that can be kept in a folder. Reading the core recommendations from such a guideline should occupy a short time (e.g. less than 10 minutes). The

---

Box 11.5   Effect of Dissemination of Information via Email
In a controlled study, half of the target group of 107 general internists received weekly emails with structured summaries of new articles in the format of a Weekly Browsing Journal Club, while the controls had access to a website with information only (Mukohara and Schwartz 2005). After three months, there was no difference between the two groups in the use of information for decisions in clinical practice or in their attitudes to evidence. A decrease was found in the intervention group in the time used for reading scientific information, while there was an increase in the control group.

Box 11.6   Use of Social Media in the Dissemination of the Safer Surgery Checklist
In a campaign named "Check a Box, Save a Life," American medical students were asked to help disseminate the World Health Organization checklist for safe surgery through Facebook (Henderson et al. 2010). The campaign staff was supported by the Institute for Healthcare Improvement and the American Medical Student Association. About 1400 students participated and introduced the innovation in their own organization. This is an example of the use of social media in the introduction of important innovations and change proposals. They may have more impact than the traditional strategies for dissemination.

Box 11.7 Social Media Release of Articles	
In one study, 16 original (open access) articles on clinical pain were blogged and released via Facebook, Twitter, LinkedIn, and Research-Blogging.org on specific dates, with other dates serving as controls (Allen et al. 2013). The primary outcomes of this dissemination program	were the rate of HTML views and PDF downloads over a seven-day period. The mean rate of HTML views after the social media release was 18 per day, in the control weeks 6 per day. The mean rate of PDF downloads was 4 per day versus 1 per day in the control weeks.

information can contain practical flow charts for diagnostics or treatment charts that can be rapidly and easily consulted. The same information can be offered via a website. Increasingly recommendations for practice, such as prescribing guidelines, are summarized into files for a hand-held device such as a personal digital assistant (PDA) or smartphone, allowing easy consultation during work (Baumgart 2005).

A summary of a proposed care process can also be presented in concise, attractive brochures that are adapted to the various target groups and are distributed on a large scale. This information should ideally be based on pre-existing questions from the relevant target groups. In addition to management recommendations, the brochure should contain scientific background information. A possible design could include:

- The presentation of a relevant question or problem in practice.
- The description of current routines: What are individuals used to doing at present?
- A summary of the new insights, highlighting the most crucial recommendations.
- An explanation of why old routines are less desirable and arguments in favor of new routines: How good is the evidence?
- Information about possible problems with changing the present management practice and how they can be solved.
- Where individuals can learn more.

The summary may be published simultaneously on the internet, for instance on the website of a professional society, and in diverse professional journals read by the target group. This step could also be accomplished in the form of an interview with a key figure who explains the proposed performance. On a local or institutional level, the proposed routines can be sent by email to the individuals involved and further distributed through internal newsletters or discussion fora.

In addition, attempts can be made to publish popularized versions of an innovation in regional or national daily newspapers, news magazines, and newsletters, and in magazines that are read by large groups of patients. Special versions for patients and policy makers are very useful. Attention from radio or television can obviously also give an extra impetus, so that patients can consult their care provider with well-founded expectations.

11.3 Personalized Approaches

Given that a mass media approach may fail to bring an innovation to the attention of the target group, particularly if it involves complex or sensitive information, personalized communication provides an alternative or additional approach. Personalized approaches may also help to prioritize a message compared to other information. Informing the target group and motivating them so that they wish to study the innovation can be achieved by applying some or all of the following options:

- Continuing medical education (CME) in courses, conferences, and educational groups.

- Use of social networks of care providers, which may be facilitated by online platforms.
- Involvement of key figures and opinion leaders in education and campaigns.
- Personal introduction by advisers and facilitators in practice settings ("academic detailing").

11.3.1 CME Courses and Conferences

Congresses, courses, and other CME programs can make an important contribution to effective information transfer with regard to new developments. This remains a popular and widely used method of dissemination of information in healthcare. Chapter 12 elaborates on educational strategies with respect to changing professional performance and healthcare delivery, thus focused on professional behaviors. Here, we elaborate the possible role of educational approaches in the dissemination of innovations and informing target groups, thus focused on awareness, knowledge, and appreciation.

A problem with courses and conferences as a method of information transfer is the fact that individuals often choose subjects that they already find interesting and, consequently, will keep up to date with them better (Sibley et al. 1982). Another problem is that the format of large courses is frequently passive, not requiring active involvement and contribution from the participants. Research showed that particularly interactive methods of education contribute to better performance. For instance, an analysis of 81 controlled studies on the impact of interactive education showed an average improvement of 6% in the desired performance (Forsetlund et al. 2009). When the participation in the interactive education is more resource intensive, the effect on performance may be more substantial. A combination of classic education (lectures) and interactive meetings proved to be more effective (on average 13.5% improvement) than these strategies alone. Although these findings concern the

improvement of actual performance in healthcare, we may assume that such educational approaches also contribute largely to the dissemination of new insights and procedures (O'Neil and Addrizzo-Harris 2009), in particular when the education takes place in a setting familiar to the target group.

With the aim of achieving successful dissemination of innovations, it appears to be important to do the following:

- Design educational programs for the innovation based on concrete, recognizable problems, questions, or cases from everyday practice (Spencer and Jordan 1999), a finding confirmed by a recent major systematic review of the CME literature in the USA (Bordage et al. 2009).
- Allow room for discussion between participants to facilitate the exchange of existing working methods. Individuals will realize that colleagues have similar problems, but may have different opinions and use different routines, which will stimulate their interest to find out more about the innovation.
- Present data on existing routines, variations in such routines, and deviations from the proposed or new working method. The basis for attracting interest often lies in confrontation with deviations from existing norms and the feeling that something actually ought to change (Grol and Lawrence 1995).

11.3.2 Social Networks

The dissemination of innovations can also occur through local networks of care providers, in which the opinions of others and those of opinion leaders can be very important (Box 11.8 provides an example). Insight into the network of relationships between colleagues and other important persons may help to enhance the spread of knowledge and behaviors (Bandura 1986; McLeroy et al. 1988). There is a growing body of research on the professional networks of care providers, which are based on patient transfer, patient sharing, and

---

Box 11.8   Conditions for Effective Dissemination of Clinical Guidelines

Vedel et al. (2018) explored whether the dissemination of new Alzheimer's disease (AD) guidelines for primary care through publication or mailing resulted in modifications in practice. Eight family medicine groups in Quebec were studied. The rate of AD diagnosis and the quality of follow-up care were monitored before and after dissemination of the guideline. Interviews and focus groups with clinicians and managers were held to explore conditions for effective dissemination. Some groups started to use the guideline recommendations, others did not. Three inter-related conditions for successful dissemination were identified: clinicians with baseline expertise and confidence in the AD field working in the group, linked to collaboration with hospital specialists; the presence of self-identified champions in the practice taking the lead; and the availability of sufficient clinical staff to enable the process.

---

professional interactions (Brunson and Laubenbacher 2018). Social networks can facilitate the exchange of information, provide individuals with access to sources of information, and help define priorities and legitimize innovations. An analysis of the networks within the target group might therefore be of importance in establishing the precise path of information flow and the identification of key figures (Rogers 2003).

The role of online networks is increasing. This refers to groups of professionals and patients, and maybe other participants (such as policy makers, managers, payers), who exchange information via online platforms. This may be an effective medium for the introduction of innovation and new procedures or routines, particularly when individuals know each other in other contexts. Experiences with the innovation can be discussed among network partners, in addition to logistical considerations and questions (Demiris 2006). Benham-Hutchins and Clancy (2010) suggest that understanding such networks can facilitate an understanding of complex systems, clearly an important aspect of healthcare delivery.

11.3.3   Influential Individuals

During the introduction of new working methods, a special role is reserved for key figures within local networks (Lomas 1993). Specific individuals, such as opinion leaders and change agents, have a key role in social networks. In the eyes of the network members, they have characteristics such as trustworthiness, expertise, and reputation (Kok 1993). They tend to have a central position in a social network. If an individual is regarded as being someone who is too far outside practice or their own profession, or as someone with revolutionary ideas, then this will make it more difficult to increase acceptance than if the presenter is regarded as being "one of us" (see Box 11.9). Therefore, the question is who has the most power of expression in a specific target group or subgroup to inform them about, and involve them in, changes in care. This is not necessarily an individual with a high position in the organizational hierarchy.

Key individuals are both the first target group for the introduction and the channel along which the introduction will be the most effective: "The heart of the diffusion process consists of interpersonal network exchanges and social modeling between individuals who had already adopted and those who then would be influenced to do so" (Rogers 2003). The term "key figures" implies respected and well-informed professionals within a target group, who filter incoming information and pass it on to the individuals around them. They are not usually the "innovators" within a group,

---

Box 11.9   Which Guidelines Do Medical Specialists Use?

Via written surveys among random samples of six groups of medical specialists in the Netherlands, data were obtained about the use of guidelines and the different sources they use to keep informed about new developments. The percentages of specialists who use the guidelines from different sources are:

Use of guidelines from: (always/often)	Cardio.	Ped.	Chest	Neuro.	Uro.
Own society	93	70	78	83	81
Independent national institute	41	52	70	52	8
College of family doctors	3	10	27	7	9
International organizations	55	40	50	35	16

Specialists used guidelines from their own society most often. In comparison with the other specialists, the chest physicians more often used guidelines from other sources. Guidelines for family physicians were not very popular among the majority of specialists. International guidelines were consulted regularly.

Box 11.10   Effect of the Use of Opinion Leaders

A systematic review of 18 studies on the effect of opinion leaders on the improvement of care provision showed an average effect of 12% improvement in a variety of process indicators (with a range of −15% to +72%). There was little difference between studies in which the opinion leaders were combined with other strategies or not (Flodgren et al. 2011).

---

but the persons who best personify the group norms and group culture. They judge new developments in the light of existing group norms. An example is a study on the impact of "local champions" on infection prevention (Damschroder et al. 2009). The literature, however, does not demonstrate a uniform positive response to the use of key figures and opinion leaders (see Box 11.10). It is not always possible to identify key figures and the mechanisms for their impact remain only partly understood.

11.3.4 Personal Introduction in Practice

Another method to bring innovations to the attention of a target group is to approach members personally and give them information and support (academic detailing or facilitation; see Box 11.11 for an example). This can be carried out by a trained colleague or an expert in a particular field who visits the target group in their own working environment and – depending on personal needs or questions – offers them support in understanding the innovation or tuition to enable training.

The influence of such a consultation (in the literature referred to as "outreach visits" or "academic detailing") on professional behaviors and the organization of care is described further in Chapter 12. There we will show that this approach has a small, but potentially relevant, impact on the patient care provided. There is evidence that personal tuition, tailored to the questions of the persons involved and given by a respected outreach visitor, can arouse interest and generate a positive attitude to innovations.

Box 11.11   Outreach Visits to Improve Smoking Cessation

A package with materials for advising patients to stop smoking was delivered to physicians in Australia in three different ways: (i) personally by a trained nurse or physiotherapist, who demonstrated the materials and encouraged the physician to use the materials; (ii) by a courier; (iii) by mail. The study showed that physicians in group (i) remembered more often that they had received the materials and that they had used more often at least one component of the package (Cockburn et al. 1992). There were no differences with respect to actual use of the minimal intervention strategy for smoking cessation or the overall attitude regarding the materials among physicians. The effects have to be assessed in the light of the costs: personal delivery by a trained person was 12 times more expensive than the courier and 24 times more expensive than mailing.

11.4   Conclusion

The literature on the dissemination of innovations shows that such dissemination may be best accomplished via various, closely linked channels:

- The target group must be presented with the innovations regularly and over a prolonged period of time via different, non-personalized mass media methods: magazines, journals, newsletters, social media, the lay press, summaries in an attractive form, or personal email.
- In addition to this, use must be made of personalized channels: interactive education via existing educational programs and local networks, with the assistance of key figures and opinion leaders. It is best to focus first on a group of relative frontrunners in the target group. Calling in the services of outreach visitors seems to be an appropriate method to accelerate the dissemination process.

It is important to realize, however, that different subgroups within the target group use different sources of information or have different preferences for sources. Some prefer scientific journals, others the internet or look to colleagues, while others might best be approached by outreach visitors or via the lay press. A good understanding of the target groups and their needs and preferences is therefore of crucial importance to the process of dissemination of innovations.

Effective dissemination and broad awareness and acceptance of an innovation are thus necessary but insufficient steps toward effective implementation. Specially designed improvement programs, tailored to the local setting, would be required to achieve that aim; this approach is discussed in the next chapters. It is ultimately of great importance to develop a "dissemination plan" in close connection with the implementation plan and to involve the target group and key figures within the target group in the development of this plan and its testing (Box 11.12).

Box 11.12   Elements of a Dissemination Plan

- Definition of the target groups.
- Description of segments of the target groups that have to be approached differently.
- The most suitable media or channels for distribution (personal and non-personal) must be established.
- Determine responsibilities: which organization takes care of informing which target group and which mediators will be used.
- A budget must be available for the development, production, and distribution of the various forms of presentation of the innovation.

References

Allen, H., Stanton, T., Di Pietro, F. et al. (2013). Social media release increases dissemination of original articles in the clinical pain sciences. *PLoS One* 8: e68914.

Bandura, A. (1986). *Social Foundations of Thought and Action*. Englewood Cliffs, NJ: Prentice-Hall.

Baumgart, D. (2005). Personal digital assistants in health care: experienced clinicians in the palm of your hand? *Lancet* 366: 1210–1222.

Benham-Hutchins, M. and Clancy, T. (2010). Social networks as embedded complex adaptive systems. *J. Nurs. Adm.* 40: 352–356.

Bordage, G., Carlin, B., and Mazmanian, P. (2009). Continuing medical education effect on physician knowledge: effectiveness of continuing medical education: American College of Chest Physicians evidence-based educational guidelines. *Chest* 135: 29S–36S.

Brunson, J.C. and Laubenbacher, R.C. (2018). Applications of network analysis to routinely collected health care data: a systematic review. *J. Am. Med. Inform. Assoc.* 25: 210–221.

Cockburn, J., Ruth, D., Silagy, C. et al. (1992). Randomised trial of three approaches for marketing smoking cessation programmes to Australian general practitioners. *BMJ* 304: 691–694.

Cook, D., Levinson, A., Garside, S. et al. (2008). Internet-based learning in the health professions: a meta-analysis. *JAMA* 300: 1181–1196.

Damschroder, L., Banaszak-Holl, J., Kowalski, C. et al. (2009). The role of the "champion" in infection prevention: results from a multisite qualitative study. *Qual. Saf. Health Care* 18: 434–440.

Demiris, G. (2006). The diffusion of virtual communities in health care: concepts and challenges. *Patient Educ. Couns.* 62: 178–188.

Dosemagen, S. and Aase, L. (2016). How social media is shaking up public health and healthcare. *Huffington Post*, Jan. 27.

Fiander, M., McGowan, J., Grad, R. et al. (2015). Interventions to increase the use of electronic health information by healthcare practitioners to improve clinical practice and health outcomes. *Cochrane Database Syst. Rev.* (3): CDCD004749. https://doi.org/10.1002/14651858.CD004749.pub3.

Flodgren, G., Parmelli, E., Doumit, G. et al. (2011). Local opinion leaders: effects on professional practice and health care outcomes. *Cochrane Database Syst. Rev.* (6): CD009255. https://doi.org/10.1002/14651858.CD000125.pub4.

Forsetlund, L., Bjørndal, A., Rashidian, A. et al. (2009). Continuing education meetings and workshops: effects on professional practice and health care outcomes. *Cochrane Database Syst. Rev.* (2): CD003030. https://doi.org/10.1002/14651858.

Greysen, S.R., Kind, T., and Chretien, K.C. (2010). Online professionalism and the mirror of social media. *J. Gen. Intern. Med.* 25: 1227–1229.

Grol, R. (2001). Successes and failures in the implementation of evidence-based guidelines for clinical practice. *Med. Care* 39 (S2): II46–II54.

Grol, R. and Lawrence, M. (1995). *Quality Improvement by Peer Review*. Oxford: Oxford University Press.

Grol, R., Zwaard, A., Mokkink, H. et al. (1998). Dissemination of guidelines: which sources do physicians use in order to be informed. *Int. J. Qual. Health Care* 10: 135–140.

Henderson, D., Carson-Stevens, A., Bohnen, J. et al. (2010). Check a box. Save a life. How student leadership is shaking up health care and driving a revolution in patient safety. *J. Patient Saf.* 6: 43–47.

Kok, G. (1993). Theorieen over verandering (Theories on change). In: *Gezondheidsvoorlichting en-opvoeding [Health Promotion]* (eds. V. Damoiseaux, V. van de Molen and G. Kok), pp. 221–235. Assen/Maastricht: Van Gorcum.

Lecouturier, J., Rodgers, H., Murtagh, M. et al. (2010). Systematic review of mass media interventions designed to improve public recognition of stroke symptoms, emergency response and early treatment. *BMC Public Health* 10: 784.

Liang, L., Safi, J.A., Gagliardi, A.R. et al. (2017). Number and type of guideline implementation tools varies by guideline, clinical condition, country of origin, and type of developer organization: content analysis of guidelines. *Implement. Sci.* 12: 136.

Lomas, J. (1993). *Teaching doctors old (and not so old) new tricks: Effective ways to implement research findings*. CHEPA working paper series 93-4. Hamilton, Ontario: McMaster University.

Lomas, J. (1997). *Beyond the Sound of Hand Clapping: A Discussion Document on Improving Health Research Dissemination and Uptake*. Sydney: University of Sydney.

Lomas, J., Anderson, G., Domnick-Pierre, K. et al. (1989). Do practice guidelines guide practice? The effect of a consensus statement on the practice of physicians. *N. Engl. J. Med.* 321: 1306-1311.

McKimm, J., Jollie, C., and Cantillon, P. (2003). Web based learning. *BMJ* 326: 870-873.

McLeroy, K., Bibeau, D., Steckle, A. et al. (1988). An ecological perspective on health promotion programs. *Health Educ. Q.* 15: 351-377.

Morgenstern, L., Staub, L., Chan, W., and Wein, T. (2002). Improving delivery of acute stroke therapy: the TLL Temple Foundation Stroke Project. *Stroke* 33: 160-166.

Mukohara, K. and Schwartz, M.D. (2005). Electronic delivery of research summaries for academic generalist doctors: a randomised trial of an educational intervention. *Med. Educ.* 39: 402-409.

Narayanaswami, P., Gronseth, G., Dubinsky, R. et al. (2015). The impact of social media on dissemination and implementation of clinical practice guidelines; a longitudinal observational study. *J. Med. Internet Res.* 17 (8): e193.

National Health and Medical Research Council (NHMRC) (2000). *How to Put the Evidence into Practice: Implementation and Dissemination Strategies*. Canberra: Commonwealth of Australia.

O'Neil, K.M. and Addrizzo-Harris, D.J. (2009). Continuing medical education effect on physician knowledge application and psychomotor skills: effectiveness of continuing medical education. *Chest* 135 (3 Suppl): 37S-41S.

Rogers, E.M. (2003). *Diffusion of Innovations*. New York: Simon and Schuster.

Sibley, J., Sackett, D., Neufeld, V. et al. (1982). A randomized trial of continuing medical education. *N. Engl. J. Med.* 306: 511-515.

Spencer, J. and Jordan, R. (1999). Learner centred approaches in medical education. *BMJ* 318: 1280-1283.

Van Everdingen, J.J., Mokkink, H.G.A., Klazinga, N.S. et al. (2003). De bekendheid en verspreiding van CBO-richtlijnen onder medisch specialisten [The acquaintance with and distribution of CBO guidelines among medical specialists]. *TSG* 81: 468-472.

Vedel, I., Le Berre, M., Sourial, N. et al. (2018). Shedding light on conditions for the successful passive dissemination of recommendations in primary care: a mixed methods study. *Implement. Sci.* 13: 129.

Ventola, C. (2014). Social media and healthcare professionals: benefits, risks and best practices. *PT* 39: 491-499.

Wagnon, J.H., Leiman, D.A., Ayers, G.D., and Schwartz, D.A. (2009). Survey of gastroenterologists' awareness and implementation of AGA guidelines on osteoporosis in inflammatory bowel disease patients: are the guidelines being used and what are the barriers to their use? *Inflamm. Bowel Dis.* 15: 1082-1089.

Wensing, M., Paech, B., Roth, C., and Schwill, S. (2019). Learning, understanding and use of information technology: a survey study in primary care physician trainees. *BMC Health Serv. Res.* 19: 728.

Wutoh, R., Boren, S.A., and Balas, E.A. (2004). eLearning: a review of internet-based continuing medical education. *J. Contin. Educ. Heal. Prof.* 24: 20-30.

12

Educational Implementation Strategies

Michel Wensing[1,2,3], *Cornelia Fluit*[4], *Jeremy Grimshaw*[5,6], *and Richard Grol*[7,8]

[1] *Faculty of Medicine, University of Heidelberg, Heidelberg, Germany*
[2] *Department of General Practice and Health Services Research, Heidelberg University Hospital, Heidelberg, Germany*
[3] *Department IQ healthcare, Radboud Institute for Health Sciences, Radboud University Medical Center, Nijmegen, The Netherlands*
[4] *Department for Research in Learning and Education, Radboudumc Health Academy, Radboud University Medical Center, Nijmegen, The Netherlands*
[5] *Clinical Epidemiology Program, Ottawa Hospital Research Institute, Ottawa, Ontario, Canada*
[6] *Department of Medicine, University of Ottawa, Ottawa, Ontario, Canada*
[7] *Radboud University, Nijmegen, The Netherlands*
[8] *Maastricht University, Maastricht, The Netherlands*

SUMMARY

- Education of health professionals is crucial for their performance, but the effects of specific educational activities (e.g. training sessions) are mixed and overall moderate.
- Determinants of increased effectiveness of education include needs assessment before the start, optimal group composition, active participation, longer educational experience, and involvement of local opinion leaders.
- Education may be particularly relevant in the context of a broader program in which it is combined with other types of strategies.

12.1 Introduction

Historically, education of health professionals has been the most widely used method to improve healthcare. The initial and continued education of health professionals is crucial for their performance and requires much time and resources, thus insight into the effectiveness of specific educational activities is important (Hutchinson 1999). The education of health professionals has become an important field of scientific research in its own right. Ideally, professional education strives to be evidence based, just like clinical practice (Petersen 1999). This chapter focuses on the effectiveness of educational strategies on healthcare professionals, aimed at better implementation of innovations or best practices, and stopping practices which are no longer recommended. Educational strategies comprise various activities aimed at improving individual competencies: knowledge, attitudes, and skills (Box 12.1 provides an example). The previous chapter focused on the *dissemination* of innovations, which may involve education that predisposes to behavior change. Here we focus on the effects of education on the actual uptake of innovations in patient care, thus on professional performance and healthcare delivery processes.

Improving Patient Care: The Implementation of Change in Health Care, Third Edition. Edited by Michel Wensing, Richard Grol, and Jeremy Grimshaw.
© 2020 John Wiley & Sons Ltd. Published 2020 by John Wiley & Sons Ltd.

Box 12.1   Learning Curves for New Surgical Techniques

When a new surgical procedure is introduced, there is a learning curve: a period during which rates of mortality and complications gradually reduce to the lowest possible. If the procedure has proven efficacy, it is important that this period is as short as possible. When a new procedure for the replacement of heart valves was introduced, surgeons from two British hospitals applied the following procedure (Hasan et al. 2000). Each surgeon participated in a training course provided in a simulated, controlled training environment. The first operation involving a live patient was done with an expert in attendance. Subsequently, operations were done by two surgeons, one with clinical responsibility, one with educational or training responsibilities. Of the 20 patients who were operated on, one died within a few weeks after the operation (5%), and most other patients had only minimal or mild complications. Previously, in the first year after the introduction of this operating procedure, about 20% of the operated-on patients died from surgical complications.

Pre-graduate education of health professionals has been studied for several decades. It has become clear that the transfer of knowledge is, by itself, often not sufficient to improve performance. Nevertheless, it is often a crucially important precondition for any implementation of change. Current thinking on the education of health professionals emphasizes self-guided, practice-based, competency-orientated, and interprofessional learning. Passive teaching methods, such as many lectures, have often been replaced by activating methods, often in small groups or on online platforms (e-learning), or a mix of online and face-to-face formats (blended learning). Training in skills (e.g. communication and surgical skills) has become a central component of many curricula.

The need for life-long learning and professional development is also conveyed in modern curricula of medicine and other health professions. As knowledge and skills correlate only moderately to professional performance in routine healthcare practice (Ram et al. 1999; Davis et al. 2006), actual performance in routine practice has increasingly become the focus of successful education. Self-assessment of professional performance is a poor assessment method, so that structured observations in clinical practice have become more central in the education of health professionals (see Box 12.2).

Educational activities may try to activate learners beyond passive consumption of knowledge, for instance by engaging them in the choice of learning goals, formats of learning, and

---

Box 12.2   360° Feedback for Medical Specialists

Feedback on professional performance is an important component of the professional development of healthcare providers. In a study with 109 medical specialists, different methods for data collection and feedback were compared (Hasan et al. 2000). These requested on average eight hours per medical specialist. In particular, feedback from non-medical co-workers was perceived to contribute to improvements. The participants indicated that factors associated with improvement included positive feedback, setting specific goals for improvement, reflection on strong and weak points with an experienced counselor, and support of both the managers and the team in which they worked.

---

commitment to change practice after education has been completed. Activating educational approaches are based on theories on learning, which assume that adults are intrinsically motivated to learn and that they can guide the learning process themselves (Newman and Peile 2002; Kaufman 2003; Koh et al. 2008). Most adults prefer to learn through problems and challenges in their daily work (Bolhuis 2016). Individuals have different learning styles: for instance, some want to understand new practices thoroughly before they act, while others want to experience the new practices first (Ruijters 2012). Educational programs need to take such differences into account. Chapter 2 provides more information on theories of education.

The chapter will first describe a variety of educational strategies and their effectiveness in health professionals. The chapter turns then to potential determinants of the effect of education, which may explain the variation in effectiveness of professional education programs. In this chapter we focus on educational strategies as single strategies; combinations with other strategies are considered in Chapter 18.

12.2 Types of Educational Strategies

There are different types of educational strategies, varying from educational materials to individual instruction. The Cochrane Effective Practice and Organisation of Care Group (EPOC 2015) distinguishes the following categories:

- *Educational materials*: publication or mailing of written recommendations for clinical care, including guidelines, audiovisual materials, electronic publications (through the internet), and educational computer programs.
- *Large-scale educational meetings*: participation of care providers in conferences and lectures attended by large groups of health professionals; participation usually has a passive character.

- *Small-scale educational meetings*: participation of care providers in workshops, skills training, educational groups, local consensus groups, and quality circles or peer review groups outside the practice setting; participation tends to be more active.
- *Outreach visits*: contact in the practice setting of care providers with a trained individual who provides information, instruction, and support, and sometimes also feedback on current practice; examples include academic detailing by pharmacists and nurses.
- *E-learning*: educational activities that use modern information and communication technologies, particularly the World Wide Web.
- *Opinion leaders*: educational activities provided by individuals who are seen as influential in a specific clinical area. This strategy is treated as a determinant of the effectiveness of education in this chapter (see Section 12.4).

While educational interventions can be categorized in different ways, the EPOC categorization has been widely used. It primarily focuses on the mode of delivery of education, rather than more analytical characteristics, such as the goals of education, active ingredients and mechanisms, or the targeted factors and processes in healthcare.

The *distribution of educational materials* can be accomplished in different ways. Several examples include published insights in journals, leaflets, and brochures that are mailed, messages via email mailing lists or social media, and broadcast educational programs on radio, the internet, or television. A larger audience can be reached in this way.

In *large group educational meetings* (for example, more than 25 persons), the focus is frequently on the presentation of information in an oral and/or visual format, with the assumption that care providers are prepared to use the information to confirm or change their performance. These meetings employ lectures or seminar methods, and are frequently described as courses, conferences, refresher programs, or symposia. Practical considerations generally limit this type of education to a teacher-orientated and passive approach. Nevertheless, conferences are the primary source of innovations in some disciplines and areas. As with written educational materials, the conference format has the potential to reach a large group of individuals.

Small-scale educational meetings have a range of functions, formats, and purposes, such as skills training to learn technical or communication skills, local consensus development, and continuing education courses in which participants work in small groups. Quality circles and supervision groups can also be seen as small-scale educational meetings, which often use additional strategies, such as feedback on practice routines (Beyer et al. 2003). Practice-based learning can be classified in this category. One classic example is the traditional "grand round," in which a small group of residents or trainee doctors and a faculty member visit hospital patients, discussing their problems and management of the case. (Note that "grand round" is actually a formal lecture in other settings.) In addition, the format of small-scale educational meetings can also be similar to large-scale meetings, but are usually more orientated toward individual needs and motivations.

Outreach visits are a specific type of education, based on the techniques used by the pharmaceutical industry to influence the prescribing patterns of physicians. Often called academic detailing, the visit comprises individual explanation, instruction, and support in the practice of the care provider by a specially trained person. The visitor may be a physician, nurse, pharmacist, or other health professional. This type of education has mainly been applied to rationalize physician prescribing behavior, but has also been used for other purposes, such as to promote prevention in primary medical care. This approach is particularly suited to tailoring a program to the individual needs of the care provider (Soumerai and Avorn 1990).

E-learning comprises educational programs that use the internet or other information technologies. Such programs may have various components, such as instruction, exchange in a virtual class or chat room, self-learning exercises, questions with direct feedback on answers, videotaped lectures and demonstrations, and skills training in virtual and augmented reality settings (Cook et al. 2008). Educational computer games ("serious gaming") may be included in this category. E-learning can use many different formats, including video-based lectures, surgical training in virtual reality, and exchanges between participants on an online platform.

12.3 Effectiveness of Education

When compared to most other strategies for the implementation of innovations and improving healthcare practice, there is a relatively large body of research evidence on the effectiveness of educational strategies. For e-learning the number of studies is lower, but quickly growing. The studies have been summarized in many systematic reviews. Table 12.1 presents a small selection of reviews of evaluations of educational strategies for changing professional behaviors. The effectiveness of educational strategies (i.e. specific educational activities) targeted at health professionals is mixed, but overall modestly positive. The available Cochrane reviews suggest average effects of 2–10% improvement of specific aspects of professional performance. While these effects are small, they can be clinically and practically relevant. Furthermore, improved knowledge, skills, and attitudes may predispose to behavior change, which occurs if other types of strategies (e.g. organizational change or financial incentives) are applied. Also, many health professionals repeatedly participate in educational activities, so that the cumulative impact may be substantial.

Table 12.1 Overview of reviews on continuing professional education.

Educational material	
Giguere et al. (2018)	Review with 64 studies (including 31 randomized trials), which suggested that printed educational material compared to no intervention may have a small beneficial effect (absolute risk difference +4%) on professional behaviors.
Grudniewicz et al. (2016)	Review with 40 studies in primary care, which reported effects in some studies, but none in a statistical meta-analysis.
Educational meetings	
Forsetlund et al. (2009)	Review with 56 studies (of 81 in total) on educational meetings (only) versus no intervention. In studies with dichotomous measures, a median absolute improvement of +6% was found (range −2 to +29%). In studies with continuous measures, the median of relative improvement was +10% (range 0–50%). The effects on patient outcomes were smaller.
Reeves et al. (2013)	Review of studies on interprofessional education: continuing education by health professionals of various disciplines. Of 15 studies, 7 found positive effects on aspects of professional behavior, while 4 found mixed effects.
Outreach visits	
O'Brien et al. (2007)	Review with 34 studies (of a total of 69) of educational outreach visits (only) versus no intervention. In studies with dichotomous measures of professional performance, improvements were 5% (median value), with a range of 1% to 20%. In studies with continuous measures, the median of relative improvement was 23% (range 0–61%).
E-learning	
Cook et al. (2008)	Review with a total of 206 studies on web-based learning for healthcare professionals versus no intervention, of which 19 included measures of professional performance or patient outcomes. The effects varied substantially: the average effect size on professional performance and skills was 0.82 and did not differ statistically from zero.

12.3.1 Educational Materials

While initial research showed that sending educational material to health professionals had little impact on professional performance, more recent research found that it has on average a small effect (Grudniewicz et al. 2016). As the costs of educational materials tend to be low (compared to other types of education), this small effect may still be relevant. Nevertheless, it is important to know that the effectiveness of educational material is variable and can also be negative (Box 12.3). Educational material is often one component in a multifaceted implementation program, so that the unique effect cannot always be determined.

It is necessary to distinguish between the dissemination of reading materials (e.g. written clinical guidelines) and engaging, interactive self-study packages (e.g. distance learning programs). Active self-study is more likely to improve professional performance, while it is less likely that simply reading materials will have such effect.

12.3.2 Educational Meetings

Educational meetings have varying effects, which are on average modest (Forsetlund et al. 2009). As compared to large educational meetings, small-scale meetings tend to have interactive, engaging components and higher responsiveness to individual participants' learning needs and learning styles, which may enhance their impact. Studies of interprofessional educational meetings (e.g. involving

---

Box 12.3 Guidelines for Head Trauma

Patients with head trauma have increased risk for brain injury due to cerebral hemorrhage. When such patients arrive at a hospital Emergency Department, this risk must be assessed at an early stage. In order to optimize practice in this area, guidelines were developed in the north of England for appropriate clinical management of these patients (Thomson et al. 1994). Specific criteria were developed for imaging tests, such as loss of consciousness, memory loss, neurological symptoms, blood from ear or nose, and so on. The guidelines were printed on posters and cards in all hospital Emergency Departments in the region. Post-intervention evaluation did not show a difference regarding appropriately managed patients between baseline (69%) and follow-up measurement (64%). Some departments had improved, but other departments had deteriorated.

Box 12.4 Guideline Implementation in Public Pharmacies

A randomized trial tested the effects of several educational strategies to implement guidelines for medication dispensing in public pharmacies (Watson et al. 2002). The focus was on medication that could be supplied with a physician's prescription. A study with 60 pharmacies compared written dissemination of guidelines (control group), attending an educational meeting, and individual instruction in the pharmacy. Participation in the educational meeting provided 2.5 hours of accreditation and the costs of traveling and a substitute pharmacist were covered. The effects were measured with simulated patients who attended the pharmacies before and after the educational interventions (they completed structured forms after each contact). The primary outcome was appropriate supply (or non-supply) of medication. No differences between the three study groups were found regarding this primary outcome or other outcomes.

---

physicians and nurses) show positive or mixed effects (Reeves et al. 2013). Box 12.4 provides an example of educational meetings. Box 12.5 shows that large-scale educational programs can also be effective.

changes which are particularly difficult to achieve. The strategy is relatively expensive, so the costs have to be carefully assessed against the effects. Box 12.6 describes a study on outreach visits.

12.3.3 Outreach Visits

The effects of outreach visits on professional performance might be expected to be strong, but reviews of published research show a large heterogeneity of effects and an average effect that is not different from other educational strategies. This variability may be explained by the complex nature of the change desired or countervailing external forces. In other words, outreach visits might be chosen for

12.3.4 E-learning

This category comprises education which uses information technology, often including the internet, among other modalities. Information technology systems provide many opportunities, such as easy access to materials, self-tests with immediate feedback, and platforms for communication with other students and teachers. E-learning has been increasingly studied, but the number of well-designed

---

Box 12.5   Quality Circles to Improve Prescribing by Primary Care Physicians

Quality circles are small-scale groups of health professionals employed for their continuing education, who learn about subjects interactively. Most frequently, data on the participant's own professional performance comprise the starting point for a discussion. Although the effectiveness of this educational strategy has been shown in randomized trials, it is less well known whether it remains effective when applied on a large scale. The effects may be diluted by a range of factors, including suboptimal fidelity of the quality circles and lowered motivation in participants (compared to the trials). A large program of quality circles included 1090 primary care physicians from three regions in Germany (Wensing et al. 2009). These were compared to 2090 other, randomly selected primary care physicians in the same regions. Measurements in 2001 and 2003 were done with on average 1201 prescriptions and 444 patients per physician. Most performance indicators showed modest, but relevant improvements, such as improved prescribing of generic medication, recommended lipid-lowering drugs, and recommended antibiotics. Mean costs per prescription were also lowered. Groups with positive views on the use of indicators, feedback, and price information showed the largest improvements.

Box 12.6   Academic Detailing to Improve the Use of Diagnostic Imaging

One-on-one academic detailing regarding guideline-supported management of shoulder pain was delivered to 87 primary care physicians in South Australia (Broadhurst et al. 2007). Additionally, three months following the initial visit, participants were offered a follow-up session. The physicians were asked to complete a 10-item questionnaire before, immediately after, and three months after the academic detailing to assess shoulder knowledge, as well as a brief survey regarding their confidence in managing shoulder complaints. The number of requests for X-rays and ultrasounds was recorded for both the intervention doctors and a corresponding group of 90 control doctors from the same region. Three months after the academic detailing, the intervention group reported having higher confidence in their abilities to properly manage shoulder pain and take meaningful histories. Requests for ultrasound imaging before the intervention were significantly higher (43.8%) than they were during the six months following the study, whereas there was no statistically significant change in X-ray request rates.

---

evaluations with measures of professional performance or patient outcomes is limited (Akl et al. 2008; Cook et al. 2008). Evaluations of e-learning in health professionals tend to focus on user satisfaction and other aspects of the user experience (Curren et al. 2017). In recent years, a combination of e-learning and face-to-face formats ("blended learning") has become popular.

12.4   Determinants of the Effectiveness of Education

There is a large number of factors that may influence the effectiveness of educational strategies to implement innovations in clinical practice. These may relate to the goals and content of the educational activities, as well as to the social and organizational context in which they are applied (Burke and Hutchins 2007). Some factors associated with the impact of continuing professional education were described in the context of theories presented in Chapter 2. In addition, many studies aimed to identify such factors. For instance, a review of (continuing) medical education with 79 studies, focused on value-based healthcare, identified three categories of determinants: (i) effective knowledge transfer, for instance on costs of services; (ii) enhanced reflection, for example reasons for diagnostic test ordering; and (iii) supportive environment, such as a culture in which the costs and benefits of professional performance are discussed (Stammen et al. 2015). An explorative meta-regression analysis of 36 studies found that the following factors were associated with higher effects of educational meetings: the degree of participation by professionals; a mix of lectures and interactive sessions (compared to only lectures or only interactive sessions); less complex or controversial content; and less severe conditions (Forsetlund et al. 2009). Analysis of small-group education and quality improvement in mental healthcare suggested that inspiring team leadership and management support were factors associated with effects on professional practice (Versteeg et al. 2012).

This chapter focuses on factors that are directly related to the educational activities themselves. They include setting targets for education, active participation, longer duration of education, the involvement of opinion leaders, and the inclusion of assessment and feedback to participants.

12.4.1 Targets for Education

A critical factor is the assessment of the subjective and objective learning needs of care providers prior to an educational activity. This fits the model for implementation described in this book, in which an analysis of the target group and setting precedes the choice of an implementation strategy. This assessment may focus both on the content of education (which topics are addressed) and on its format (how the content is delivered). Using the results of the assessment, the program can be tailored to the needs and preferences of the target group (e.g. knowledge deficits, learning styles, logistics organization). Ideally, needs are related to the working place of the target group.

Despite the intuitively plausible importance of needs assessment, research demonstrates a mixed picture (Box 12.7). Some large reviews of the literature suggested that it has no consistent effects (Beaudry 1989; Burke and Hutchins 2007). An explanation may be that clinicians cannot accurately assess the quality of their performance, particularly physicians with much experience and high confidence (Davis et al. 2006). Also, they may choose learning objectives in domains in which they are experts already, although they are less likely to improve their knowledge and skills in those domains (Sibley et al. 1982). Nevertheless, learning seems more likely when the educational content is perceived to be relevant and when explicit goals and specific learning targets have been articulated (Burke and Hutchins 2007).

Box 12.7   Effect of Needs Assessment before Continuing Education

A controlled trial with 100 physicians examined the effect of (interactive) continuing education that was tailored to the results of an assessment of knowledge and skills (Hobma 2005). The control group received written educational materials only. Measures concerned prescribing in patients with nose, ear, or throat symptoms as well as doctor–patient communication. The educational program improved communication but not prescribing. A potential explanation is that physicians were not motivated for this particular clinical domain, but found doctor–patient communication highly relevant.

12.4.2 Active Participation

Active participation of professionals in the educational program and control over the learning process are also expected to improve the effectiveness of education (Burke and Hutchins 2007). For instance, case-based discussions and exercises lead to behavior changes in practice (Mazmanian and Davis 2002). Health professionals have a variety of reasons to participate in continuing education (see Box 12.8) and education may be most effective if these are taken into account. A meta-analysis on continuing education showed that the effectiveness is higher if it comprises active participation by participants (Mansouri and Lockyer 2007). Active participation can enhance motivation and tailor the program to individual learning needs (Frisby et al. 2014). Furthermore, knowledge is organized in a meaningful way (Emke et al. 2016). Active participation may be enhanced by interaction, but also by stimulating individual tasks.

12.4.3 Duration of Education

It is plausible that an educational program may be more effective if more time is invested in it, since participants have more exposure, perhaps with repetition, to what is being taught. This "inconvenient truth" may be ignored by busy people, who prefer "quick fixes" (e.g. a short course on a new and complex topic), although these often do not have an effect on performance. This observation does not permit unlimited time on one topic, however, particularly for busy clinicians. One review demonstrated that continuing education lasting one day is less effective than education over several days, but there was little difference between education of two days and education of longer duration (Beaudry 1989). Educational spread over several sessions facilitates the development of collaboration and networks, which may increase the effectiveness (Steinert et al. 2006).

12.4.4 Opinion Leaders

The use of opinion leaders in educational activities may influence their effectiveness (Box 12.9 provides an example). Opinion leaders are individuals who are seen by colleagues as those with a commitment to clinical improvements; as recognized clinical authorities in a specific area; and as altruistic role models. Role modeling is a component of education (Burke and Hutchins 2007). There are structured methods to identify these persons by interviewing healthcare professionals in a specific setting or discipline. The opinion leaders may have different roles, varying from signing a letter that accompanies educational material to delivering lectures

---

Box 12.8 Why Do Care Providers Participate in Continuing Education?

The literature suggests a range of motivations in professionals to participate in education:

- Education is seen as part of the profession; they are interested in the subject; they think that continuing education can confirm or change behavior that they have learned; they have specific objectives (knowledge of behavior); they feel it is an escape from routine and an opportunity to meet colleagues (Richards and Cohen 1980).
- An educational program is more likely to be chosen if it contributes to accreditation, the subject is important, presenters have a good reputation, there are no conflicting social/family obligations, and the traveling distance is not too large (Slotnick et al. 1994).
- Professionals participate in continuing education because they like to learn new things, want to develop as a professional, experience external pressure, expect social interaction, and want to escape from routine and boredom (Tassone and Heck 1997).

Box 12.9   Implementation of Dementia Guidelines by Neurologists Using Opinion Leaders

A written survey was performed among a sample of neurologists in six areas in the USA to identify 12 local opinion leaders, who were then used in an educational program on guidelines for dementia from the American Academy of Neurology (Gifford et al. 1999). The educational strategy included a mailed self-learning package, a questionnaire for depression in dementia patients, a chart with factual information for patients and caregivers, and several reminders of the messages. In addition, neurologists in the intervention group were invited to a seminar lasting three hours, during which they attended lectures by opinion leaders. A randomized trial showed that neurologists in the intervention group were more adherent to three of six recommendations compared to those in the control group as measured by paper-based scenarios. This effect was stronger in those neurologists who actually attended the seminar (about half of the total number invited).

---

during educational meetings, chairing a local group session, or visiting care providers in their practice. A Cochrane review (with 24 studies) showed that education with the involvement of opinion leaders probably improves health professionals' compliance with evidence-based practice; the absolute improvement was 10.8% on average (Flodgren et al. 2019). The variation of effects, however, was substantial (interquartile range of 3.5–14.6%).

12.4.5   Assessment and Feedback

Assessment and feedback are powerful means to influence learning by participants (Rust 2002). Assessment influences how content is learned (e.g. remember, reproduce, apply) and also when it is learned (e.g. shortly before an exam, throughout a time period). Assessment can be used before an educational meeting in order to raise the motivation for learning specific content (Mazmanian and Davis 2002). Such feedback may be based on structured audits of aspects of clinical performance, such as medication prescribing (see Chapter 13). However, in most educational settings it is based on direct observation and reflection on situations in training and education sessions. It seems particularly important for those who are low performers at the start (Cherry et al. 2010).

12.5   Discussion and Conclusions

Education of care providers can lead to change of professional behavior, but the effects of most types of education are modest (less than 10% change on measures of performance). The small changes may nevertheless be clinically and practically relevant. Many health professionals participate repeatedly in continuing education activities, so that the overall impact of education in the healthcare system over a long period of time is substantial. Insight into the determinants of effectiveness can help to optimize the effectiveness of educational activities for improving healthcare.

There are indications that education which is interactive and personal (small-scale educational meetings and educational outreach visits) is more effective than passive education (for example written material or large-scale, didactic educational meetings). Interactive education can be facilitated by online platforms and even in well-prepared sessions with large audiences. The social interaction element may motivate health professionals and facilitate learning processes. However, the effects of all types of education are mixed and written material can also be effective, particularly if it implies active self-study by using knowledge tests, needs assessments, and practical exercises. Modern information technology provides many new ways to integrate activating components in an educational intervention. More research on e-health can be expected in the coming years.

Health professionals learn in many ways other than formal education, particularly through contacts with colleagues, patients, and others (Owen et al. 1989). While education of health professionals is probably a necessary component of any implementation strategy, it is likely that additional strategies are needed to effect a sizable change in behavior on the part of professionals. Other types of implementation strategies will be discussed in subsequent chapters.

References

Akl, E.A., Kairouz, V.F., Sackett, K.M. et al. (2008). Educational games for health professionals. *Cochrane Cochrane Database Syst Rev* 1: CD006411. https://doi.org/10.1002/14651858.CD006411.pub4.

Beaudry, J.S. (1989). The effectiveness of continuing medical education: a quantitative synthesis. *J. Contin. Educ. Heal. Prof.* 9: 285–307.

Beyer, M., Gerlach, F.M., Flies, U. et al. (2003). The development of quality circles/peer review groups as a tool for quality improvement in Europe. Results of a survey in 26 European countries. *Fam. Pract.* 20: 443–451.

Bolhuis, S. (2016). *Leren en veranderen. Emotie, gedrag en denken [Learn and Change. Emotion, Behaviour, and Thinking].* Bussum: Coutinho.

Broadhurst, N.A., Barton, C.A., Rowett, D. et al. (2007). A before and after study of the impact of academic detailing on the use of diagnostic imaging for shoulder complaints in general practice. *BMC Fam. Pract.* 8: 12.

Burke, L.A. and Hutchins, H.M. (2007). Training transfer: an integrative literature review. *Hum. Resour. Dev. Rev.* 6: 263–296.

Cherry, M., Brown, J., Neal, T., and Shaw, N. (2010). What features of educational interventions lead to competence in aseptic insertion and maintenance of CV catheters in acute care? BEME Guide No. 15. *Med. Teach.* 32: 198–218.

Cook, D.A., Levinson, A.J., Garside, S. et al. (2008). Internet-based learning in the health professions: a meta-analysis. *JAMA* 300: 1181–1196.

Curren, V., Matthews, L., Fleet, L. et al. (2017). A review of digital, social, and mobile technologies in health professional education. *J. Contin. Educ. Heal. Prof.* 37: 195–206.

Davis, D.A., Mazmanian, P.E., Fordis, M. et al. (2006). Accuracy of physician self-assessment compared with observed measures of competence: a systematic review. *JAMA* 296: 1137–1139.

Emke, A., Butler, A., and Larsen, D. (2016). Effects of team-based learning on short-term and long-term retention of factual knowledge. *Med. Teach.* 38: 306–311.

EPOC (2015). *EPOC Taxonomy of Strategies.* Effective Practice and Organisation of Care (EPOC) at Cochrane Collaboration https://epoc.cochrane.org/epoc-taxonomy.

Flodgren, G., O'Brien, M.A., Parmelli, E., and Grimshaw, J.M. (2019). Local opinion leaders: effects on professional practice and health care outcomes. *Cochrane Database Syst. Rev.* (1): CD000125. https://doi.org/10.1002/14651858.CD000125.pub4.

Forsetlund, L., Björndal, A., Rashidian, A. et al. (2009). Continuing education meetings and workshops: effects on professional practice and health care outcomes. *Cochrane Database Syst. Rev.* (6): CD003030. https://doi.org/10.1002/14651858.

Frisby, B., Weber, K., and Beckner, B. (2014). Requiring participation: an instructor strategy to influence student interest and learning. *Commun. Q.* 62: 308–322.

Gifford, D.R., Holloway, R.G., Frankel, M.R. et al. (1999). Improving adherence to dementia guidelines through education and opinion leaders. A randomized controlled trial. *Ann. Intern. Med.* 131: 237–246.

Giguere, A., Auguste, D.U., Carmichael, P.H. et al. (2018). Printed educational materials: effects on professional practice and health care outcomes. *Cochrane Database Syst. Rev.* (3): CD004398. https://doi.org/10.1002/14651858. CD004398.pub3.

Grudniewicz, A., Kealy, R., Rodseth, R.N. et al. (2016). What is the effectiveness of printed educational materials on primary care physician knowledge, behavior, and patient outcomes: a systematic review and meta-analysis. *Implement. Sci.* 10: 164.

Hasan, A., Pozzi, M., and Hamilton, J.R.L. (2000). New surgical procedures: can we minimise the learning curve? *BMJ* 320: 171–173.

Hobma, S. (2005). *Directed self-learning*. Thesis. Maastricht: Maastricht University.

Hutchinson, L. (1999). Evaluating and researching the effectiveness of educational interventions. *BMJ* 318: 1267–1269.

Kaufman, D.M. (2003). Applying educational theory in practice. *BMJ* 326: 213–216.

Koh, G.C.H., Khoo, H.E., Wong, M.L., and Koh, D. (2008). The effects of problem-based learning during medical school on physician competency: systematic review. *CMAJ* 178: 34–41.

Mansouri, M. and Lockyer, J. (2007). A meta-analysis of continuing medical education effectiveness. *J. Contin. Educ. Heal. Prof.* 27: 6–15.

Mazmanian, P.E. and Davis, D. (2002). Continuing medical education and the physician as a learner. *JAMA* 288: 1057–1060.

Newman, P. and Peile, E. (2002). Valuing learner's experience and supporting further growth: educational models to help experienced adult learners in medicine. *BMJ* 325: 200–202.

O'Brien, M.A., Rogers, S., Jamvedt, G. et al. (2007). Educational outreach visits: effects on professional practice and health care outcomes. *Cochrane Database Syst. Rev.* (4): CD000409. https://doi.org/10.1002/14651858.CD000409. pub2.

Owen, P.A., Allerly, L.A., Harding, K.G. et al. (1989). General practitioners' continuing medical education within and outside their practice. *BMJ* 299: 238–240.

Petersen, S. (1999). Time for evidence based medical education. Tomorrow's doctors need informed educators and not amateur tutors. *BMJ* 318: 1233–1234.

Ram, P., Grol, R., Rethans, J.J. et al. (1999). Assessment of general practitioners by video observation of communicative and medical performance in daily practice: issues of validity, reliability and feasibility. *Med. Educ.* 33: 447–454.

Reeves, S., Perier, L., Goldman, J. et al. (2013). Interprofessional education: effects on professional practice and healthcare outcomes. *Cochrane Database Syst. Rev.* (3): CD002213. https://doi.org/10.1002/14651858. CD002213.pub3.

Richards, R.K. and Cohen, R.M. (1980). Why physicians attend traditional CME programs. *J. Med. Educ.* 55: 479–485.

Ruijters, M. (2012). *Liefde voor leren. Over diversiteit van leren en ontwikkelen in en van organisaties [Love to Learn. On Diversity of Learning and Development in and of Organizations]*. Alphen aan den Rijn, Netherlands: Kluwer.

Rust, C. (2002). The impact of assessment on student learning. *Learn High Educ.* 3: 145–158.

Slotnick, H.B., Raszokowski, R.R., Jensen, C.E. et al. (1994). Physician preferences in CME including insights into education versus promotion. *J. Contin. Educ. Heal. Prof.* 14: 173–186.

Soumerai, S.B. and Avorn, J. (1990). Principles of educational outreach ("academic detailing") to improve clinical decision making. *JAMA* 263: 549–556.

Spiby, H., McCormick, F., Wallace, L. et al. (2009). A systematic review of education and evidence-based practice interventions with health professionals and breast feeding counsellors on duration of breast feeding. *Midwifery* 25: 50–61.

Stammen, L.A., Stalmeijer, R.E., and Paternotte, E. (2015). Training physicians to provide high-value, cost-conscious care. A systematic review. *JAMA* 314: 2384–2400.

Steinert, Y., Mann, K., Centeno, A. et al. (2006). A systematic review of faculty development initiatives designed to improve teaching effectiveness in medical education: BEME Guide No. 8. *Med. Teach.* 28: 497–526.

Tassone, M.R. and Heck, C.S. (1997). Motivational orientations of allied health care professionals participating in continuing education. *J. Contin. Educ. Heal. Prof.* 17: 97–105.

Thomson, R., Gray, J., Madhok, R. et al. (1994). Effect of guidelines on management of head injury on record keeping and decision making in accident and emergency departments. *Qual. Health Care* 3: 86–91.

Versteeg, M.H., Laurant, M.G.H., Franx, G.C. et al. (2012). Factors associated with the impact of quality improvement collaborative in mental health care: an explorative study. *Implement. Sci.* 7 (1).

Watson, M.C., Bond, C.M., Grimshaw, J.M. et al. (2002). Educational strategies to promote evidence-based community pharmacy practice: a cluster randomized controlled trial. *Fam. Pract.* 19: 529–536.

Wensing, M., Broge, B., Riens, B. et al. (2009). Quality circles to improve prescribing of primary care physicians. Three comparative studies. *Pharmacoepidemiol. Drug Saf.* 18: 763–769.

13

Clinical Performance Feedback and Decision Support

Noah Ivers[1,2,3], Benjamin Brown[4], and Jeremy Grimshaw[5,6]

[1] *Women's College Research Institute and Family Practice Health Centre, Women's College Hospital, Toronto, Ontario, Canada*
[2] *Department of Family and Community Medicine, University of Toronto, Toronto, Ontario, Canada*
[3] *Dalla Lana School of Public Health, University of Toronto, Toronto, Ontario, Canada*
[4] *Centre for Primary Care and Centre for Health Informatics, University of Manchester, Manchester, UK*
[5] *Clinical Epidemiology Program, Ottawa Hospital Research Institute, Ottawa, Ontario, Canada*
[6] *Department of Medicine, University of Ottawa, Ottawa, Ontario, Canada*

SUMMARY

- Feedback of performance data, which are delivered extemporaneously to the clinical encounter, can lead to behavior change by drawing the attention of the individual or team of recipients to gaps between ideal and actual practice, where improvement efforts may be warranted.

- Decision support involves providing clinically relevant information for a specific patient, typically at the point of care. It works by reminding and prompting the individual health professional to take specific actions during a patient encounter.

- Both feedback and decision support have been found to improve healthcare delivery and outcomes, but their effectiveness is highly variable.

- The impact of feedback and decision support depends on a range of factors. These include the relevance and quality of the underlying evidence that supports the recommendations targeted by the feedback or decision support, the level of baseline performance, and the capacity of the recipient to take action.

- Feedback seems most effective when it is perceived as accurate and relevant, when it comes from a credible source repeatedly over time, or when it includes specific targets and action plans.

- Decision support seems most effective when it requires a response and when reminder fatigue is avoided.

13.1 Introduction

Health professionals are typically highly motivated to provide the best care and achieve the best outcomes for their patients (Payne and Hysong 2016). However, often their work environment is characterized by organized chaos, many tasks, and little time. Consider, for instance, the average primary care provider: estimates suggest that to implement all guideline-recommended preventive activities for an average-size practice would take more than seven hours per day, leaving little or no time for the management of other issues of immediate concern to patients (Korownyk et al. 2017). Similar challenges exist in hospitals and community care settings, especially where there are staff and resource shortages, such as in developing countries. In such circumstances, prioritization is necessary and gaps between recommended and actual care inevitable. Healthcare organizations and jurisdictions can leverage data to support health professionals to identify and address these gaps (Baker et al. 1999).

Two of the most common strategies used to support health professionals to reliably implement evidence-based practice are feedback (see Box 13.1 for an example) and decision support (see Box 13.2 for an example). Both these strategies take routinely collected health data and attempt to turn it into actionable information for providers. Perfect information does not automatically result in perfect practice, as the effectiveness of both feedback and decision support vary widely across studies. In this chapter, we summarize the evidence regarding these strategies, consider best practices for each, and explore areas of uncertainty. This chapter focuses on clinical performance feedback and decision support to professionals, teams, practices, and institutions in the context of improving patient care. Using feedback in the context of "external evaluation" (e.g. professional accreditation) or for accountability purposes (e.g. public reporting) are discussed in Chapter 7. Feedback of patient-reported measures and decision aids for patients are covered under patient-mediated interventions in Chapter 14.

Box 13.1 Example of Feedback to Improve Diagnostic Test Ordering in Primary Care

This diagram is from the "DRAM" randomized controlled trial of audit and feedback to 85 general practices in the north-east of Scotland to reduce nine unnecessary laboratory tests (Thomas et al. 2006).

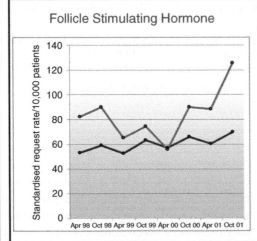

Follicle Stimulating Hormone (FSH) is released by the pituitary gland and acts to stimulate sex hormone production and reproductive processes. In general, FSH testing is of limited value in the assessment of menopausal status in women over 40 years of age, and so should not be requested for this purpose.

Menopausal/Peri-menopausal status is best confirmed retrospectively based on clinical symptoms, signs and frequency or absence of menstruation. Biochemical measurement adds little to this classification, and may mislead.

Box 13.2 Example of Decision Support That Interrupts Workflow and Requires a Response

This is an example of a clinical decision support system that is alerting a user to a possible drug–drug interaction while they are prescribing medication in an electronic health record (http://inspiredehrs.org/designing-for-clinicians/drug-alerts.php).

The alert interrupts their workflow of prescribing medication until they acknowledge the alert and choose an action (top image). Once they make a choice, the alert allows them to proceed (bottom image).

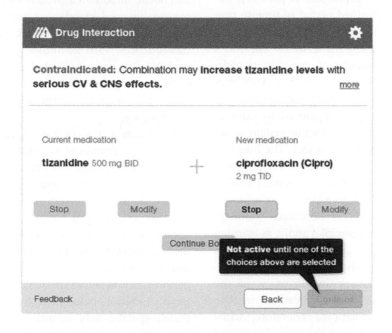

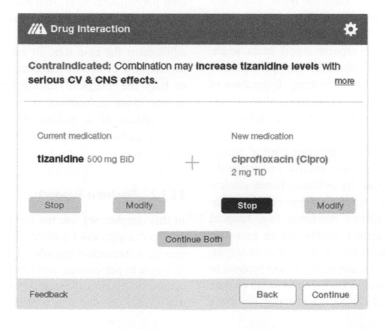

13.2 Definitions, Characteristics, and Components

13.2.1 Feedback

In this chapter, we use the term *feedback* as shorthand for delivering information about clinical performance provided to patient populations over a specified period of time to professionals, practices, or institutions, for the purpose of increasing the team's or clinician's insight into the quality of care they provide, and improving it when possible. This may occur in the context of mandatory or voluntary initiatives and may be organized by external groups (such as the healthcare system or an insurer) or internal/local teams. The information provided is typically based on a clinical "audit." The literature separates such clinical audits from feedback provided as part of continuing professional development, although many of the same principles apply, as learning from feedback is a fundamental human learning strategy (Shute 2008). Many clinical performance feedback initiatives avoid the term "audit" due to the perceived negative or punitive connotations. Therefore, while the literature often uses the term "audit and feedback," in practice the common terminology for these initiatives includes performance feedback, practice reports, report cards, scorecards, quality dashboards, key performance indicators, and benchmarking. Regardless of the terminology, the importance of the measurement aspect of the strategy cannot be underestimated.

An audit involves measuring clinical performance against explicit criteria or standards, usually informed by evidence-based clinical guidelines (e.g. avoiding inappropriate or wasteful tests) or patient outcomes (e.g. hospital admission or death). Audits can be based on routinely available information, such as administrative databases, electronic patient records, or medical registries, or they may be based on data collected specifically for this purpose. Feedback may also be based on patient-reported measures (based on their experience of care or based on the completion of validated scales to assess clinical outcomes). Sometimes, feedback incorporates clinical audit, patient-reported measures, plus peer or staff input, an approach known as 360° feedback. Regardless of the data sources for the audit, it should be recognized that not all important aspects of care are readily measurable, and in selecting some aspects of care to be measured there is a risk of unintended consequences, such as tunnel vision (Gulberg et al. 2010) or gaming (Yi et al. 2013). Measurement is always to some extent flawed, but is often still useful for learning and improving performance.

The feedback itself includes a number of key features (Colquhoun et al. 2017). Information about aspects of clinician performance, about patients' experiences, about the organization of care, its outcomes, and/or the costs of care may be summarized in written, graphical, and/or verbal format. It may be delivered to the recipient electronically, on paper, or in person. In terms of content, the recipient's own performance is summarized using aggregated population-level data, though there may be patient-specific data as well. The recipient's own performance over time may be compared to a target and/or to the performance of peers, and there may or may not be a description or adjustment for case mix. In addition, recommendations or action plans may be provided to help the recipient improve their performance. Usually, feedback is provided outside the context of a patient interaction, and usually delivered outside of clinician–patient consultations.

13.2.2 Decision Support

In this chapter, we use the term *decision support* to describe brief patient- or consultation-specific information intended to prompt a professional to perform or avoid a specific clinical action, or make a ("correct") decision (e.g. a diagnosis). The decision support often acts as a prompt, typically given *immediately before* or *during* contact with patients, and thus may be seen as a prospective or real-time approach – in contrast to feedback that provides a retrospective view of past performance. In other words, the decision support is presented to the provider within the context of a patient interaction and is typically "pushed" automatically to the recipient, without requiring them to "pull" the information.

Decision support provides additional information at the point of care (e.g. noting a drug–drug interaction, or the cost of certain diagnostic tests). In addition to the alert, there may also be a specific recommendation (e.g. suggesting alternative medication or testing options). Decision support may address potential errors of omission (e.g. forgetting to order a test for which the patient is due) or of commission (e.g. ordering a treatment for a patient with a known contra-indication). The clinical action can also take place before the patient contact, such as hand washing before surgery or preparing drugs in a clinical department. Other types of strategies may seek to "remind" providers about required tasks, such as generic posters in the clinic room, but here we focus on patient-specific decision support, which may do more than just "remind," they may provide novel information to "support" evidence-based actions. Typically, these point-of-care decision supports are provided through computerized systems (Wright et al. 2011). Thus, in this chapter we will refer frequently to the evidence for the effectiveness of computerized decision-support systems (CDSS).

Electronic health records are increasingly supported by knowledge management systems, through which clinical practice guideline recommendations or predictions from machine learning and artificial intelligence systems can be turned into automated prompts (Musen et al. 2014). Data from the patient chart is analyzed using a set of algorithms, which trigger on-screen prompts when a recommended clinical action is recommended or contra-indicated. These prompts may or may not be programmed

such that they require a response from the provider to over-ride the recommendation.

13.3 Effectiveness of Feedback and Decision Support

The effectiveness of feedback and decision support is well studied and is generally small to moderate, and highly variable (Table 13.1). Key systematic reviews examining the effects of feedback are Ivers et al.'s (2012) Cochrane review and the Tuti et al. (2017) review assessing electronic audit and feedback. The Cochrane Review included 140 randomized controlled trials (RCTs) where feedback was tested alone or deemed a core, essential element of a multifaceted intervention, and summarized the effects of these trials using the "median of medians" approach.

Key systematic reviews examining the effects of decision-support systems are Kwan et al. (2019) and a set of reviews covering the role of CDSS in preventive care, acute care, chronic disease management, diagnostic test ordering, prescribing, and drug monitoring (see Table 13.2). Reviews have also been published on specific disease topics, including antimicrobial prescribing (Rawson et al. 2017) and asthma (Fathima et al. 2014).

Little is known about the sustainability of effects for feedback or decision support. Current studies vary in the duration of time under analysis (ranging from months to years). It is unclear how long the feedback and decision support must continue after a change in processes of care or an improvement in the quality indicator has been achieved. Often professionals relapse to the old level of functioning after an intervention ends (Munchin et al. 2018). To consolidate the desired performance, it appears necessary to maintain the feedback or decision support for a long time or to accompany the process with other interventions. Ideally, the feedback or decision support should be

Table 13.1 Overview of reviews on performance feedback.

Ivers et al. (2012)	Audit and feedback containing interventions with other co-interventions versus usual care: studies with dichotomous outcomes (82 comparisons from 49 studies) included 2310 clusters/groups of health providers (from 32 cluster trials), and 2053 health professionals (from 17 trials allocating individual providers). The analysis found median 4.3% improvement in guideline-concordant care (interquartile range [IQR] 0.5–16%). Studies with continuous outcomes (26 comparisons from 21 studies) included 661 groups of healthcare providers (from 13 cluster trials) and 605 healthcare professionals (from 8 trials allocating individual providers). These showed median 1.3% improvement in guideline-concordant care (IQR 1.3–23.2%).
Ivers et al. (2012)	Audit and feedback alone versus usual care: studies with dichotomous outcomes (32 comparisons from 26 studies) included 759 groups of health providers (from 12 cluster trials) and 1617 health professionals (from 14 trials allocating individual providers). They showed a median 3% improvement in guideline-concordant care (IQR 1.8–7.7%). Studies with continuous outcomes (14 comparisons from 13 studies) included 348 groups of health providers (from 8 cluster trials) and 494 health professionals (from 5 trials allocating individual providers). The analysis showed a median 1.3% improvement in guideline-concordant care (IQR 1.3–11%).
Tuti et al. (2017)	Electronic audit and feedback: the review looks at 7 studies comprising 81 700 patients being cared for by 329 healthcare professionals/primary care facilities. Odds ratio for compliance with desired practice: 1.93 (95% CI 1.36–2.73) (very high heterogeneity was observed, $I^2 = 99\%$).

Table 13.2 Overview of reviews on computerized decision support systems (CDSS).

Jaspers et al. (2011)	This overview of reviews up to 2009 found evidence that CDSS significantly impacted practitioner performance in 52 out of 91 unique studies of the 16 systematic reviews (SRs) examining this effect (57%). Only 25 out of 82 unique studies of the 16 SRs reported evidence that CDSS positively impacted patient outcomes (30%).
Jia et al. (2016)	This overview of reviews on CDSS for medication safety found evidence that CDSS significantly impacted process of care in 108 out of 143 unique studies of the 16 SRs examining this effect (75%). Only 18 out of 90 unique studies of the 13 SRs reported significant evidence that CDSS positively impacted patient outcomes (20%). Ratings for the overall scores of AMSTAR resulted in a mean score of 8.3, with a range of scores from 7.5 to 10.5.
Kwan et al. (2019)	The review includes 106 studies reporting 120 comparisons. Adherence to target processes improved by 6.2% (95% CI 4.3–8.2%). In a sensitivity analysis using the best improvement from each study, improvements of 8.5% (95% CI 6.8–10.3%) were observed.
Roshanov et al. (2011a)	This review of CDSS for chronic disease management included 55 trials. 87% (n = 48) measured system impact on the process of care and 52% (n = 25) of those demonstrated statistically significant improvements. 65% (36/55) of trials measured impact on, typically, non-major (surrogate) patient outcomes, and 31% (n = 11) demonstrated benefits.
Sahota et al. (2011)	This review of CDSS for acute care management included 36 studies. The CDSS improved process of care in 63% (22/35) of studies, including 64% (9/14) of medication dosing assistants, 82% (9/11) of management assistants using alerts/reminders, 38% (3/8) of management assistants using guidelines/algorithms, and 67% (2/3) of diagnostic assistants. 20 studies evaluated patient outcomes, of which 3 (15%) reported improvements, all of which were medication dosing assistants.

Table 13.2 (Continued)

Roshanov et al. (2011b)	This review of CDSS for diagnostic test ordering included 33 trials. 55% (18/33) of CDSS improved testing behavior overall, including 83% (5/6) for diagnosis, 63% (5/8) for treatment monitoring, 35% (6/17) for disease monitoring, and 100% (3/3) for other purposes. Four of the systems explicitly attempted to reduce test ordering rates and all succeeded.
Hemens et al. (2011)	This review of CDSS for drug prescribing and management included 65 studies. Methodological quality was generally high and unchanged with time. CDSS improved process of care performance in 64% (37/59) studies assessing this type of outcome. 21% (6/29) of trials assessing patient outcomes reported improvements.

built into a system for continuous monitoring and improvement of the quality of care. This system can be used to determine whether improvements are still necessary and what progress has been made. Thus, these interventions should not be conceptualized as an intervention with a start and end point, but as a permanent service or structure subject to change to align with the needs of the recipients.

13.4 Factors Associated with Effects

13.4.1 Underlying Assumptions, Relevant Theories, and Mechanisms

Both feedback and decision support start from the assumption that the health professional is both motivated to optimize performance and has the skills and resources to reliably implement the targeted clinical action (Lock and Latham 2005). That is, they assume an existing belief among recipients that the targeted clinical action is desirable because it is likely to benefit patients (or otherwise aligned with their professional priorities), perceived as part of their professional role, or motivated by external factors (e.g. financial incentives for the implementation of practices).

An assumed mechanism of action for feedback is through the creation of cognitive dissonance (Festinger 1957). This concept describes the psychological discomfort experienced by health professionals when they learn that they are not reliably implementing best practices for their patients in the way that they had planned. The discomfort is addressed through (i) rationalizing a change (reduction) in the goal/target performance level; (ii) discrediting the results by, for instance, questioning the validity of the audit; or (iii) making plans to improve. Often, health professionals who interact with feedback will seek to validate the data in some manner before attempting to change their practice – especially if it implies they are performing "suboptimally." If they do accept the results, they may decide to change their practice in some fashion. Formal psychological theories that help explain the mechanism of action for feedback of clinical performance measures include goal-setting theory (Lock and Latham 2005) and control (self-regulation) theory (Carver and Scheier 1982), which emphasize the cyclical, iterative process described earlier and highlight, among other things, the role of self-efficacy in taking action to reach goals. In addition, feedback intervention theory (Kluger and DeNisi 1996), developed from a review of studies from the industrial and educational literatures, emphasizes the need to focus the recipient's attention on the task targeted by the feedback, and the potentially problematic role that emotions can play in this process. However, in randomized trials of interventions involving audit and feedback, very few used theory of any sort to plan or interpret their studies (Colquhoun et al. 2013). Those involved in the study of these initiatives did not seem to systematically unearth and address potential predictors of feedback effectiveness, limiting the ability of new interventions to achieve maximal impact (Ivers et al. 2014).

In addition, organizational constraints often influence the opportunities to adapt clinical behaviors after receiving feedback. Taking action in response to feedback may involve "trying harder" with each patient they see in future or, if they have the required skills and resources, attempting to implement new system-wide processes, often at the team or organizational level, to address the problem (Ivers et al. 2014). Ideally, feedback initiatives should be crafted to enable these steps so they are more appealing for health professionals than the other options of reducing cognitive dissonance already outlined. This means understanding the steps required to achieve higher performance and enabling them. Principles of user-centered design are relevant for both feedback and decision support. With feedback, there is the challenge of ensuring that the recipient's attention is directed to the key message (i.e. the area where improvement efforts are needed and the suggested actions for improvement in that area).

For decision support, the mechanism of action involves a prompt which may interrupt the usual workflow, asking the health professional to conduct a specific clinical action (Fox et al. 2010). Thus, ensuring the interruption is acceptable and compatible with the needs of the health professional whose goals it is meant to support is essential.

Future health professionals might develop workflows, which naturally involve the use of computerized decision support. Nevertheless, "reminder fatigue" is a major risk when decision-support systems overwhelm users with frequent, low-priority reminders (Ancker et al. 2017). Additionally, if a decision is already made when the reminder is presented, for instance in the case where a delegate (or a medical student) is carrying out the action on behalf of the true clinical decision maker, the potential benefits of CDSS may be lost. Those developing decision support should seek input from users about the types of clinical interactions when the potential decision support would be useful, and about both how and when to present the decision support in a way that is most likely to be helpful.

For both feedback and decision support, users may provide helpful insights during the development phase on a variety of design decisions (Brunner et al. 2017). Key points to consider include the optimal quantity of data to report, how data presentation is designed, how to strike the right tone (not too strict, engaging for the reader), and how to tailor the information to the individual or local needs of users. However, user-informed design does not require implementing all user preferences, especially if users indicate a preference that contradicts best established evidence regarding behavior change (Bravo et al. 2018). Careful preparation and piloting of the chosen format are desirable before the strategy is implemented on a large scale.

13.4.2 Factors Associated with Effects

The variable effects in studies of feedback and decision supports are not surprising, and can partially be explained by the heterogeneity of the studies in terms of the methods used and the interventions themselves. The reviews referenced earlier cover a wide range of clinical actions and target groups, and the interventions vary widely in their form and content. If the purpose of an audit is to determine whether clinical changes are needed (and further, to help convince health professionals that they should change; Baker et al. 1999), the audit should be carried out carefully, with attention to the reliable collection of data with face, construct, and content validity, and it should focus on areas where process improvement is both feasible and meaningful for patient outcomes (Willis et al. 2016). The same is true when considering topics for the creation of decision support.

Multivariate meta-regression in the Cochrane review of feedback (Ivers et al. 2012) indicated that feedback is more effective when baseline performance is low, the source is a supervisor or colleague, it is provided more than once, it is delivered both verbally and in writing, and it includes both explicit targets and an action plan.

In the meta-regressions for the latest review of decision support, only one characteristic was significantly associated with larger effects: "acknowledgment + documentation" (Kwan et al. 2019). This means that, when users had to enter a reason or click on a menu supplying a reason for complying/not complying, the improvements were more substantial. This may work by increasing the attention paid to the content of the decision support. A prior meta-regression (Roshanov et al. 2013) identified additional important covariates: (i) reminders that included advice for patients (by possibly making the reminder more actionable) or (ii) that were presented separately from electronic chart (by possibly being presented earlier in the decision-making process or avoiding alert fatigue; Kawamoto et al. 2005) were more effective. Evaluations by the developers of the reminder rather than a third party also found greater effects (Roshanov et al. 2013). These results were generally supported by another systematic review of head-to-head trials of CDSS, except that requiring acknowledgment and including specific recommendations or advice was not observed to be more effective in the head-to-head studies (Van de Velde et al. 2018a). Box 13.3 provides an example of a feedback strategy, which was combined with co-intervention to encourage use of the data.

Recently, increasing effort has been devoted to understanding the moderators and mediators of effect size for feedback and for decision support, with an eye to developing best practices for each. For example, Brehaut et al. (2016) interviewed experts from a range of fields to develop hypotheses and develop suggestions to optimize effectiveness for feedback (Table 13.3). Many of these may be just as relevant to decision support as they are to feedback.

In addition, Brown et al. (2019) conducted a meta-synthesis of qualitative studies of over 70 different feedback interventions to understand the factors that seemed to explain variation in their effectiveness. They ultimately used their findings to develop a detailed clinical performance feedback intervention theory (CP-FIT; Figure 13.1). CP-FIT states that effective feedback is a cyclical process of goal setting, data collection and analysis, feedback, recipient interaction, perception, and acceptance of the feedback, followed by intention, behavior, and clinical performance improvement (the feedback cycle). Feedback becomes less effective if any individual process fails, causing progress round the cycle to stop. This is influenced by several factors operating via a set of common explanatory mechanisms: feedback method used; health professional receiving feedback; and context in which feedback takes place. CP-FIT also highlights that feedback can have unintended outcomes such as *gaming*, where health professionals may manipulate clinical data or change their patient population to artificially improve their measured clinical performance, or *tunnel vision*, where they excessively focus on the topic against which clinical performance is measured to the detriment of other clinical areas. In the discussion of their findings, the authors posit that many of CP-FIT's hypotheses may also be relevant to CDSS.

For both feedback and reminders, the *source* and the *agent of delivery* may be important. This may help the user of the information trust that the data are valid and reliable. Ideally, the provider of the information is a respected organization or colleague, or a person more highly placed in the work hierarchy. The person who is responsible for clinical decision making should directly receive the information, as should, preferably, those who exercise control over an organization's quality improvement activities. To help recipients of feedback perceive comparisons as fair, consider adjusting for relevant variables such as the differences in underlying *case mix*. However, the

---

Box 13.3 Example of Primary Care Practice-Level Feedback with Patient-Specific Data, Along with Co-Interventions to Encourage Use of the Data to Make Changes

---

This was an intervention of web-based feedback conducted in Scotland to reduce high-risk prescribing (Dreischulte et al. 2016). Primary care practices were initially given an educational session on the topic, then access to a web-based tool that provided practice-level feedback on the proportion of patients receiving targeted high-risk prescriptions. The tool also provided patient-level information about the type of high-risk prescriptions received by patients. Practices received an initial fixed payment of £350 (US$600) and £15 ($25) for every patient for whom the targeted high-risk prescribing was reviewed. Targeted high-risk prescribing was significantly reduced, from a rate of 3.7–2.2% (adjusted odds ratio 0.63; 95% confidence interval [CI], 0.57–0.68; P < 0.001).

5. **Example text from an 8 weekly newsletter sent 24 weeks after the practice started the intervention where little initial change in prescribing**

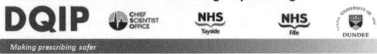

Dear GP/PM,

Six months have now passed since your practice has started the DQIP programme, with 6 months remaining. We are writing to you today in order to give you an update on your progress with the DQIP work.

Trends in high-risk prescribing

The run chart below (screenshot from the DQIP tool) shows that the total numbers of patients affected by any high-risk NSAID or antiplatelet prescribing have dropped to some extent since the last update 8 weeks ago, but the overall level of high-risk prescribing has remained similar to that seen before you've started DQIP. Figure 2 shows an update of the run chart of a practice who have successfully minimised their high-risk prescribing over 6 months.

Figure 1: Run chart for your practice   **Figure 2:** Run chart for a practice with comparable numbers of patients affected at DQIP start

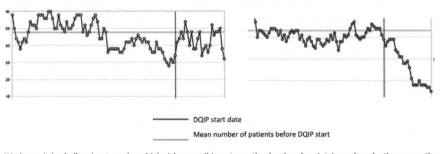

—————— DQIP start date

—————— Mean number of patients before DQIP start

We know it is challenging to reduce high-risk prescribing at practice level and maintain such reductions over time, because it requires not only stopping high-risk prescriptions in patients who have been flagged up by the DQIP tool, but also avoiding new high-risk prescriptions in patients with risk factors. This is especially the case when not all prescribers in the practice are involved in conducting the DQIP reviews. Where it is not possible to involve all prescribers in the review work, alerting colleagues when high-risk prescriptions have been issued may be crucial to increase awareness of future high-risk situations, in which NSAIDs and antiplatelets should be avoided or risk mitigating strategies implemented (if avoidance is not possible).

Can we help?

Please let us know if there is anything we can do to help (including a further practice visit if you think this would be helpful). You can contact us via email at dqip@dundee.ac.uk or by phone under 01382-420000.

Medication reviews

The practice has reviewed a total of 42 patients since the beginning of the DQIP trial corresponding to a payment of £630. There are currently 8 patients in your practice, who have yet to be reviewed. Please note that because we are measuring high-risk prescribing in the last 8 weeks, the *full* impact of any medication changes made may take a few weeks to show up in the run chart.

Kind regards,
The DQIP team

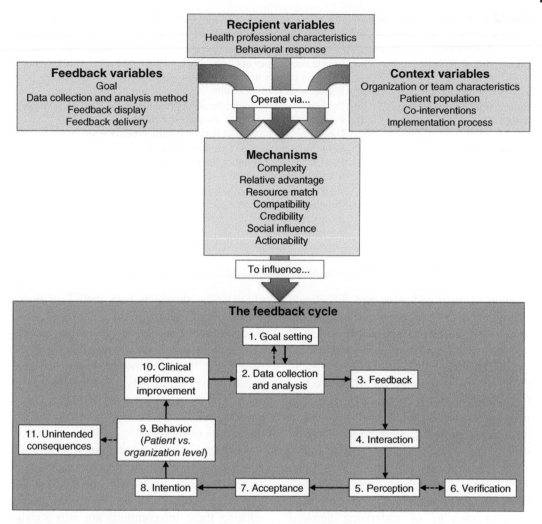

Figure 13.1 Clinical performance feedback intervention theory (CP-FIT).

comparison in feedback is there to motivate improvement effort and should be selected accordingly. In an RCT by Kiefe et al. (2001), the use of achievable benchmarks significantly enhanced the effectiveness of physician performance feedback.

For CDSS, an evidence synthesis coupled with input from international experts was used to produce a checklist for best practices in design and implementation (Van de Velde et al. 2018b). The checklist, known as GUIDES, recommends consideration of four domains. The first domain is the *context* (e.g. Does it address factors that predict the relevant behaviors? Is valid data available to construct decision support? Will users receive it positively? Can it be implemented within existing systems?). The second domain is the *content* (e.g. Is the evidence base valid? Is it pertinent? Are the recommendations clear and actionable?). The third domain is the *system* (e.g. Is usability optimized? Does the right information get to the right recipient at the right time?). The fourth domain is *implementation* (e.g. Are training and supports and co-interventions adequate? Can the system adapt or improve based on user input?).

It is important to consider the other initiatives that may be vying for the time and

Table 13.3 Suggestions for optimizing the effectiveness of audit and feedback.

Feedback domain	Best practices
Nature of desired action	Ensure consistency of feedback with established goals and priorities Focus on actions that can be improved Recommend specific actions
Nature of data available for feedback	Provide >1 instance of feedback; provide feedback as soon as possible Provide individual rather than general data Use credible comparators that recipients identify with
Visual display	Link visual displays to summary messages Provide feedback in more than one way Minimize cognitive load
Delivering the feedback intervention	Address barriers to using feedback Provide short actionable message followed by optional detail Assess credibility of information Prevent defensive reactions to feedback Construct feedback through social interaction

Source: Data from Brehaut et al. (2016).

attention of these end-users, and this should inform the selection of topics and quality indicators. In some environments, reminder fatigue is posited as a factor that might mitigate the potential benefits of CDSS (Backman et al. 2017). Finally, it is important to ensure that if multifaceted interventions are attempted, these are developed thoughtfully – as seen in the evidence summary, multifaceted interventions do not always achieve greater results and may not warrant investment (see Chapter 18). Selection of complementary (rather than redundant) co-interventions should be based on (i) knowledge of underlying barriers/facilitators for the desired behavior changes; and (ii) mapping of intervention strategies to address those barriers and facilitators. See Box 13.4 for an example of a strategy that combines feedback and decision support.

13.5 Discussion and Conclusions

The science of using routinely collected data and turning it into actionable information, through performance reporting (feedback) and decision support systems, is evolving. Those seeking to use these strategies to support the reliable implementation of best practices by health professions have a wealth of evidence upon which they can base their initiatives. The evidence highlights that these initiatives tend to have a positive impact, but the answer to the questions "how big an effect will it have?" and "how can the effect size be maximized?" are "it depends." This chapter lays out a series of tentative best practices and issues for consideration when developing or refining these types of strategies.

Feedback and decision-support interventions are commonly tested in randomized trials and even more commonly implemented in healthcare settings, but the best practices for utilizing these interventions are only slowly emerging. The situation has been described as "growing literature but stagnant science" (Ivers et al. 2014) and has led to initiatives to enhance the science of audit and feedback (Grimshaw et al. 2019). The studies conducted so far tell us relatively little about the right quantity of data or the optimal form in which the feedback or reminder should be presented. In the latest Cochrane review, feedback was most often provided in a written form, such as a printout of a computer file, but *web-based* feedback is, of course, increasingly seen. As of yet we know little about effective methods to report web-based feedback, and evaluative studies are needed to learn more about the most effective methods. Thus, there are unanswered questions as far as the design of

---

Box 13.4   Example of Electronic Audit and Feedback Plus Clinical Decision Support

The Performance Improvement plaN GeneratoR (PINGR) is an electronic feedback system with embedded CDSS (Brown et al. 2018). It is primarily used to support the treatment of patients with chronic diseases in primary care in the UK National Health Service. These images show how PINGR provides population-level feedback (top), lists of patients whose care requires improvement (middle), and individual patient-level data (bottom). It suggests tailored actions to improve clinical performance, which could be taken by healthcare teams and by clinicians for individual patients, on the left-hand side of the screen. Users have the option to provide responses for why they may disagree with a suggested action, which in turn is used to learn and improve the system's algorithms.

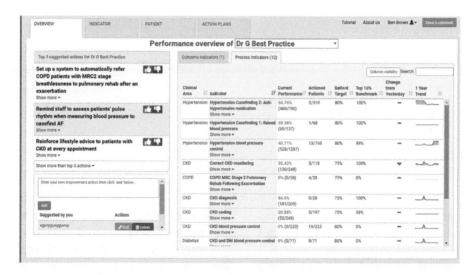

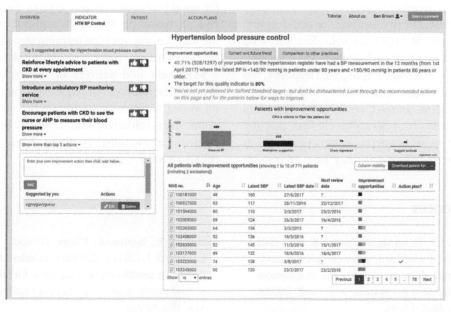

(Continued)

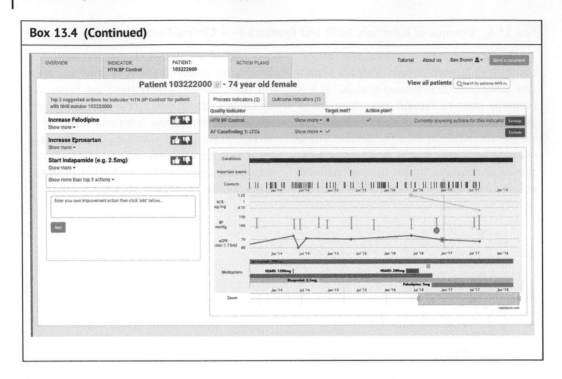

feedback or reminders is concerned: Do the targets of an intervention prefer information on a computer screen or on paper? Should it be a narrative report, an overview of figures, or a schematic representation?

The *timing* of the feedback or decision support is another important consideration. With the almost universal uptake of electronic health records and computerized feedback, this presents unique opportunities and platforms on which to conduct randomized controlled experiments in real-world clinical practice. Similar to e-commerce companies such as Amazon and Google, it may now be possible for users to conduct A/B tests to understand how varying the design and delivery of feedback and reminders could be optimized. Also like these large corporations, there is room for novel methods that aim to tailor the intervention based on the needs and patterns of the user (i.e. via machine learning techniques). We recommend that those involved in the development and delivery of feedback and/or decision-support strategies partner with interested academics to iteratively test and refine their initiatives and to report broadly rigorous evaluations resulting from these collaborations.

References

Ancker, J.S., Edwards, A., Nosal, S. et al. (2017). Effects of workload, work complexity, and repeated alerts on alert fatigue in a clinical decision support system. *BMC Med. Inform. Decis. Mak.* 17: 36.

Backman, R., Bayliss, S., Moore, D., and Litchfield, I. (2017). Clinical reminder alert fatigue in healthcare: a systematic literature review protocol using qualitative evidence. *Syst. Rev.* 6: 225.

Baker, R.H., Hearnshaw, H.M., and Robertson, N. (1999). *Implementing Change with Clinical Audit.* Hoboken, NJ: Wiley.

Bravo, C.A., Llovet, D., Witteman, H.O. et al. (2018). Designing emails aimed at increasing family physicians use of a web-based audit and feedback took to improve cancer screening rates: cocreation process. *JMIR Publ.* 5: 3.

Brehaut, J.C., Colquhoun, H.L., Eva, K.W. et al. (2016). Practice feedback interventions: 15 suggestions for optimizing effectiveness. *Ann. Intern. Med.* 164: 435–434.

Brown, B., Balatsoukas, P., Williams, R. et al. (2018). Multi-method laboratory user evaluation of an actionable clinical performance information system: implications for usability and patient safety. *J. Biomed. Inform.* 77: 62–80.

Brown, B., Gude, W.T., Blakeman, T. et al. (2019). Clinical Performance Feedback Intervention Theory (CP-FIT): a new theory for designing, implementing, and evaluating feedback in health care based on a meta synthesis of qualitative research. *Implement. Sci.* 14: 40.

Brunner, J., Chuang, E., Goldzweig, C. et al. (2017). User-centered design to improve clinical decision support in primary care. *Int. J. Med. Inform.* 104: 56–64.

Carver, C.S. and Scheier, M.F. (1982). Control theory: a useful conceptual framework for personality—social, clinical and health psychology. *Psychol. Bull.* 92: 111–135.

Colquhoun, H.L., Brehaut, J.C., Sales, A. et al. (2013). A systematic review of the use of theory in randomized controlled trials of audit and feedback. *Implement. Sci.* 8: 66.

Colquhoun, H., Michie, S., Sales, A. et al. (2017). Reporting and designing elements of audit and feedback interventions: a secondary review. *BMJ Qual. Saf.* 26: 54–60.

Dreischulte, T., Donnan, P., Grant, A. et al. (2016). Safer prescribing – a trial of education, informatics and financial incentives. *N Engl. J. Med.* 374: 1053–1046.

Fathima, M., Peiris, D., Naik-Panvelkar, P. et al. (2014). Effectiveness of computerized clinical decision support systems for asthma and chronic obstructive pulmonary disease in primary care: a systematic review. *BMC Pulm. Med.* 14: 189.

Festinger, L. (1957). *A Theory of Cognitive Dissonance.* Stanford, CA: Stanford University Press.

Fox, J., Glasspool, D., Patkar, V. et al. (2010). Delivering clinical decision support services: there is nothing as practical as good theory. *J. Biomed. Inform.* 43: 831–843.

Grimshaw, J.M., Ivers, N., Linklater, S. et al. (2019). Reinvigorating stagnant science: implementation laboratories and a meta-laboratory to efficiently advance the science of audit and feedback. *BMJ Qual. Saf.* 28: 416–423.

Gulberg, T.L., Vedsted, T., Lauritzen, V., and Zoffman, V. (2010). Suboptimal quality of type 2 diabetes care discovered through electronic feedback led to increased nurse–GP cooperation: a qualitative study. *Prim. Care Diabetes* 4: 33–39.

Hemens, B.J., Holbrook, A., Tonkin, M. et al. (2011). Computerized clinical decision support systems for drug prescribing and management: a decision-maker–researcher partnership systematic review. *Implement. Sci.* 6: 89.

Ivers, N., Grimshaw, J., Jamtvedt, G. et al. (2014). Growing literature, stagnant science? Systematic review, meta-regression and cumulative analysis of audit and feedback interventions in health care. *J. Gen. Intern. Med.* 29: 1534–1541.

Ivers, N., Jamtvedt, G., Flottorp, S. et al. (2012). Audit and feedback: effects on professional practice and healthcare outcomes. *Cochrane Database Syst. Rev.* (6): CD000259.

Jaspers, M.W., Smeulers, M., Vermeulen, H., and Peute, L.W. (2011). Effects of clinical decision-support systems on practitioner performance and patient outcomes: a synthesis of high-quality systematic review findings. *J. Am. Med. Inform. Assoc.* 18: 327–334.

Jia, P., Zhang, L., Chen, J. et al. (2016). The effects of clinical decision support systems on medical medication safety: an overview. *PLoS One* 11: e0167683.

Kawamoto, K., Houlihan, C.A., Balas, A.E., and Lobach, D.F. (2005). Improving clinical practice using clinical decision support systems: a systematic review of trials to identify features critical to success. *Br. Med. J.* 330: 765.

Kiefe, C., Allison, J., and Williams, D. (2001). Improving quality improvement using achievable benchmarks for physician feedback. A randomized controlled trial. *JAMA* 285: 2871–2879.

Kluger, A.N. and DeNisi, A. (1996). The effects of feedback interventions on performance. A historical review, a meta-analysis, and a preliminary feedback intervention theory. *Psychol. Bull.* 119: 254–284.

Korownyk, C., McCormack, J., Kolber, M.R. et al. (2017). Competing demands and opportunities in primary care. *Can. Fam. Physician* 63: 664–668.

Kwan, J.L., Lo, L., Ferguson, J. et al. (2019). How well do clinical decision support systems improve care? A meta-analysis of controlled clinical trials. Toronto: University of Toronto and Mount Sinai Hospital.

Lock, E.A. and Latham, G.P. (2005). Building a practically useful theory of goal setting and task motivation. A 35-year odyssey. *Am. Psychol.* 57: 705–717.

Munchin, M., Roland, M., Richardson, J. et al. (2018). Quality of care in the United Kingdom after removal of financial incentives. *N. Engl. J. Med.* 379: 948–957.

Musen, M.A., Middleton, B., and Greenes, R.A. (2014). Clinical decision-support systems. In: *Applied Health Care Biomedical*, 4e (eds. E.H. Shortliffe and J. Cimino), 643–647. London: Springer-Verlag.

Payne, V.L. and Hysong, S. (2016). Model depicting aspects of audit and feedback that impact physicians' acceptance of clinical performance feedback. *BMC Health Serv. Res.* 16: 260.

Rawson, T.M., Moore, L.S.P., Hernandez, B. et al. (2017). A systematic review of clinical decision support systems for antimicrobial management: are we failing to investigate these interventions appropriately? *Clin. Microbiol. Infect.* 23: 524–532.

Roshanov, P.S., Fernandes, N., Wilczynski, J.M. et al. (2013). Features of effective computerized clinical decision support memory systems: meta-regression of 162 randomized trials. *Br. Med. J.* f657: 346.

Roshanov, P.S., Misra, S., Gerstein, H.C. et al. (2011a). Computerized clinical decision support systems for chronic disease management: a decision-maker–researcher partnership systematic review. *Implement. Sci.* 9: 92.

Roshanov, P.S., You, J.J., Dhaliwal, J. et al. (2011b). Can computerized clinical decision support systems improve practitioners' diagnostic test ordering behaviour? A decision-maker–researcher partnership systematic review. *Implement. Sci.* 6: 88.

Sahota, N., Lloyd, R., Ramakrishna, A. et al. (2011). Computerized clinical decision support systems for acute care management: a decision-maker–researcher partnership systematic review of effects on process of care and patient outcomes. *Implement. Sci.* 6: 91.

Shute, V. (2008). Focus on formative feedback. *Rev. Educ. Res.* 78: 153.

Thomas, R.E., Croal, B.L., Ramsay, C. et al. (2006). Effect of enhanced feedback and brief educational reminder messages on laboratory test requesting in primary care: a cluster randomised trial. *Lancet* 367: 1990–1996.

Tuti, T., Nzinga, J., Njoroge, M. et al. (2017). A systematic review of electronic audit and feedback: intervention effectiveness and use of behaviour change theory. *Implement. Sci.* 12: 61.

Van de Velde, S., Heselmans, A., Delvaux, N. et al. (2018a). A systematic review of trials evaluating success factors of interventions with computerized clinical decision support. *Implement. Sci.* 13: 114.

Van de Velde, S., Kunnamo, I., Rashanov, P. et al. (2018b). The GUIDES checklist: development of a tool to improve the successful use of guideline-based computerized clinical decision support. *Implement. Sci.* 13: 86.

Willis, T.A., Heartley, S., Glidewell, L. et al. (2016). Action to Support Practices Implement Research Evidence (ASPIRE): protocol for a cluster-randomised evaluation of adaptable implementation packages targeting "high impact" clinical practice recommendations in general practice. *Implement. Sci.* 11: 25.

Wright, A., Sittig, D.F., Ash, J.S. et al. (2011). Development and evaluation of comprehensive clinical decision support taxonomy: comparison of front-end tools in commercial and internally developed electronic health systems. *J. Am. Med. Inform. Assoc.* 18: 232–242.

Yi, S.G., Wrat, N.P., Jones, S.L. et al. (2013). Surgeon-specific performance reports in general surgery: an observational study of initial implementation and adoption. *J. Am. Coll. Surg.* 217: 636–647.

14

Engaging Patients in Healthcare Improvement and Innovation

Glyn Elwyn[1] and Amy Price[2]

[1] *Dartmouth Institute for Health Policy and Clinical Practice, Geisel School of Medicine at Dartmouth College, Lebanon, NH, USA*
[2] *Stanford Medicine X, Stanford University School of Medicine, Stanford, CA, USA*

SUMMARY

- There are multiple levels to the engagement of patients in healthcare design, improvement, and innovation, from interpersonal decision making to policy development.
- Engaging patients in decision making in clinical encounters leads to significant change in knowledge, more accurate risk perception, and influence on intervention choice.
- The work involved in engaging and activating patients in their own care is highly dependent on factors such as attitudes, incentives, and organizational workflows.
- Implementing high-intensity patient engagement activity at organizational and policy levels is rare compared to lower-intensity efforts, such as conducting surveys.

14.1 Introduction

Healthcare in any nation can only be successful by building on the core principles of communication, compassion, and co-production with patients. All this takes is for clinicians and patients to build relationships together, independent of resource limitations. Most successful service industries rely on ensuring that customers are kept entirely satisfied and, where possible, free from experiencing delays, faults, or errors. Healthcare can learn from the service industry. Paying attention to satisfaction and convenience, and to the views and preferences of end-users – namely, patients and their carers – may be one way in which healthcare providers and healthcare systems can improve and grow. With higher literacy, internet access, and open access to research publications, the roles of patients are changing, with the role of patients finding recognition at multiple levels (Christensen et al. 2008). The publication of a number of conceptual frameworks from around the world is an indication that the roles of clinicians and patients are changing in relation to decision making, at both interpersonal, organizational, and policy levels.

At the community level, engagement and involvement have become an area of considerable debate since the 1960s. Arnstein's "ladder of citizen participation" made provocative distinctions between non-participation, tokenism, and citizen power (Arnstein 1969). Using an economics lens, Ostrom (1996) instead studied collaboration when communities faced the

Improving Patient Care: The Implementation of Change in Health Care, Third Edition. Edited by Michel Wensing, Richard Grol, and Jeremy Grimshaw.

task of making sustainable use of common resources, such as forests and fishing areas, and developed the concept of co-production, a concept that has been adapted for healthcare service design (Bate and Robert 2006; Batalden et al. 2016). An overarching framework describing the elements of patient and family engagement and how to develop interventions was constructed using a multistakeholder process, as illustrated by Figure 14.1 (Carman et al. 2013). The framework provides a matrix covering the continuum of engagement, from consultation to shared responsibility and leadership, on one dimension, and on the other illustrates how these can be achieved at different levels of care, such as face-to-face encounters, organizational design, or policy development. This chapter uses this framework to summarize the evidence about the influence of patient engagement on healthcare innovation. When you mix communication, compassion, and co-production with courtesy, curiosity, and evidence, our proposition is that shared values and preferences naturally emerge.

14.2 Impact of Patient Engagement on Direct Care

14.2.1 Well-Established Conceptual Frameworks

From the late 1970s onward, clinicians shared ideas about a different way of practicing medicine (Engel 1979; Katz 1984): an approach where the patient's views and opinions were sought, respected, and, indeed, might become the guiding principle for how treatment decisions are made. Some 40 years later, after a cascade of differing terms such as patient-centered care, person-centered care, patient activation, and shared decision making (SDM), the debate continues about the wisdom or otherwise of putting more emphasis on the goals and priorities of patients, how to achieve this end, and whether this approach leads to better clinical outcomes. In the interim, patient-centered care has grown as an educational model for clinical practice (Silverman et al. 2016). Many clinicians have been trained in patient-centered communication skills.

Continuum of engagement					
Levels of engagement	**Consultation**		**Involvement**		**Partnership and shared leadership**
Direct care	Patients receive information about a diagnosis	→	Patients are asked about their preferences in a treatment plan	→	Treatment decisions are made based on medical evidence, patients' preferences, and clinical judgment
Organizational design and governance	Organization surveys patients about their care experiences	→	Hospital involves patients as advisors or advisory council members	→	Patients co-lead hospital safety and quality improvement committees
Policy making	Public agency conducts focus groups with patients to ask opinions about a healthcare issue	→	Patients' recommendations about research priorities are used by a public agency to make funding decisions	→	Patients have equal representation on agency committee that makes decisions about how to allocate resources to health programs

Factors influencing engagement:
- **Patient, Family and Clinician** (beliefs about patient role, health literacy, education)
- **Organization** (policies and practices, culture)
- **Society** (social norms, regulations, policy)

Figure 14.1 A framework for patient and family engagement. *Source:* Carman et al. (2013).

14.2.2 Persistent Theory–Practice Gap

Despite the dominance of the conceptual model, empirical studies that assess the communication practices of clinicians find a theory–practice gap, where practitioners are found to fall short of behaving according to patient-centered ideals, and overestimate their skills at informing patients, eliciting their views and preferences, and tailoring interventions accordingly (Couët et al. 2015). By focusing patient engagement in terms of SDM, it is possible to examine the results of multiple studies. Efforts have been made to promote SDM, using tools called patient decision aids, designed to support SDM. These efforts are largely successful in tightly controlled research settings (Stacey et al. 2017; Box 14.1), where patient decision aids successfully help patients become better informed and able to participate in decisions. However, challenges arise for successful implementation in everyday clinical settings (Légaré et al. 2018), and it is difficult to ensure that the style of patient-centered communication advocated during training can be maintained in busy work settings (Elwyn et al. 2013; Box 14.2).

In an effort to assess whether patient engagement during direct care has an impact on health outcomes, Clayman et al. (2016) reported that while the ethical and moral arguments for involving patients and respecting their views are compelling, declaring definitively that adopting such a process leads to improved outcomes is difficult. A systematic review searched for studies focused on assessing the impact of patient participation in medical decisions on patient outcomes (Clayman et al. 2016) – see Box 14.3. Its conclusion was that there was a lack of measurement consistency, which made comparison between studies difficult, and that few high-quality studies have addressed the relationship between patient engagement in decision making and other outcomes. Such an analysis would need to assess the process of working toward shared goals and decisions, as well as the degree to which the patient had become informed.

Box 14.1   The Impact of Using Patient Decision Aids – Summarizing a Systematic Review

Across 105 studies, involving 31 043 participants:

- Patients gained knowledge about the attributes relating to the choices described (mean difference 13/100).

- Patients accurately reported the perceived risks.
- Patients reported greater congruence between their informed values and their care choices.

Source: Data from Stacey et al. (2017).

Box 14.2   Shared Decision Making in Routine Care

One study used observations of consultations and qualitative content analysis to explore decision making in routine cancer care in a hospital in Germany (Hahlweg et al. 2017). It found that one physician or a group of physicians made treatment decisions in most cases. Patients who were active (i.e. asked questions, demanded participation, opposed treatment decisions) facilitated SDM. Time pressure, frequent change of responsible physicians, and poor coordination of care were the main barriers observed. The authors concluded that strategies are needed to enhance SDM.

Box 14.3 Summary of Studies on Impact of Patient Participation on Health Outcomes

The goal of this review was to assess the extent to which patient participation in clinical encounters is associated with measured patient outcomes:

- 116 studies were analyzed, of which 11 were randomized trials.
- In 10 of these 11 trials, the interventions led to increased patient participation in decision making.
- In 5 of these 10 trials, at least one positive patient outcome was detected.

Source: Data from Clayman et al. (2016).

- However, the trials typically had many outcomes, thus reducing statistical power and resulting in a lower ratio of positive outcomes.

Few trials have examined the relationship between patient participation in medical decision making and patient outcomes. The results are mixed.

Another systematic review focused on the association of SDM measurement with other patient outcomes, such as knowledge, satisfaction, and other affective-cognitive constructs (Shay and Lafata 2015). After analyzing 39 studies, the review reported that "52% of outcomes assessed with patient-reported SDM were significant and positive." When observer-based measures of SDM were used, the rate was lower, at 21%, suggesting that patients are inclined to give positive appraisals compared to judges who examine audio or videotape representations of clinical encounters.

Might the search for significant beneficial biomedical outcomes and related patient behaviors be misguided? For instance, one study found no difference in clinical outcomes for patients with a diagnosis of Parkinson's disease when seen at home using videoconferencing technology compared to them attending an outpatient clinic (PCORI 2014). The patients far preferred being advised at home, and avoiding the high burden and cost of travel.

14.2.3 Broader Impacts

There is a broader way to consider patient engagement, which has come to increasing attention over the last few years. It has been described using the term co-production, and can be viewed as "[t]he interdependent work of users and professionals to design, create, develop, deliver, assess and improve the relationships and actions that contribute to the health of individuals and populations" (Batalden et al. 2016). Again, other terms are often used, such as co-creation or partnering with patients. Despite the many labels, the direction of change is clear. Passive patienthood and professional direction give way to collaboration, where compliance with professional recommendations is replaced by engagement, the conferment of agency, and self-management (Swensen et al. 2010; Coulter 2012; Elwyn et al. 2012; Nelson et al. 2014).

Without using the term, Wagner pioneered co-production by proposing the "chronic care model." This model relies (among other things) on an informed and activated patient engaging with a proactive clinical care team to strive for the best possible health outcomes (Coleman et al. 2009). Wagner's model can be summarized by the saying: "It's like having two experts in the room" (Tuckett et al. 1985). The patient has expertise on their personal resources, goals, functioning, symptoms, well-being, and treatment burden, whereas the clinician has expertise in pathophysiology, biomedical science, and which treatments might be best able to reduce the burden of illness. Co-production focuses on the skill of blending and balancing patient goals, preferences, and experience against the pursuit of biomedical targets (Reuben and Tinetti 2012).

The key concept for a full engagement of patients is the co-creation of value, or what Ostrom called co-production (Ostrom 1996). The co-creation of value already lies at the heart of leading-edge organizations and of some service sectors such as banking, travel, and financial services. Co-production is made even more powerful by the facilitation of service networks (i.e. facilitated networks), where many people form an alliance to solve problems, generate solutions, and share resources. Facilitated networks offer a powerful, transformative strategy that has been adopted by many innovative organizations to increase access to quality services while lowering costs of production (Christensen et al. 2008).

Facilitated networks have transformed many aspects of our life. In transport, for example, Uber and Lyft have radically changed the experience of traveling in urban areas, because more people have shared their vehicles and time using a platform that connects users with providers in real time. Airbnb has changed how people use their spare accommodation; eBay has changed the way people buy and sell belongings; and Wikipedia has surpassed all printed encyclopedias as the source of up-to-date information. All of these are examples of how facilitated networks have been leveraged to co-create valuable services, albeit not without adverse effects as well.

Despite innovative work by pioneers who have advanced aspects of healthcare co-production, such as Wagner's chronic care model (Wagner et al. 1996), Coulter's advocacy for patient engagement (Coulter 2012), Lorig's approach to evidence-based self-care (Lorig 2001), and the SDM approach itself (Makoul and Clayman 2006), healthcare providers have yet to consider co-production principles for developing facilitated networks to support healthcare provision. Some organizations such as Patients Like Me have pooled the experience of patients with a specific illness, but so far we have not witnessed rapid extensive use of facilitated networks in healthcare services. Such developments could serve as the means to shift services from being defined and delivered by professionals to services that are co-created in partnership with patients (Rozenblum and Bates 2013; Batalden 2018).

Healthcare managers often use the term "service lines," as if they were in a business characterized by industrial-style assembly lines for producing (and billing for) standard "products" such as diagnostic tests, injections, infusions, and surgical procedures. There is some truth in this healthcare as "product" perspective, especially when the evidence base clearly supports "doing this for that condition under these circumstances if the patient desires doing this for that." The Aravind Clinic in India provides a good example of the value of the service line approach for doing cataract surgery with high quality and low production costs, and thereby provides access to better vision even for those living in poverty, where the "focused factory" approach enables 600 eye operations a day, and by using an income-based pricing system enables cost-effective quality solutions for even the poorest people (Kasturi 2003).

However, there is increasing evidence from many settings – rheumatology (Hvitfeldt et al. 2009; Essén and Lindblad 2013), inflammatory bowel disease (Crandall et al. 2011), oncology (Basch et al. 2016, 2017), and primary care (Fernandopulle 2017) – that it is entirely possible to use co-production principles to add value to healthcare services, to help patients reduce the burden of illness and treatments, and to reduce the overall cost to society.

14.3 Impact of Patient Engagement on Organizational Design and Governance

Many healthcare organizations have become well accustomed to measuring the satisfaction of patients with the care they have received, and in some countries the measurement of patient satisfaction levels has been linked to payment and incentives. More recently, there has been a trend to measure more directly patients' experience of care and to engage patients in the planning, design, or delivery of care. There are a number of studies that report that engaging patients leads to improved processes and outcomes, such as efficiency and effectiveness. For example, a systematic review of five randomized trials and seven comparative studies found that involving users as employees of mental health services led to clients having "greater satisfaction with personal circumstances and less hospitalization" (Simpson and House 2002).

It is difficult to assess the state of the literature in this domain. As the framework in Figure 14.1 suggests, many different approaches to patient and family engagement are possible. Surveys, interviews, and focus groups are ways to seek views, but such methods risk being superficial, with little impact on the actual design of care processes. It is also likely that a very large number of organizations conduct consultations with patients and families about perceived needs, deficits, and plans, and that these exercises will never be published in peer-reviewed articles, irrespective of how successful they might have been at transforming care. With these caveats in mind, a systematic review conducted by Bombard and colleagues addressed the strategies and contextual factors that enable the optimal engagement of patients in the design, delivery, and evaluation of health services (Bombard et al. 2018).

The Bombard review focused on the organizational design and governance layer of Carman et al.'s framework; that is, on studies that consulted, involved, partnered, or co-designed health services with patients. Their search identified 20 957 studies, of which 20 909 were excluded because they did not report outcomes related to healthcare delivery, design, or evaluation, a result that in itself indicates that although there has been enormous interest in patient engagement activities, evaluative work in this domain is scarce and of low intensity, and runs the risk of being tokenistic. The results are summarized in Box 14.4.

In addition to summarizing the results, Bombard et al. described key strategies for optimal patient engagement (see Box 14.5).

In terms of outcomes, the studies could be categorized as being directed to the development of either "discrete products" (educational material, tools, policy, or planning documents) or toward the development or refinement of a new "care process" or a new service. The authors concluded that discrete products were more likely to use lower levels of engagement, such as consultation or surveys. The development of new care processes, however, was more likely to make use of higher levels of engagement, involving collaboration over time and co-design methods. These methods were also more likely to have an impact on the institution itself, in terms of shifts in organizational culture.

This review indicates that there is limited high-quality research that proves beyond doubt

---

Box 14.4   A Review of Studies on Patients' Engagement in Organizational Design

Of the 48 studies included in the review, 27 were qualitative studies. Half of the articles (n = 24) engaged patients using low-level consultative methods such as surveys or requests for comments on pre-prepared documents. The other half used higher-level engagement strategies, such as collaborative longer-term processes involving multiple steps and discussions. Most studies were from the UK (n = 26) and the USA (n = 11).

Source: Data from Bombard et al. (2018).

Box 14.5   Strategies for Optimal Patient Engagement

Techniques for enhancing patient input	• Enable patients to set agenda • Clarify goals and roles • Early participation and at all stages • Ensure diverse/multiple patient representation
Creating a receptive context	• Facilitate dialogue/discussion • Use skilled facilitators • Consider preparation and training
Leadership actions	• Secure institutional commitment • Involve institutional leaders • Engage before decisions are made

Source: Data from Bombard et al. (2018).

---

that engaging patients leads to improved clinical outcomes for patients; very few studies have been designed to evaluate such a goal. However, there is a growing body of literature to show that engaging patients leads to services that better meet the needs of patients (Coulter 2012) and improve patient-reported outcomes and experiences (Hunter et al. 2009). Perhaps patients might prioritize aspects such as access, convenience, and low opportunity costs over and above some clinical outcomes, which might well be the end-result of engaging patients in defining how value is created in healthcare delivery processes.

14.4   Impact of Patient Engagement in Policy Making

Enthusiasm for involving patients in many other aspects of healthcare has witnessed significant acceleration in the last few years, so much so that it seems increasingly difficult to develop a policy, a guideline, or a research proposal, or publish a paper in some journals, without first ensuring that a plan or process exists for meaningful patient and public involvement (PPI).

The earliest work in this domain was in the area of clinical practice guidelines (CPGs). When Boivin consulted over 50 CPG developers in 2009 (Boivin et al. 2010), he found that many had set up PPI methods that included training initiatives. At that time, there was limited understanding of which PPI strategies were likely to support patient engagement in the development of CPGs. In 2011, the Institute of Medicine set standards for the development of trustworthy guidelines that included structured PPI processes. When undertaking a review of guideline development processes in 101 organizations in the US National Guideline Clearinghouse, Armstrong and Bloom (2017) reported that less than 10% had required PPI in their published guidelines, suggesting significant room for increased patient engagement in this area of work. Guideline production methods would do well to develop and adopt standards on how to produce guidance that includes as a necessity the engagement of end-users; that is, the patients who are affected by such decisions.

Research funders are increasingly recommending, or requiring, PPI in the development of research proposals, the conduct of research, and the dissemination of results.

Box 14.6   Involving Patients in Setting Priorities for Healthcare Improvement

Patients are increasingly involved in priority setting for healthcare improvement. This cluster randomized trial examined the impact of patient involvement on the agreement of patients' and professionals' priorities, costs, and professionals' intention to use the results of the priority-setting activity (Boivin et al. 2014). A total of 172 individuals from 6 communities in Canada were involved. The study found that the study arm with patient involvement had a higher percentage of shared priorities. Costs were higher in the arm with patient involvement, while the intention to use the results was similar in the two study arms. The authors concluded that patient involvement can change priority setting, but that further research is required to examine the generalizability of the findings.

A prime example of this approach has been that taken by the Patient Centered Outcomes Research Institute in the USA, where applications will fail unless they can demonstrate evidence of significant patient engagement. Strong advocates will argue that patients' priorities should shape research agendas (Chalmers et al. 2013), and that research is always best done by following co-production principles (Hickey et al. 2018).

Over the last few years, the number of evaluations of PPI has grown significantly (Jagosh et al. 2012; Domecq et al. 2014). Nevertheless, there will be questions about the added value of engaging patients, and a need to evaluate whether or not the added work and cost are justified (Becker et al. 2010). A systematic review by Crocker provides welcome evidence that PPI leads to enhanced patient recruitment into research studies (Crocker et al. 2018). Boivin suggests a pragmatic approach to ensure that evaluation is not paralyzed by claims that PPI is too "controversial or complex" to be studied (Boivin et al. 2018). Box 14.6 provides an example.

14.5   Conclusion

In industry, end-user roles have evolved from that of a passive recipient to one that evaluates, provides feedback, and, in the most innovative enterprises, co-designs the experience and product. And so it is in healthcare: patients and their families are increasingly considered by innovative organizations as partners and collaborators, whether this is at the level of direct care, delivery design, or policy and research. While there is a need to evaluate the value of engaging patients in healthcare service improvement and innovation, healthcare providers and decision makers need to be acutely sensitive to how to define that value. It might be wise to temper the natural urge to demand superior biomedical outcomes before adopting health service delivery innovations. Lower treatment burden, lower cost, and less impact on quality of life are high priorities for many patients, and they may well trade marginal medical benefits for such outcomes. It is at least important for clinicians and patients to use the principles of co-production to align on the outcomes that make sense to both parties.

References

Armstrong, M.J. and Bloom, J.A. (2017). Patient involvement in guidelines is poor five years after Institute of Medicine Standards: review of guideline methodologies. *Res. Involv Engagem.* 3: 19.

Arnstein, S.R. (1969). A ladder of citizen participation. *J. Am. Inst. Plann.* 35: 216–224.

Basch, E., Deal, A.M., Kris, M.G. et al. (2016). Symptom monitoring with patient-reported outcomes during routine cancer treatment: a randomized controlled trial. *J. Clin. Oncol.* 34: 557–565.

Basch, E.A.M., Deal, A.M., Dueck, A.C. et al. (2017). Overall survival results of a trial assessing patient-reported outcomes for symptom monitoring during routine cancer treatment. *JAMA* 318: 197–198.

Batalden, P. (2018). Getting more health from healthcare: quality improvement must acknowledge patient coproduction—an essay by Paul Batalden. *BMJ* 362: k3617.

Batalden, M., Batalden, P., Margolis, P. et al. (2016). Coproduction of healthcare service. *BMJ Qual. Saf.* 25: 509–517.

Bate, P. and Robert, G. (2006). Experience-based design: from redesigning the system around the patient to co-designing services with the patient. *Qual. Saf. Health Care* 15: 307–310.

Becker, S., Sempik, J., and Bryman, A. (2010). Advocates, agnostics and adversaries: researchers' perceptions of service user involvement in social policy research. *Soc. Policy Soc.* 9: 355–366.

Boivin, A., Currie, K., Fervers, B. et al. (2010). Patient and public involvement in clinical guidelines: international experiences and future perspectives. *Qual. Saf. Health Care* 19: e22.

Boivin, A., Lehoux, P., Lacombe, R. et al. (2014). Involving patients in setting priorities in healthcare improvement: a cluster randomized trial. *Implement. Sci.* 9: 24.

Boivin, A., Richards, T., Forsythe, L. et al. (2018). Evaluating patient and public involvement in research. *BMJ* 363: k5147.

Bombard, Y.G., Baker, R., Orlando, E. et al. (2018). Engaging patients to improve quality of care: a systematic review. *Implement. Sci.* 13: 98.

Carman, K.L., Dardess, P., Maurer, M. et al. (2013). Patient and family engagement: a framework for understanding the elements and developing interventions and policies. *Health Aff.* 32: 223–231.

Chalmers, I., Atkinson, P., Fenton, M. et al. (2013). Tackling treatment uncertainties together: the evolution of the James Lind initiative, 2003–2013. *J. R. Soc. Med.* 106: 482–491.

Christensen, C.M., Grossman, J.H., and Hwang, J. (2008). *The Innovator's Prescription: A Disruptive Solution for Health Care*. McGraw-Hill Professional: New York.

Clayman, M.L., Bylund, C.L., Chewning, B., and Makoul, G. (2016). The impact of patient participation in health decisions within medical encounters: a systematic review. *Med. Decis. Making* 36: 427–452.

Coleman, K., Austin, B.T., Brach, C., and Wagner, E.H. (2009). Evidence on the chronic care model in the new millennium. *Health Aff.* 28: 75–85.

Couët, N., Desroches, S., Robitaille, H. et al. (2015). Assessments of the extent to which health-care providers involve patients in decision making: a systematic review of studies using the OPTION instrument. *Health Expect.* 18: 542–561.

Coulter, A. (2012). Patient engagement—what works? *J. Ambul. Care Manage.* 35: 80–89.

Crandall, W., Kappelman, M.D., Colletti, R.B. et al. (2011). ImproveCareNow: the development of a pediatric inflammatory bowel disease improvement network. *Inflamm. Bowel Dis.* 17: 450–457.

Crocker, J.C., Ricci-Cabello, I., Parker, A. et al. (2018). Impact of patient and public involvement on enrolment and retention in clinical trials: systematic review and meta-analysis. *BMJ* 363: k4738.

Domecq, J.P., Prutsky, G., Elraiyah, T. et al. (2014). Patient engagement in research: a systematic review. *BMC Health Serv. Res.* 14: 89.

Elwyn, G., Frosch, D., Thomson, R. et al. (2012). Shared decision making: a model for clinical practice. *J. Gen. Intern. Med.* 27: 1361–1367.

Elwyn, G., Scholl, I., Tietbohl, C. et al. (2013). "Many miles to go ...": a systematic review of the implementation of patient decision support interventions into routine clinical practice. *BMC Med. Inform. Decis. Mak.* 13 (Suppl 2): S14.

Engel, G.L. (1979). The biopsychosocial model and the education of health professionals. *Gen. Hosp. Psychiatry* 1: 156–165.

Essén, A. and Lindblad, S. (2013). Innovation as emergence in healthcare: unpacking change from within. *Soc. Sci. Med.* 93: 203–211.

Fernandopulle, R. (2017). Primary care needs a complete rebuilding and not just more renovations. *J. Ambul. Care Manage.* 40: 121–124.

Hahlweg, P., Haerter, M., Nestoriuc, Y., and Scholl, I. (2017). How are decisions made in cancer care? A qualitative study using participant observation of current practice. *BMJ Open* 7: e016360.

Hickey, G., Richards, T., and Sheehy, J. (2018). Co-production from proposal to paper. *Nature* 562: 29–31.

Hunter, R., Cameron, R., and Norrie, J. (2009). Using patient-reported outcomes in schizophrenia: the Scottish schizophrenia outcomes study. *Psychiatr. Serv.* 60: 240–245.

Hvitfeldt, H., Carli, C., Nelson, E.C. et al. (2009). Feed forward systems for patient participation and provider support: adoption results from the original US context to Sweden and beyond. *Qual. Manag. Health Care* 18: 247–256.

Jagosh, J., Macaulay, A.C., Pluye, P. et al. (2012). Uncovering the benefits of participatory research: implications of a realist review for health research and practice. *Milbank Q.* 90: 311–346.

Kasturi, R.V. (2003). *The Aravind Eye Hospital, Madurai, India: In Service for Sight*. Boston, MA: Harvard Business School.

Katz, J. (1984). *The Silent World of Physician and Patient*. New York: Free Press.

Légaré, F., Adekpedjou, R., Stacey, D. et al. (2018). Interventions for increasing the use of shared decision making by healthcare professionals. *Cochrane Database Syst. Rev.* (7): CD006732. https://doi.org/10.1002/14651858. CD006732.pub4.

Lorig, K. (2001). *Patient Education: A Practical Approach*. Sage: Thousand Oaks, CA.

Makoul, G. and Clayman, M.L. (2006). An integrative model of shared decision making in medical encounters. *Patient Educ. Couns.* 60: 301–312.

Nelson, E.C., Meyer, G., and Bohmer, R. (2014). Self-care: the new principal care. *J. Ambul. Care Manage.* 37: 219–225.

Ostrom, E. (1996). Crossing the great divide: coproduction, synergy, and development. *World Dev.* 24: 1073–1087.

PCORI (2014). Do video house calls with a specialist help get care to people with Parkinson's disease? Patient-Centered Outcomes Research Institute. https://www.pcori.org/research-results/2013/do-video-house-calls-specialist-help-get-care-people-parkinsons-disease (accessed November 7, 2019).

Reuben, D.B. and Tinetti, M.E. (2012). Goal-oriented patient care--an alternative health outcomes paradigm. *N. Engl. J. Med.* 366: 777–779.

Rozenblum, R. and Bates, D.W. (2013). Patient-centred healthcare, social media and the internet: the perfect storm? *BMJ Qual. Saf.* 22: 183–186.

Shay, L.A. and Lafata, J.E. (2015). Where is the evidence? A systematic review of shared decision making and patient outcomes. *Med. Decis. Making* 35: 114–131.

Silverman, J., Kurtz, S., and Draper, J. (2016). *Teaching and Learning Communication Skills in Medicine*. Boca Raton, FL: CRC Press.

Simpson, E.L. and House, A.O. (2002). Involving users in the delivery and evaluation of mental health services: systematic review. *BMJ* 325: 1265.

Stacey, D., Légaré, F., Lewis, K. et al. (2017). Decision aids for people facing health treatment or screening decisions. *Cochrane Database Syst. Rev.* (4): CD001431. https://doi.org/10.1002/14651858.CD001431.pub5.

Swensen, S.J., Meyer, G.S., Nelson, E.C. et al. (2010). Cottage industry to postindustrial care—the revolution in health care delivery. *N. Engl. J. Med.* 362: e12.

Tuckett, D., Boulton, M., Olson, C., and Williams, A. (1985). *Meetings Between Experts*. London: Tavistock.

Wagner, E.H., Austin, B.T., and Von Korff, M. (1996). Organizing care for patients with chronic illness. *Milbank Q.* 74: 511–544.

15

Organizational Implementation Strategies

Michel Wensing[1,2,3], Miranda Laurant[3,4], and Richard Grol[5,6]

[1] *Faculty of Medicine, University of Heidelberg, Heidelberg, Germany*
[2] *Department of General Practice and Health Services Research, Heidelberg University Hospital, Heidelberg, Germany*
[3] *Department IQ healthcare, Radboud Institute for Health Sciences, Radboud University Medical Center, Nijmegen, The Netherlands*
[4] *University of Applied Sciences Arnhem-Nijmegen, Nijmegen, The Netherlands*
[5] *Radboud University, Nijmegen, The Netherlands*
[6] *Maastricht University, Maastricht, The Netherlands*

SUMMARY

- Organizational strategies for improving healthcare can be directly targeted at patient care (e.g. revision of professional roles, enhanced teams for patient care, knowledge management) or at the organization of healthcare delivery (e.g. integrated care programs, quality and safety management).

- Research showed that organizational strategies can influence a range of outcomes, including aspects of quality of care and uptake of recommended practices. The effects are mixed and difficult to summarize, because the strategies and the settings of application are heterogeneous.

- The implementation of organizational strategies is a challenge by itself, which requires targeted activities.

15.1 Introduction

Many strategies for improving healthcare focus directly on individual health professionals. Examples include continuing education, audit and feedback, reminders, and decision support. On average, absolute improvements in professional behaviors of 5–10% can be achieved in this way (see Chapters 12 and 13). While such change can be clinically and financially relevant, more consistent and potentially larger changes would be desirable. Changes in healthcare organizations may contribute to this. Health system strategies, such as changes in reimbursement of healthcare providers (see Chapter 17), can stimulate and facilitate quality improvement and implementation of innovations in practice. Their impact is often mediated by organizational strategies, for instance a healthcare delivery model or an information technology (IT) infrastructure. Thus, organizational factors and strategies can have important impacts on processes and outcomes of change. Planned changes in the organization of healthcare can therefore contribute to more successful implementation of innovations, often in combination with interventions targeted at individual healthcare providers and/or healthcare system strategies.

Organizational implementation strategies may be applied relatively close to the delivery of patient care (Box 15.1 provides an example)

Improving Patient Care: The Implementation of Change in Health Care, Third Edition. Edited by Michel Wensing, Richard Grol, and Jeremy Grimshaw.
© 2020 John Wiley & Sons Ltd. Published 2020 by John Wiley & Sons Ltd.

Box 15.1   Multidisciplinary Rounds in Internal Medicine Departments

A large American hospital introduced multidisciplinary rounds in its internal medicine departments as part of a large quality improvement program (Curley et al. 1998). The effects were tested in a randomized trial, in which patients were randomly allocated to one of six teams: three teams used multidisciplinary rounds and three teams did not use this method. The authors reported that patients in the multidisciplinary rounds groups had on average a shorter hospital stay (5.46 versus 6.06 days) and lower costs (US$6681 versus $8090). Not all teams and departments showed the same changes.

Box 15.2   Organizational Implementation Strategies

- *Revision of professional roles*: changes in the professional roles of healthcare professionals, such as enhanced clinical activities of nurses, pharmacists, or psychologists.
- *Enhanced patient care teams*: increased coordination activities or clinical competence in patient care teams.
- *Knowledge management*: use of IT to support patient care, such as electronic patient records and decision-support systems.
- *Integrated care system*: enhanced structuring of patient care for specific patient groups, also known as disease management; case management is often one component.
- *Quality and safety management*: comprehensive system approaches to improve the quality and safety of care, such as accreditation, patient safety culture, and change of leadership.

---

or be more at a distance and initiated by the management of a healthcare organization. This chapter provides an overview of various organizational change strategies and their effects on professional behaviors, costs, and patient outcomes. It will also explore which factors influence the uptake of organizational changes. Box 15.2 lists the types of organizational implementation strategies that will be distinguished. In this chapter, the emphasis will be on changes made by health professionals and managers within existing healthcare organizations.

15.2   Revision of Professional Roles

Many studies have focused on a revision of professional roles, which often comprises the transfer of traditional physician tasks to non-physicians, such as pharmacists and nurses.

In some cases, new professions have been defined, such as nurse practitioners and physician assistants. The activities and professional autonomy of non-physician healthcare providers vary substantially between healthcare systems (Freund et al. 2015). In many countries, nurses take on activities of primary care physicians (Maier and Aiken 2016). In some countries, specific clinical tasks in primary care have been delegated to practice assistants (who are usually not nurses), which can enhance patient satisfaction with care (Szecsenyi et al. 2011).

A distinction can be made between substitution (replacement) and supplementation (addition) of physician tasks. In practice, it often comprises a mix of the two. Another distinction is between delegated tasks (tasks performed by non-physicians under the supervision of physicians) and referred tasks (tasks performed by non-physicians who are professionally autonomous). The revision of professional roles can contribute to the implementation of innovations, if it helps address gaps between recommended and provided healthcare. An example is offered in Box 15.3, in which nurses took on activities which are recommended, yet underperformed in the management of patients with chronic diseases in primary care.

Table 15.1 presents selected reviews of studies on the revision of professional roles. Overall, nurses and pharmacists achieve similar or better healthcare utilization, quality of care, patient experiences with care, and patient health status outcomes compared to physicians, at least in the context of research projects. The impact on health costs was mixed or absent. Substitution of primary care physicians by nurses, often in chronic illness care, results in lowered mortality (Martinez-Gonzalez et al. 2014; Laurant et al. 2018). A potential explanation is that non-physicians provide more patient education, adhere better to guidelines, and document their activities more extensively compared to physicians. At the same time, they use more time for consultations, perhaps because they tend to receive less support, and they may induce more follow-up contacts compared to physicians (Van der Biezen et al. 2016).

Box 15.3 Nurses in Primary Care Practices

A cluster randomized trial examined the effect of the introduction of nurses to substitute physicians in providing primary care (Laurant et al. 2004). The nurses were experienced community nurses, who had received additional training in chronic obstructive pulmonary disorder (COPD), asthma, dementia, and cancer. Patients could be referred to nurses, who then independently managed them. They had access to medical records and could consult the physician at any time if necessary. The study included 48 physicians, of whom 35 reported on their workload. The study showed that the number of consultations increased in the intervention group, particularly for patients with COPD. No changes of physician workload were found.

Table 15.1 Overview of reviews on revision of professional roles.

Author (number of studies)	Content	Main results
Blalock et al. (2013) (n = 21)	Patient care by community pharmacists	37% of all outcomes showed improvement, including blood pressure values, patient safety indicators, and patients' quality of life.
Laurant et al. (2018) (n = 18)	Substitution of general practitioners by nurses	Lowered mortality (relative risk [RR] 0.77). Similar or slightly better outcomes for nurses for aspects of health status, patient satisfaction, quality of care, and healthcare utilization. The effects on costs remain uncertain.
Martinez-Gonzalez et al. (2014) (n = 26)	Substitution of general practitioners by nurses	Lowered mortality (RR 0.89), lowered risk of hospitalization (RR 0.76), and higher patient satisfaction were found. Effects on cost and quality of life were inconsistent.
Stokes et al. (2015) (n = 36)	Case management in primary care for patients at risk for hospitalization	Small effects on patient reported health status (effect size [ES] 0.07) and patient satisfaction (ES 0.26). No effects on mortality, costs, or healthcare utilization were found.

Box 15.4   Care Coordination Delivered by Practice Assistants

In some countries, primary care is provided by physicians in office-based practice, supported by practice assistants (who are usually not nurses). In a project in Baden-Wuerttemberg, Germany, these practice assistants were trained to take on tasks in primary care for patients with multiple chronic conditions (Freund et al. 2016). In this way, primary care practices developed a team for delivering care. Patients of these practices received additional monitoring and education with a view on improving their quality of life and avoiding hospitalization. The effects were tested in a randomized trial, which involved 2076 patients from 115 practices; they had type 2 diabetes, COPD, or chronic heart failure. All-cause hospitalizations – the primary outcome – did not differ between groups at 12 and 24 months. Quality of life (measured with the SF-12 and EQ-5D instruments) improved significantly at 24 months. Intervention costs were US$10 per patient per month.

Various factors can influence the effects of the revision of professional roles. Martinez-Gonzalez et al. (2014) reported that the effects seemed most consistently large for nurse practitioners (nurses with extensive training and large professional autonomy) compared to registered or licensed nurses. Blalock et al. (2013) found that a number of factors may influence the effects in relation to pharmacists, such as the quality of relations between pharmacists and physicians, staffing of pharmacies, communication between pharmacy technicians, and financial reimbursement. Stokes et al. (2015) found in secondary analyses that the effects of case management may be higher if it is delivered by a multidisciplinary team, when a social worker was involved, and when delivered in a setting with a low strength of primary care. Barriers for substitution of physician tasks were found in four domains: negative attitudes in patients and professionals; restrictive laws and regulations; adverse financial incentives; and suboptimal training of non-physician clinicians (Laurant et al. 2009).

15.3   Enhanced Patient Care Teams

Patient care teams can be adapted in different ways, including enhanced coordination (e.g. different logistics of processes) and extended competency (e.g. adding a pharmacist; Bosch et al. 2009). Teams can also be enhanced by training in communication and collaboration skills, which influence teamwork, and by the implementation of checklists and other tools. Besides team composition, communication processes in teams are in many ways crucial for achieving team outcomes (Boxes 15.4 and 15.5 provide examples). However, research on the impact of team characteristics on healthcare delivery has not provided consistent clues on which factors are predictably influential (Holleman et al. 2009).

A range of studies have examined the effects of interventions on patient care teams (Table 15.2). For instance, a review of studies on multidisciplinary teams in hospital care distinguished two categories of interventions: changes in team composition and changes in team logistics. Most studies did not show effects on hospital stay, readmissions, or mortality, but half of the studies found a positive effect on prevention of complications (Pannick et al. 2015). Prevention of infections by the involvement of an infection specialist in the team was highly prevalent among the effective enhanced patient care teams. Enhanced teams in oncology were found to improve the process and outcomes of care (Prades et al. 2015). A review of interventions to improve interprofessional care remained inconclusive (Reeves et al. 2017).

Box 15.5   Network Analysis of Teams in a Neonatal Intensive Care Unit

In a neonatal intensive care unit, a total of 168 nurses cared for 3891 infants, who stayed an average of 9 days in the unit. As nurses work in shifts, hand-offs can be used to define a network structure based on notes routinely made by nurses. A study found that team size per patient (number of different nurses) grew with increasing length of stay (Gray et al. 2010). For each infant, the percentage of newcomers (nurses they had not seen before) dropped from more than 80% to 20% after about 120 shifts. Team size was not linked to family perceptions of nursing quality, but to the team structure. More nursing problems were reported in infants who stayed longer in the unit. The authors suggested that these hand-off networks can be visualized as a chain rather than a circle, or a more complex network structure with the same nurses in several shifts.

Table 15.2   Overview of reviews on enhanced patient care teams and team-orientated interventions.

Author (number of studies)	Content	Main results
Pannick et al. (2015) (n = 30)	Multidisciplinary teams in intramural hospital care	Positive effects were found on hospital stay in 30% of studies, which measured this outcome, and on rehospitalization in 20%, on mortality in 7% of studies. 50% of studies reported a lowered number of complications.
Prades et al. (2015) (n = 51)	Multidisciplinary teams in oncology care	Multidisciplinary teams showed positive effects on clinical and process aspects of care. Survival was higher in some cancers.
Reeves et al. (2017) (n = 9)	Interventions to improve interprofessional collaboration	Several effects were found, but no clear conclusions could be drawn from the studies. Collaborative working enhanced in 4 studies and the use of healthcare resources may be slightly improved in 3 studies.

15.4 Knowledge Management (Use of IT)

This section focuses on strategies for knowledge management by healthcare providers which use IT systems. Reminders generated by computerized decision-support systems are covered by Chapter 13. Knowledge management aims to support decision makers in retrieval, storage, and access to relevant information. In healthcare, this covers both patient-specific data and generic guidance (e.g. clinical guidelines and decision aids for patients). Examples of knowledge management strategies are computerized patient records and systems for online exchange of patient data. Some healthcare systems have integrated IT reasonably well, while uptake seems more limited in other systems. For instance, primary care practices in the Netherlands in 2020 have elaborate patient record systems, which integrate clinical decision support, facilitate exchange of data with pharmacists and hospitals, and may provide patients with access to their patient records and online booking of contacts. Box 15.6 illustrates that not all computerized information systems are effectively implemented and achieve the expected outcomes.

Table 15.3 summarizes the results of selected reviews on IT systems in healthcare. Electronic

---

Box 15.6   Implementation of Hospital Information System

In the province of Limpopo, South Africa, a large program was set up to implement a computerized information system in 42 hospitals in the region (Littlejohns et al. 2003). The aim was to improve the efficiency and effectiveness of healthcare by using a computer system for clinical, administrative, and evaluative purposes. A study was done to evaluate the introduction, benefits, and costs. This study was constructed as a randomized trial, but the implementation of the information system failed, so a mixed-methods case study was done to identify the determinants of this result. Many contributing factors for the failure were found, including:

- Education of workers had focused on "how" the system worked rather than "why" it had to be used.

- The use of the system disrupted interactions in daily practice and did not fit well with the complex flow of patients through the healthcare system.
- Few teams were consistent throughout the time period.
- Stopping the implementation was a difficult decision to make.

The authors suggest that these problems are similar to those in other cases of the implementation of IT. Lessons from the case should be learned in order to prevent waste of resources in the future.

Table 15.3 Overview of reviews on the use of information technology in healthcare.

Author (number of studies)	Content	Main results
Campanella et al. (2015) (n = 47)	Electronic patient records	Meta-analysis showed increased guideline adherence (relative risk [RR] 1.33) and lowered number of medication errors (RR 0.46), and fewer adverse outcomes (RR 0.66). No effect on mortality was found.
Flodgren et al. (2015) (n = 93)	Interactive telemedicine applications, such as monitoring and videoconferencing	Positive effects were found on quality of life (mean deviation [MD] -4.39) and clinical parameters (e.g. blood pressure). Effects on hospital admissions were mixed (range of 64% reduction to 60% increase). No effect on mortality was found.
Fiander et al. (2015) (n = 6)	Strategies to enhance use of information technology by health professionals	Training can enhance health professionals' use of information technology, although this does not necessarily translate into improved healthcare. One study did not find an effect of a customized versus generic interface.
Menachemi et al. (2018) (n = 24)	Health information exchange	All studies reported some positive benefits, and none reported adverse effects. For instance, 9 of 10 analyses found a positive effect on quality of care.
Varghese et al. (2017) (n = 70)	Computerized decision support in hospital inpatient care	Positive effects were found on mortality (7% of studies), life-threatening events (23%), and non-life-threatening events (40%). Almost a third (29%) of studies found no effect on patient outcomes.

patient records were found to be associated with positive impacts on healthcare delivery (Campanella et al. 2015). Interactive telemedicine applications had positive effects on quality of life and clinical parameters, and mixed effects on hospital admissions (Flodgren et al. 2015). In the years to come, much development of IT applications and their integration in patient care can be expected. Training of health professionals can help to increase their use of IT systems, although this does not necessarily translate into improved health outcomes (Fiander et al. 2015).

A qualitative synthesis of 65 studies on decision making regarding the adoption of medical technologies (Varabyova et al. 2017) suggested that three types of decision making can be distinguished: medical-individualistic (physicians are the main actors), fiscal-managerial (department and institutional heads are the main actors), and strategic-institutional (chief executives and governing boards are most important). Many determinants influence these types of decision making, for instance hospital size, resources availability, technology leadership, hospital competition, and urbanization. The various types of factors (individual, organizational, environmental, innovation related) have differential weights in the different modalities of decision making. For instance, the highest number of organizational and innovation-related determinants was found in medical-individualistic decision making, while the number of environmental determinants was highest in fiscal-managerial decision making.

15.5 Integrated Care Systems

There is no uniform definition of "integrated care." Related concepts include clinical pathways, disease management, collaborative care, coordinated care, shared care, and case management. Integrated care can address various aims, often including higher continuity of care, better uptake of recommended practices, higher efficiency, and better patient experiences in care. In essence, integrated care means the structuring of healthcare delivery for a defined patient population, for instance individuals with diabetes, and the involvement of healthcare professionals with various disciplinary backgrounds in a multiprofessional healthcare delivery model. A review identified the following components of integrated care: patient education and self-management support, structured follow-up and case management, a multidisciplinary patient care team, multidisciplinary clinical pathways, feedback, reminders, and continuing education for health professionals (Ouwens et al. 2005). The implementation of integrated care is a challenge in itself. In practice, case managers (who may be nurses or others) often have a key role in the translation of recommended practices to individual patients in the context of integrated care programs. Box 15.7 provides an example of an integrated care system in one hospital.

Box 15.7   Integrated Care for Patients with Head and Neck Cancer

An integrated care program for patients with head and neck cancer was developed at a university hospital (Ouwens et al. 2009). Using a step-wise model, current performance was measured and barriers to improvement were identified, followed by planning and implementation of improvements in the integrated care system. Components of the improvement program were the design of an optimal clinical pathway, feedback to health professionals, and an information package for patients. Chart audits and surveys were used to assess the impact. Results included a shortened waiting time for diagnostic tests and start of treatment, better support for attempts to stop smoking and for dietary changes, more involvement of a specialized radiologist for assessment of computed tomography (CT) and magnetic resonance imaging (MRI) scans, and more contact with specialized nurses.

Table 15.4 provides a number of reviews on integrated care programs. Several focus on ambulatory or primary care for patients with chronic diseases (Tricco et al. 2012; Reynolds et al. 2018). Self-management support seems the single most influential component of programs, but other components were found to have impact as well on outcomes such as healthcare utilization, clinical parameters, and patient experiences. Other reviews of the literature focus on strategies to enhance admission to and discharge from hospital (Leppin et al. 2014; Gonsalvez-Bradley et al. 2016). This research showed that strategies can result in fewer readmissions, lowered use of emergency care, and better patient experiences. More intensive strategies and strategies that support patient self-care seemed to be most effective (Leppin et al. 2014). The implementation of structured management of patients with chronic diseases in primary care is influenced by a range of factors, which relate to organizational culture, structural characteristics, networks and communication, implementation climate and readiness, presence of supportive leadership, and provider attitudes and beliefs (Kadu and Stolee 2015).

While integrated care systems enhance the implementation of recommended practices in patient care, the implementation of these

Table 15.4 Overview of reviews on integrated care programs.

Author (number of studies)	Content	Main results
Gonsalvez-Bradley et al. (2016) (n = 30)	Hospital discharge planning	Interventions led to shorter length of stay (mean deviation [MD] -0.73) and fewer readmissions (relative risk [RR] 0.87). Patient satisfaction with care may be improved. Effects on costs were unclear.
Leppin et al. (2014) (n = 42)	Strategies to reduce hospital readmissions	Strategies effectively reduced hospital readmissions (RR 0.82). Most effective seemed to be strategies which included more components, involved more individuals, and supported patient self-care.
Reynolds et al. (2018) (n = 157)	Strategies to improve chronic disease management	Studies were mapped onto the Chronic Care Model. Self-management support most frequently showed improvements in patient outcomes. Delivery system redesign showed improvement in professional practice and patient outcomes for a narrow range of diseases. Decision support had impacts on professional practice, in particular use of medications. Clinical information systems had positive impacts on both professional practice and patient outcomes.
Smith et al. (2017) (n = 42)	Shared care (primary care and specialist care) for various conditions	Mental health outcomes improved, particularly response to treatment (RR 1.40) and recovery (RR 2.59) in depression. Various other health outcomes and patient behaviors showed little or mixed change.
Tricco et al. (2012) (n = 142)	Strategies to improve diabetes care	A wide range of strategies improved diabetes care. Highest effects were found for strategies that included self-management support and case management.

systems themselves may require targeted activities. Relevant factors include acceptance by patients and health professionals, sufficient resources, and well-organized practices (Davy et al. 2015). An analysis of research on the implementation of integrated care programs in mental healthcare identified six strategies: continuing professional education, quality improvement processes, technical support, stakeholder involvement in the design and conduct of programs, enlarged role of nurses, and financial incentives (Franx et al. 2013). The impact of integrated care depends on successful and sustained implementation in healthcare practice.

15.6 Quality and Safety Management

Healthcare organizations can improve the quality and safety of healthcare in various ways, which are summarized here broadly as quality and safety management. Examples include accreditation, certification, lean management, value-based healthcare, total quality management, continuous quality improvement, and patient safety programs. These strategies may target implementation of innovations (e.g. evidence-based clinical guidelines), but also other aims, such as higher efficiency or improved patient experiences. Strategies for quality management generally focus on organizations, rather than individuals, and tend to emphasize short-cycle improvement, performance measurement, organizational culture, and leadership. Box 15.8 presents an example of a study on quality management in healthcare. The implementation of quality management in healthcare organizations is influenced by a range of contextual factors (Kringos et al. 2015).

The evidence base for many quality and safety management strategies comprises largely observational studies. A review of studies on practice accreditation found that it was associated with substantial costs and unclear benefits (Mumford et al. 2013). Changes in organizational culture and leadership are specific components of quality management that potentially have an impact on a wide range of clinical activities. Aspects of organizational culture were found to be associated with quality of care (Scott et al. 2003). Reviews on changing safety culture found effects for some strategies (Morello et al. 2013). Many of these successful strategies comprised team training, multidisciplinary rounds, tools for effective communication, or small-scale improvement projects.

Hospital, department, and practice leaders can obviously influence the implementation of innovations in several ways. Leadership can be characterized in many ways, including

---

Box 15.8 Impact of Total Quality Management and Organizational Culture in Patients after Coronary Bypass Surgery

A prospective cohort study measured outcomes in 3045 coronary artery bypass graft patients from 16 hospitals, including clinical parameters, functional status, costs, and satisfaction with care. Substantial variation in outcomes was found across hospitals, of which only a small part could be attributed to measures of implementation of quality management and organizational culture. In hospitals with high total quality management (TQM) scores, patients were more satisfied with nursing care, but more likely to have a hospital stay of over 10 days. A supportive group culture was associated with shorter post-surgery intubation, better functional status after six months, but also with longer stays in hospital. Thus, few effects of TQM or organizational culture on outcomes were found.

charismatic, transformational (focused on culture change), or transactional (focused on individual interests; see also Chapter 2). A review of observational studies of leadership suggested that leadership characteristics may be associated with quality and safety of healthcare delivery (Millar et al. 2013). Nevertheless, it remains difficult to indicate which type of leadership is associated with what outcomes.

15.7 Conclusions

Many organizational strategies to improve healthcare practice are available. Given the heterogeneity of strategies and settings, it is difficult to summarize the literature. Studies found positive effects on a range of outcomes for most approaches, but the hypothesized causality of associations is often uncertain and the generalizability of findings remains unclear. Having an impact on quality of care and health outcomes involves a long causal chain for organizational strategies. The implementation of organizational changes is often a challenge by itself, which requires targeted activities. For instance, research identified many barriers and facilitators for the implementation of the chronic care model, an integrated care system (Kadu and Stolee 2015), and the implementation of computer systems in the exam room (Patel et al. 2017). The healthcare system and organizational context are likely to influence the implementation, effectiveness, sustainability, and scalability of organizational strategies.

The chapter did not consider all types of organizational strategies. For instance, we did not consider increase of staffing. Increasing the number of nurses per patient is associated with lowered mortality, particularly in departments for intensive care and post-surgical care (Shekelle 2013). Reallocation of care between sectors (e.g. from hospital to primary care) was not discussed, neither were leadership interventions that may impact on the implementation of innovations (Gifford et al. 2018). Many organizational strategies are multifaceted and it remains largely unclear which of their components actually contributed to their impact. Organizational strategies are not necessarily tailored to locally relevant barriers to change (Bosch et al. 2007), a fact that probably reduces their impact. Finally, organizational strategies tend to have a wide range of objectives, of which improved professional performance and outcomes are just one. These strategies may also be targeted at reducing costs, at increasing the volume of patients that can be treated, at meeting specific societal expectations, or at solving problems of physician workload. This means that their success is also related to the extent to which they achieve those other objectives – which were not considered in this chapter.

References

Blalock, S.J., Roberts, A.W., Lauffenburger, J.C. et al. (2013). The effect of community pharmacy-based interventions on patient health outcomes. *Med. Care Res. Rev.* 70: 235–266.

Bosch, M., Faber, M.J., Cruijsberg, J. et al. (2009). Effectiveness of patient care teams and the role of clinical expertise and coordination: a literature review. *Med. Care Res. Rev.* 66: S5–S35.

Bosch, M., van der Weijden, T., Wensing, M., and Grol, R. (2007). Tailoring quality improvement interventions to identified barriers: a multiple case analysis. *J. Eval. Clin. Pract.* 13: 161–168.

Campanella, P., Lovoto, E., Marone, C. et al. (2015). The impact of electronic health records on the healthcare quality: a systematic review and meta-analysis. *Eur. J. Pub. Health* 26: 60–64.

Curley, C., McEachern, E., and Sperof, T. (1998). A firm trial of interdisciplinary rounds on the inpatient medical wards. An intervention designed using continuous quality improvement. *Med. Care* 36: AS4–AS12.

Davy, C., Bleasel, J., Liu, H. et al. (2015). Factors influencing the implementation of chronic care models: a systematic literature review. *BMC Fam. Pract.* 16: 102.

Fiander, M., McGowan, J., Grad, R. et al. (2015). Interventions to increase the use of electronic health information by health practitioners to improve clinical practice and health outcomes. *Cochrane Database Syst. Rev.* (3): CD004749. https://doi.org/10.1002/14651858. CD004749.pub3.

Flodgren, G., Rachas, A., Farmer, A.J. et al. (2015). Interactive telemedicine: effects on professional practice and health care outcomes. *Cochrane Database Syst. Rev.* (9): CD002098. https://doi.org/10.1002/14651858. CD002098.pub2.

Franx, G., Dixon, L., Wensing, M., and Pincus, H. (2013). Implementation strategies for collaborative primary care-mental health models. *Curr. Opin. Psychiatry* 26: 502–510.

Freund, T., Everett, C., Griffiths, P. et al. (2015). Skill mix, roles and remuneration in the primary care workforce: who are the healthcare professionals in the primary care teams across the world? *Int. J. Nurs. Stud.* 52: 727–743.

Freund, T., Peters-Klimm, F., Boyd, C.M. et al. (2016). Medical assistant-based care management for high-risk patients in small primary care practices: a cluster randomized clinical trial. *Ann. Intern. Med.* 164: 323–330.

Gifford, W.A., Squires, J.E., Angus, D.E. et al. (2018). Managerial leadership for research use in nursing and allied health professions: a systematic review. *Implement. Sci.* 13: 127.

Gonsalvez-Bradley, D.C., Lannin, N.A., Clemson, L.M. et al. (2016). Discharge planning from hospital. *Cochrane Database Syst. Rev.* (6): CD000313. https://doi.org/10.1002/14651858.

Gray, J.E., Davis, D.A., Pursley, D.M. et al. (2010). Network analysis of team structure in the neonatal intensive care unit. *Pediatrics* 125: e1460–e1467.

Kadu, M.K. and Stolee, P. (2015). Facilitators and barriers of implementing the chronic care model in primary care: a systematic review. *BMC Fam. Pract.* 16: 12.

Kringos, D.S., Sunol, R., Wagner, C. et al. (2015). The influence of context on the effectiveness of hospital quality improvement strategies: a review of systematic reviews. *BMC Health Serv. Res.* 15: 277.

Laurant, M., Harmsen, M., Wollersheim, H. et al. (2009). The impact of nonphysician clinicians: do they improve the quality and cost-effectiveness of health care services? *Med. Care Res. Rev.* 66: S36–S89.

Laurant, M.G.H., Hermens, R.P.M.G., Braspenning, J.C.C. et al. (2004). Impact of nurse practitioners on workload of general practitioners: randomised controlled trial. *BMJ* 328: 927–930.

Laurant, M., Van der Biezen, M., Wijers, N. et al. (2018). Nurses as substitutes for doctors in primary care. *Cochrane Database Syst. Rev.* (7): CD001271. https://doi.org/10.1002/14651858. CD001271.pub3.

Leppin, A.L., Gionfridda, M.R., Kessler, M. et al. (2014). Preventing 30-day hospital readmissions. A systematic review and meta-analysis of randomized trials. *JAMA Intern. Med.* 174: 1095–1107.

Littlejohns, P., Wyatt, J.C., and Garvican, L. (2003). Evaluating computerised health information systems: hard less still to be learnt. *BMJ* 326: 860–863.

Maier, C.B. and Aiken, L.H. (2016). Task shifting from physicians to nurses in primary care in 39 countries: a cross-country comparative study. *Eur. J. Pub. Health* 26: 927–934.

Martinez-Gonzalez, N., Djalali, S., Tandjung, R. et al. (2014). Substitution of physicians by nurses in primary care: a systematic review and meta-analysis. *BMC Health Serv. Res.* 13: 214.

Menachemi, N., Rahurkar, S., Harle, C.A., and Vest, J.R. (2018). The benefits of health information exchange: an updated systematic review. *J. Am. Med. Inform. Assoc.* 25: 1259–1265.

Millar, R., Mannion, R., Freeman, T., and Davies, H.T.O. (2013). Hospital board oversight of quality and patient safety: a narrative review and synthesis of recent empirical research. *Milbank Q* 91: 738–770.

Morello, R.T., Lowthian, J.A., Barker, A.L. et al. (2013). Strategies for improving patient safety culture in hospitals: a systematic review. *BMJ Qual. Saf.* 22: 11–18.

Mumford, V., Forde, K., Greenfield, D. et al. (2013). Health services accreditation: what is the evidence that the benefits justify the costs? *Int. J. Qual. Health Care* 25: 606–620.

Ouwens, M.M., Hermens, R.R., Hulscher, M.M. et al. (2009). Impact of an integrated care program for patients with head and neck cancer on the quality of care. *Head Neck* 31: 902–910.

Ouwens, M., Wollersheim, H., Hermens, R. et al. (2005). Integrated care programmes for chronically ill patients: a review of systematic reviews. *Int. J. Qual. Health Care* 17: 141–146.

Pannick, S., Davis, R., Ashrafian, H. et al. (2015). Effects of interdisciplinary team care interventions on general medical wards a systematic review. *JAMA Intern. Med.* 175: 1288–1298.

Patel, M.R., Vichich, J., Lang, I. et al. (2017). Developing an evidence base of best practices for integrating computer systems into the exam room: a systematic review. *J. Am. Med. Inform. Assoc.* 24: e207–e215.

Prades, J., Remue, E., Van Hoof, E., and Borras, J.M. (2015). Is it worth reorganizing cancer services on the basis of multidisciplinary teams (MDTs)? A systematic review of the objectives and organization of MDTs and their impact on patient outcomes. *Health Policy* 119: 464–479.

Reeves, S., Pelone, F., Harrison, R. et al. (2017). Interprofessional collaboration to improve professional practice and healthcare outcomes. *Cochrane Database Syst. Rev.* (6): CD0000072. https://doi.org/10.1002/14651858. CD000072.pub3.

Reynolds, R., Dennis, S., Hasan, I. et al. (2018). A systematic review of chronic disease management interventions in primary care. *BMC Fam. Pract.* 19: 11.

Scott, T., Mannion, R., Marshall, M., and Davies, H. (2003). Does organisational culture influence healthcare performance? A review of the evidence. *J. Health Serv. Res. Policy* 8: 105–117.

Shekelle, P.G. (2013). Nurse–patient ratios as a patient safety strategy. *Ann. Intern. Med.* 158: 404–409.

Smith, S.M., Cousins, G., Clyne, B. et al. (2017). Shared care across the interface between primary and secondary care in management of long term conditions. *Cochrane Database Syst. Rev.* (6): CD004910. https://doi.org/10.1002/14651858.CD004910.pub3.

Stokes, J., Panagioti, M., Alam, R. et al. (2015). Effectiveness of case management for 'at risk' patients in primary care: a systematic review and meta-analysis. *PLoS One* 10: e0132340.

Szecsenyi, J., Goetz, K., Campbell, S. et al. (2011). Is the job satisfaction of primary care team members associated with patient satisfaction? *BMJ Qual. Saf.* 20: 508–514.

Tricco, A.C., Ivers, N.M., Grimshaw, J.M. et al. (2012). Effectiveness of quality improvement strategies on the management of diabetes: a systematic review and meta-analysis. *Lancet* 379: 2252–2261.

Van der Biezen, M., Schoonhoven, L., Wijers, N. et al. (2016). Substitution of general practitioners by nurse practitioners in out-of-hours primary care: a quasi-experimental study. *J. Adv. Nurs.* 72: 1813–1824.

Varabyova, Y., Blankart, C.R., Greer, A.L., and Schreyögg, J. (2017). The determinants of medical technology adoption in different decisional systems: a systematic literature review. *Health Policy* 121: 230–242.

Varghese, J., Kleine, M., Gessner, S.I. et al. (2017). Effects of computerized decision support system implementations on patient outcomes in inpatient care: a systematic review. *J. Am. Med. Inform. Assoc.* 25: 593–602.

16

Patient Safety Strategies

Marieke Zegers[1,2], Mirelle Hanskamp-Sebregts[2,3], Hub Wollersheim[2], and Charles Vincent[4]

[1] Department Intensive Care, Radboud Institute for Health Sciences, Radboud University Medical Centre, Nijmegen, The Netherlands
[2] Department IQ healthcare, Radboud Institute for Health Sciences, Radboud University Medical Center, Nijmegen, The Netherlands
[3] Institute for Quality Assurance, Radboud Institute for Health Sciences, Radboud University Medical Center, Nijmegen, The Netherlands
[4] Department of Surgery and Cancer, Imperial College, London, UK

SUMMARY

- Research showed that about 10% of patients in hospital are harmed as a result of adverse events. In primary care, about 12% of patients experience patient safety incidents, although these do not necessarily lead to actual harm. Half of the adverse events in hospitals and primary care are preventable.

- Factors associated with patient safety incidents are, for example, inadequate training, problems in communication between health professionals, stressful situations, and problems with equipment.

- A range of strategies is available to measure and improve patient safety, including teamwork training, improved handover, and interventions to prevent infections, falls, pressure ulcers, and adverse drug events.

- Strategies to assure patient safety include efforts to enhance clinical leadership, improve safety culture, and improve governance.

- The research on these strategies shows mixed and overall moderately positive impacts.

16.1   Introduction

Alongside patient-centeredness, timeliness, efficacy, efficiency, and equity, patient safety is an important aspect of quality of healthcare. The World Health Organization (WHO) describes patient safety as: "The freedom for a patient from unnecessary harm or potential harm caused by adverse events in any healthcare setting" (Runciman et al. 2009). Attention for patient safety has increased in the last few decades, but some pioneers addressed it much earlier (Box 16.1). This chapter elaborates on patient safety in healthcare with a focus on strategies for improvement and assurance. Although there are overlaps with other chapters in this book, patient safety is a somewhat separate domain that is characterized by specific topics and approaches.

An analysis from the Harvard Medical Practice Study in 1991 showed that 4% of the patients admitted to hospitals in New York State suffered from adverse events (Brennan et al. 1991). A number of similar studies followed in several countries and showed that the median incidence of adverse events was 9.2%

Improving Patient Care: The Implementation of Change in Health Care, Third Edition. Edited by Michel Wensing, Richard Grol, and Jeremy Grimshaw.
© 2020 John Wiley & Sons Ltd. Published 2020 by John Wiley & Sons Ltd.

Box 16.1   Safety in Surgery

Ernest Codman (1869–1940) was a pioneer in the field of safety in surgery. He set up a method to measure surgical outcomes at the Massachusetts General Hospital and publicly discussed complications during so-called morbidity and mortality conferences. His colleagues and superiors became very anxious with his intention to publish a study on 123 incidents in 337 discharged patients. As a result, he was deprived of his staff position. After his rehabilitation he was appointed chairman of the American College of Surgeons. The work of Codman inspired the foundation of the Joint Commission in 1951, the world's first institute for quality of healthcare.

Table 16.1 Incidence of in-hospital adverse events across the world.

Study	Incidence of adverse events (%)
New York State (Brennan et al. 1991)	3.7
Australia (Wilson et al. 1999)	16.6
Utah/Colorado (Thomas et al. 2000)	2.9
UK (Vincent et al. 2001)	10.8
Denmark (Schiøler et al. 2001)	9.0
New Zealand (Davis et al. 2002)	12.9
Canada (Baker et al. 2004)	7.5
Spain (Aranaz-Andres et al. 2008)	8.4
Brazil (Mendes et al. 2009)	7.6
The Netherlands (Zegers et al. 2009)	5.7
Sweden (Soop et al. 2009)	12.3
Argentina, Colombia, Costa Rica, Mexico, and Peru (Aranaz-Andres et al. 2011)	10.5
Norway (Deilkås et al. 2015)	13.0
Ireland (Rafter et al. 2017)	10.3
Portugal (Sousa et al. 2018)	12.5

(de Vries et al. 2008). About half of these incidents (44%) were thought to be preventable. The adverse events which occurred most frequently were those entailing procedures (operations, deliveries, intervention radiology), prescribing or giving medication, wrong or delayed diagnoses, and events related to particular clinical problems (hospital infections, falls, pain, pressure ulcers, thrombosis, and bleeding;

de Vries et al. 2008). Rates of in-hospital adverse events across a number of studies are shown in Table 16.1.

A substantial number of consultations and treatments are realized in primary care, which is a separate sector in most healthcare systems. A recent systematic review (Madden et al. 2018) showed that the mean number of safety incidents per 100 patient records in primary care was 12.6. Within studies, a mean of 30.6% of incidents was associated with severe harm (range 8.6–50%), and a mean of 55.6% of incidents was considered preventable (range 32.7–93.5%). Poor communication and coordination between professionals and missing links between the health and social care system are among the primary causes of many of the problems identified in primary care (Vincent and Amalberti 2016). In addition, inadequate training and experience of individual professionals may cause adverse events such as delayed diagnosis and inadequate treatments.

16.2   Definition of Patient Safety Concepts

The WHO Alliance for Patient Safety produced an International Patient Safety Event Taxonomy (see Box 16.2; Runciman et al. 2009). The aim of the taxonomy is to enable the global healthcare community to analyze, evaluate, and learn from near miss and adverse event data at the international level, as well as

---

Box 16.2 Definitions for Key Concepts Related to Patient Safety

- *Incident*: an unintended event or circumstance that could have resulted, or did result, in unnecessary harm to a patient ("unnecessary" implies that it is potentially avoidable).
- *Near miss*: an incident which did not reach the patient.
- *Adverse event*: an incident that resulted in temporary or permanent harm to a patient, death, or prolonged hospital stay, caused by healthcare management rather than the underlying disease or injury.
- *Complication*: an unintended event or calculated risk that resulted in extra treatment or permanent harm arising during or after the provision of healthcare.

- *Harm*: impairment of the structure or function of the body and/or any deleterious effect arising therefrom, including disease, injury, suffering, disability, and death, which may be physical, social, or psychological.
- *Error*: a failure to carry out a planned action as intended or the application of an incorrect plan.
- *Preventable*: an incident that is being accepted by the community as avoidable in the particular set of circumstances.
- *Contributing factor*: a circumstance, action, or influence which is thought to have played a part in the origin or development of an incident or to increase the risk of an incident.

---

develop evidence-based preventive strategies in a consistent way across sources of safety data (such as reporting systems, claims data, patient-reported data, and medical record studies), the entire spectrum of healthcare, disciplines, time, cultures, and languages.

Measurement, improvement, and assurance of patient safety are necessary steps to prevent or mitigate patient harm in all kind of healthcare settings. In this chapter, we give an overview of strategies to measure, improve, and assure patient safety.

16.3 Strategies to Measure Patient Safety

Measuring and analyzing patient safety incidents are crucial steps in recognizing and learning to deal with unsafe situations. There are a number of methods that rely on different sources of data (see also Chapter 7). The different methods have different purposes and each of the methods has particular advantages and disadvantages (Table 16.2).

Medical record review is by far the most widely applied and thoroughly studied method for measuring adverse events. This method often has two stages. In the first stage, reviewers use a trigger tool to select records for a detailed review of adverse events in the second stage. A *trigger* is a risk indicator for an adverse event (Zegers et al. 2007), such as unplanned admission to the intensive care unit (ICU).

Indicators are used to measure incidents and adverse events in clinical and administrative data. Specific patient safety indicators have been developed (SimPatIE 2007; OECD 2009). The most-used indicator is the *hospital standardized mortality ratio* (HSMR). The HSMR is the ratio of observed and expected mortality of in-hospital patients based on patient factors such as age, sex, primary diagnosis, co-morbidities, and admission status. It is therefore an indicator for preventable deaths in hospitals. A higher HSMR suggests lower safety of care. However, the validity of this HSMR is disputed: both the correct and complete input of data and the way risks are adjusted are the subject of debate (Lilford and Pronovost 2010).

Table 16.2 Methods for measuring incidents and adverse events.

Methods	Advantages	Disadvantages
Record review	Commonly used, well-defined, and standardized method (experience in many previous studies) Almost no workload for clinical staff No inconvenience for departments or interruptions of the healthcare process	Potential information bias, e.g. incomplete or inadequate patient records, and hindsight bias Less appropriate for assessment of causal factors and preventability Expensive and time consuming Poor to moderate reliability
Analysis of routinely collected administrative data using indicators	Inexpensive Can be easily computerized Covers large populations	Low reliability of routinely collected information: data collected for other purposes (coding irregularities) and may therefore be incomplete or inaccurate Low sensitivity, fair specificity
Active clinical surveillance	Potentially accurate and precise	Time consuming and expensive
Morbidity and mortality conferences and autopsy	Can suggest latent errors Familiar to healthcare providers	Hindsight bias Reporting bias Focused on diagnostic errors Infrequently utilized
Litigation (liability claims) and complaints data	Provides multiple perspectives (patients, provider, lawyers)	Reporting bias: under-reporting of minor adverse outcomes Hindsight bias Non-standardized source of data
Voluntary (anonymous) incident reporting by healthcare providers and administrative personnel	Involvement of healthcare workers raises the awareness about patient safety and the development of a patient safety culture	Time consuming Under-reporting of severe adverse events, and some classes of adverse events by the willingness to report Low reliability Hindsight bias
Direct observation of patient care	Potentially accurate and precise Provides data otherwise unavailable; more insight into causes and preventability of adverse events Detects more active errors than other methods	Time consuming, expensive and resource intensive Difficult to train reliable observers Possible to be overwhelmed with information Hawthorne effect

Source: Battles and Lilford (2003); Lilford et al. (2003); Thomas and Petersen (2003); Zhan and Miller (2003).

A potentially more valid method of measuring adverse events is clinical surveillance. An example is a system of registration of postoperative myocardial infarctions with administration of electrocardiograms and measurement of cardiac enzymes in a standardized manner for all patients at a specified time and place. This method is ideal for assessing the effectiveness of specific interventions to decrease explicitly defined adverse events, but it is costly (Thomas and Petersen 2003).

Other methods are incident reporting systems, analysis of claims and complaints, and direct observation. The main problem of these methods is that single events – numerators – are assessed that are not systematically linked to denominators, thereby restricting the ability to estimate incidence rates (Pronovost et al. 2004).

There are several *incident reporting systems* at local level (ward or hospital) and at national level. Examples are the National Reporting and Learning System of the UK's National Patient Safety Agency (NPSA) and the Central Registration of Medication Incidents for pharmacists in the Netherlands. A weakness of incident reporting is under-reporting due to feelings of shame, fear of disapproval, time pressure, insufficient feedback on how the report was dealt with, and insufficient involvement of the reporter in the learning process. Practical experience shows that most incidents are reported by nurses (Leape 2002). "Autopsy analyses" and morbidity and mortality conferences are classic methods with which physicians analyze mostly diagnostic shortcomings and complications, often from a pathophysiologic perspective (Shojania et al. 2003; Deis et al. 2008).

For systematic, retrospective analysis of the underlying causes of incidents and adverse events, so-called *root cause analysis* is used. Several versions are available, for example *PRISMA* (Prevention and Recovery Information System for Monitoring and Analysis) and *SIRE* (Systematic Incident Reconstruction and Evaluation; Snijders et al. 2009; Leistikow et al. 2016). In these analyses, a "tree of causes" or a "herringbone analysis" is constructed, clustering causes. Vincent et al. (1998) developed the *London protocol*: a framework for analyzing and classifying incidents and causal factors. The system analysis of incidents tries to capture the wide variety of all contributory factors leading up to the incident, including all aspects of the healthcare system like professional and team-, patient-, organization-, and technique-related factors (see Table 16.3). *Health failure mode and effect analysis* (HFMEA)

Table 16.3 Factors influencing incidents.

Level of healthcare pyramid	Factors of influence	Examples
System	Finances, rules, legislation	Safety not in the legislation on quality of care, phased inspection
Organization	Budget, organizational structure, priorities, targets, attitude, safety culture	Safety not on the agenda of board of directors or heads of departments
Working environment	Staff (number, professions), design and maintenance of equipment, administrative and management support	High workload, overdue maintenance of equipment, messy administration
Team	Interprofessional and interdepartmental oral and written communication, supervision, leadership, team structure, and team morale	No, insufficient, incomplete, or wrong (or misunderstood) information, juniors overestimating themselves, poor supervision of managers
Duties	Complexity of duties, availability of protocols, job description and job clarity, accuracy and availability of diagnostic tests	Unclear or badly coordinated care processes, no or contradictory protocols
Healthcare provider	Knowledge, experience, competencies, physical, and mental health	Insufficient knowledge and experience of physicians, fatigue, stress, being addicted
Patient	Complexity of the disorder, language and communication problems, psychosocial circumstances, personality characteristics	Language barrier, illiteracy, lack of assertiveness

Source: Vincent et al. (1998).

is a prospective process analysis, originating from space travel. Experts are asked to analyze a high-risk process in their work in terms of risky steps, and to subsequently study the reduction of these risks. These suggestions are then entered into the process in question (Shebl et al. 2009). There are indications that fewer mistakes occur after HFMEA has been applied to medication, blood product, and biochemical laboratory analysis chains (Chiozza and Ponzetti 2009).

16.4 Patient Safety Improvement Strategies

Patient safety interventions aim to prevent or mitigate unintended patient harm stemming from the process of healthcare and to improve the safety of healthcare for patients (Dy et al. 2011). Because a wide variety of factors are associated with incidents, patient safety improvement interventions are often multitargeted, with strategies aimed at different levels (micro level, meso level, and macro level) within healthcare. A review of systematic reviews summarized the evidence for the effectiveness of safety interventions in hospital care (Zegers et al. 2016a). Little research has been done into specific safety-improving interventions in primary care and other non-hospital sectors. This section offers an overview of patient safety strategies that are proven to be effective and/or those that are widely used in daily practice. Effective interventions and factors that influence their effectiveness are summarized in Table 16.4. Box 16.3 provides an example of a multifaceted patient safety program (Health Foundation 2011).

16.4.1 Teamwork Training

Breakdown in team processes, such as coordination, leadership, or communication, has frequently been associated with adverse events and patient harm (Schmutz and Manser 2013). Aviation-based crew resource management

(CRM) training has been introduced to improve teamwork, communication, and patient safety in highly dynamic domains of healthcare, such as operating rooms, intensive care, or emergency medicine settings. Efforts to improve communication, in addition to CRM team training, include tools for standardization such as SBAR (see Box 16.4; Müller et al. 2018).

Simulation-based learning is increasingly used by healthcare professionals as a safe method to learn and practice non-technical skills, such as communication and leadership, required for effective CRM. CRM simulation-based training for interprofessional and interdisciplinary teams shows better results in teaching CRM in the simulator when compared to didactic case-based CRM education (Boet et al. 2014; Fung et al. 2015; MacDonald 2016). CRM skills learned at the simulation center are transferred to clinical settings, and lead to improved safety knowledge and attitudes of staff and patient outcomes, including a decrease in mortality (Boet et al. 2014; Hesselink et al. 2016).

Facilitators that improve the implementation of CRM are the perception of implementation leaders as a new and promising way to improve patient safety, as well as educating the whole staff. The costs of CRM and a lack of implementation expertise are important barriers during the orientation and the change phase, respectively (Kemper et al. 2017).

16.4.2 Improved Handovers

Multiprofessional cooperation is important, particularly in the light of the aging population and related increase of complex patients (multiple co-morbidities and poly-pharmacy), increasing specialization, and shift to more outpatient care. Patients are confronted with an ever-increasing number of healthcare providers. Misunderstandings, lack of clarity, and mistakes often arise at points of transitions (i.e. a patient moves from one healthcare provider or healthcare setting to another), and are therefore vulnerable moments in healthcare

Table 16.4 Overview of reviews on strategies to improve patient safety.

Strategies	Author, year (number of studies)	Effectiveness	Facilitators (F) and barriers (B) for implementation
Team training	Hesselink et al. (2016) (n = 18) Fung et al. (2015) (n = 12) Boet et al. (2014) (n = 9) Schmutz and Manser (2013) (n = 28)	Improved safety knowledge and attitudes of staff Improved patient outcomes, including a decrease in mortality	Implementation leaders (F) Educating the whole staff (F) Costs of CRM (B) Lack of implementation expertise (B)
Improved handover in hospitals	Luu et al. (2016) (n = 20) Stelfox et al. (2015) (n = 224) Rennke et al. (2013) (n = 47) Hesselink et al. (2012) (n = 36) Hansen et al. (2011) (n = 43) Øvretveit (2011) (n = 105)	Positive effects on patient safety outcomes, including hospital readmissions	Training of physicians (F) Structuring the handover process (F) Use of an electronic documentation template (F)
Improved handovers in intensive care units	Wibrandt and Lippert (2017) (n = 8)	Improved continuity of care (e.g. reduced discharge delay) Reduced adverse events	Checklist to structure discharge communication (F) Lack of feedback culture (B) Absence of ICU discharge criteria (B) Overestimation of ICU capabilities by general wards (B) Patient and family anxiety (B) Limited availability of ICU and ward resources (B)
Surgical safety checklist	Bergs et al. (2015) (n = 7)	Association with increased detection of potential safety hazards; reduction of post-operative complications, mortality, and surgical-site infections Improved communication among operating staff	Lack of clear written implementation guidelines (B) Absence of a safety culture, leadership, and teamwork (B) Conflicting priorities and different perspectives and motives of stakeholders (B)
Rapid response teams	McGaughey et al. (2017) (n = 105) Maharaj et al. (2015) (n = 29) Winters et al. (2013) (n = 43)	Reduction of cardiopulmonary arrests outside the ICU	Experienced staff with sufficient skills mix (F) Flexible use of EWS protocols (F) Access to ongoing, competency-based multiprofessional education for staff (F) Ward cultures (B) Hierarchic referral systems (B) Workload (B) Staffing resources (B)
Prevention of infections	Gould et al. (2017) (n = 26) Damiani et al. (2015) (n = 53) Luangasanatip et al. (2015) (n = 41) Zingg et al. (2015) (n = 92) Huis et al. (2012) (n = 41)	Reduction of infection and mortality rate	Infection control organization at hospital level (F) Materials and equipment availability (F) Appropriate use of guidelines (F) Education and training (F) Auditing; surveillance and feedback (F) Engagement of champions (F) Positive organizational culture (F)

(Continued)

Table 16.4 (Continued)

Strategies	Author, year (number of studies)	Effectiveness	Facilitators (F) and barriers (B) for implementation
Prevention of delirium	Bannon et al. (2019) (n = 15) Herling et al. (2018) (n = 12) Siddiqi et al. (2016) (n = 39) Martinez et al. (2014) (n = 7) Reston and Schoelles (2013) (n = 19)	Multicomponent interventions prevent delirium in hospitalized patients	Unknown
Prevention of falls	Cameron et al. (2018) (n = 95) Miake-Lye et al. (2013) (n = 19) Tricco et al. (2017) (n = 283)	Significant association between fall-prevention programs and reductions in injurious falls	Leadership support (F) Engagement of frontline clinical staff in intervention design (F) Guidance by a multidisciplinary committee (F) Pilot testing of the intervention (F) Providing data about falls and adherence by information systems (F) Education and training of clinical staff (F)
Prevention of pressure ulcers	Joyce et al. (2018) (n = 4) McInnes et al. (2015) (n = 59) Sullivan and Schoelles (2013) (n = 26)	Standard medical sheepskins prevent pressure ulcers	Simplification and standardization of specific interventions and documentation (F) Involvement of multidisciplinary teams (F) Leadership (F) Designated skin champions (F) Ongoing staff education (F) Sustained audit and feedback (F)
Prevention of pain/pain management	Meissner et al. (2015) (n = NA)	Pain management teams improved assessment and use of analgesics, no effect on pain outcomes	Deficient knowledge (B) Lack of instructions (B)
Medication safety	Korb-Savoldelli et al. (2018) (n = 14) Khalil and Roughead (2017) (n = 9) Christensen and Lundh (2016) (n = 10) Mekonnen et al. (2016) (n = 10) Prgomet et al. (2017) (n = 20) Lainer et al. (2015) (n = 43) Wang et al. (2015) (n = 4) Nuckols et al. (2014) (n = 16) Davey et al. (2013) (n = 221) Kwan et al. (2013) (n = 18) Lainer et al. (2013) (n = 10)	Participation of a pharmacist in physician rounds is associated with a reduced adverse drug event rate	Pharmacy staff involvement (F) Electronic tool (F) Safety culture in primary care (B)

CRM = crew resource management; EWS = early warning system; ICU = intensive care unit; NA = not applicable.

Box 16.3   System Interventions: Large-Scale Organizational Intervention to Improve Patient Safety in UK Hospitals

In 2004, the Safer Patients Initiative (SPI) program was launched: a large-scale, two-year initiative addressing patient safety in the UK. It had the overall aim of halving the number of adverse events within hospitals across the UK with an organization-wide program, based on experiences of the US Institute for Healthcare Improvement (IHI). The SPI focused on improving the reliability of specific frontline care processes and ensuring safety was a strategic priority by involving the chief executives and senior executive teams. The program consisted of generic elements focused on improving the culture of safety and good leadership (walkrounds), training for identifying safety problems and using methods to reduce risks (education on performing Plan–Do–Study–Act [PDSA] and HFMEA), and fostering an understanding of the principles of safe practice (formation of a collaborative learning community). In addition, the program included specific interventions focused on identifying and responding to deteriorating patients (Early Warning Score System [EWSS] and rapid response team), reducing medication error (ME; HFMEA, e.g. anti-coagulant prescribing; medication reconciliation on admission), improving communication between staff (Situation–Background–Assessment–Recommendation [SBAR] and safety briefings), and infection control (evidence-based practice, e.g. following ventilator guidelines to reduce ventilator-acquired pneumonia and improving hand hygiene; Health Foundation 2011). The results of the program evaluation were disappointing. A small improvement was found in staff attitudes to organizational climate. On a range of other measures (guideline compliance, quality of medical history taking, medication prescription errors, safety culture) and outcomes related to patient safety (adverse events, mortality, patient satisfaction), an additive effect attributable to SPI was not detected (Benning et al. 2011). The evaluators proposed potential reasons why there was no improvement in practice:

- Compliance was already high at baseline (such as use of steroids in over 85% of cases).
- Results may not have achieved statistical significance because of lack of statistical power.
- The intervention may have been insufficient to create the anticipated changes.
- Improvement may surface in the longer term.

Box 16.4   SBAR to Improve Communication between Healthcare Professionals

Communication errors are a common cause of adverse patient safety events in the healthcare field. The SBAR communication tool was introduced (Leonard et al. 2004) to guide the communication of critical patient care information.

- S = Situation (a concise statement of the problem)
- B = Background (pertinent and brief information related to the situation)
- A = Assessment (analysis and considerations of options – what you found/think)

- R = Recommendation (action requested/ recommended – what you want)

SBAR is useful for framing any conversation, especially critical ones, requiring a clinician's immediate attention and action. It allows for an easy and focused way to set expectations for what will be communicated and how between members of the healthcare team, which is essential for developing teamwork and fostering a culture of patient safety.

delivery and associated with medical errors, adverse events, increased mortality, and poor patient satisfaction with care (Stelfox et al. 2015). There are several interventions for improving handovers at hospital discharge that had positive effects on patient safety outcomes, including a discharge protocol, early discharge planning, patient education, organizing post-discharge services or follow-up, (early) assessment of follow-up needs and resources, electronic structured formats for discharge summaries, a dedicated transition provider, medication reconciliation, use of fax and email to transmit discharge summaries in a timely manner, or web-based access to discharge information for general practitioners (Hansen et al. 2011; Øvretveit 2011; Hesselink et al. 2012; Rennke et al. 2013). Training of physicians, structuring the handover process (e.g. dedicated time and place, avoidance of interruptions), and the use of an electronic documentation template facilitate safe and effective handovers (Kripalini 2011).

Handover of intensive care unit (ICU) patients from ICU to a different hospital ward is a high-risk episode in patient care for extra-vulnerable patients. Effective interventions include liaison nurses to improve communication and coordination of care; forms to facilitate timely, complete, and accurate handover information; and giving patients and their families a supplementary written or verbal status report before transfer (van Sluisveld et al. 2015; Zegers et al. 2016b; Wibrandt and Lippert 2017). These interventions resulted in improved continuity of care (e.g. reduced discharge delay) and reduced adverse events.

The *surgical safety checklist* (SSC) was developed to improve the handover of surgical patients through the complete peri-operative trajectory. Several studies showed that the implementation of the surgical checklist was associated with increased detection of potential safety hazards; a reduction of post-operative complications, mortality, and surgical-site infections; and improved communication among operating staff (de Vries et al. 2010; Bergs et al. 2014). Box 16.5 provides an example of a multidisciplinary SSC. Aspects that increase the effect of surgical checklists are improved perception of teamwork and safety climate among respondents (Bergs et al. 2014). Factors that impede the effect of the SSC include, for instance, the length, design, and content of the checklist, the implementation process (e.g. lack of clear written implementation guidelines), and the local context (e.g. the absence of a safety culture, leadership and teamwork; Bergs et al. 2015). Furthermore, conflicting

---

Box 16.5   Improved Patient Safety by Implementing a Multidisciplinary Surgical Checklist

A large number of preventable adverse events are encountered during hospital admission and in particular around surgical procedures. The multidisciplinary SURPASS (SURgical PAtient Safety System) checklist accompanies the patient during each step of the surgical pathway until discharge, and is completed by different healthcare professionals involved in the surgical process. Therefore, the SURPASS checklist is more comprehensive than the WHO SSC, which covers the immediate peri-operative period. Each component checklist requires signing off (and dating) by the appropriate person(s). Implementing a surgical checklist that targets the entire surgical pathway, rather than just the operating room, reduces in-hospital mortality by nearly a half and the total number of surgical complications by a third in hospitals that already had a high standard of care (De Vries et al. 2010). The use of the SURPASS checklist leads to better compliance with regard to the timing of antibiotic prophylaxis administration and covers the entire surgical experience for a patient.

priorities and different perspectives and motives of stakeholders complicate checklist implementation. Enlisting institutional leaders as local champions facilitates team learning to foster the mutual understanding of perspectives and motivations, and the realignment of routines (Bergs et al. 2015).

16.4.3 Rapid Response Team

Ward patients may deteriorate to the point of unexpected ICU admission or even cardiac arrest and death. Rapid response systems (RRSs) were introduced in hospital to improve recognition of and response to deteriorating patients, to ultimately prevent cardiopulmonary arrest and mortality (Maharaj et al. 2015). Cardiopulmonary arrests outside the ICU reduced after the implementation of rapid response teams. Important components of successful RRSs include activation criteria, a system for notifying and activating the response team, and an administrative and quality improvement component to train staff, collect and analyze event data, provide feedback, coordinate resources, and ensure improvement or maintenance over time (Winters et al. 2013). Additionally, RRSs achieved desired outcomes when there was a sufficient skills mix of experienced staff, early warning system protocols were used flexibly alongside clinical judgment, and staff had access to ongoing, multiprofessional, competency-based education. However, ward cultures, hierarchical referral systems, workload, and staffing resources had a negative impact on the implementation of the RRS (McGaughey et al. 2017).

16.4.4 Infection Prevention

Healthcare-associated infections (HCAIs), including central line–associated bloodstream infection, catheter-associated urinary tract infection (CAUTI), ventilator-associated pneumonia, and surgical-site infection, are acquired during (hospital) care. HCAIs have been associated with a significant impact on morbidity and mortality and pose major threats to patient safety (Gould et al. 2017). In the USA, HCAIs are responsible for over 90 000 deaths each year and rank among the leading causes of death. The total annual number of patients with an HCAI in European acute care hospitals was recently estimated at 3.2 million.

Implementing interventions, such as checklists and care bundles, reduced infection and mortality rates significantly (de Vries et al. 2010; Bergs et al. 2014; Meddings et al. 2014; Damiani et al. 2015). The use of a reminder and/or stop order to prompt removal of unnecessary urinary catheters led to a 53% reduction of CAUTI episodes per 1000 catheter days (Meddings et al. 2014). The implementation of a program to improve compliance to sepsis care bundles led to a statistically significant decreased mortality rate (Damiani et al. 2015).

Key components to reduce HCAIs are the organization of infection control at the hospital level, availability of and ease of access to materials and equipment and optimum ergonomics, appropriate use of guidelines, education and training, auditing, surveillance and feedback, multimodal and multidisciplinary prevention programs for behavioral change, engagement of champions, and positive organizational culture (Zingg et al. 2015). Programs should be planned by multidisciplinary groups, take into account local guidelines, follow a multimodal intervention strategy that emphasizes hands-on training, and be regularly assessed and adjusted if necessary (Zingg et al. 2015).

Hand hygiene is widely thought to be the most important activity for the prevention of HCAIs. In 2005, the WHO launched the campaign "Clean Care Is Safer Care," aimed at improving hand hygiene in healthcare (WHO 2009). It is a multifaceted hand hygiene intervention consisting of five components: system change, training and education, observation and feedback, reminders in the hospital, and a hospital safety climate. These interventions are associated with improved compliance with hand hygiene among healthcare workers in hospital compared with standard practice (Luangasanatip et al. 2015; Gould et al. 2017;

Box 16.6   A National Approach: Australian National Hand Hygiene Initiative

The Australian National Hand Hygiene Initiative (NHHI) is a standardized culture-change program for hospitals based on the WHO Multimodal Hand Hygiene Improvement Strategy, with a focus on system change, healthcare worker education, and audit and feedback (Grayson et al. 2018). The NHHI aims to improve hand hygiene compliance among Australian healthcare workers and reduce the risk of HCAIs. Eight years after implementation, the NHHI has been associated with a significant sustained improvement in hand hygiene compliance and a decline in the incidence of healthcare-associated *Staphylococcus aureus* bacteremia (HA-SAB). For every 10% increase in hand

hygiene compliance, the incidence of HA-SAB decreased by 15%. Key contributors to NHHI success include leadership from the government agency Australian Commission on Safety and Quality in Health Care, a standardized national approach with collaboration and engagement between federal and jurisdictional authorities, adoption of the WHO methodology, participation in the NHHI as mandatory for hospital accreditation, public reporting of hospital hand hygiene compliance data, and considerable efforts from frontline infection control practitioners who develop, implement, coordinate, and evaluate a hospital-wide infection control program.

Box 16.6). However, it is unclear whether the interventions reduce infection and colonization rates (Gould et al. 2017). The addition of goal setting, reward incentives, performance feedback, and accountability strategies may lead to further improvements of hand hygiene compliance and reduction of infection rates. Placement of alcohol-based hand rub close to the point of use probably slightly improves hand hygiene compliance (Gould et al. 2017).

The most frequently addressed determinants of behavior change that prompted good hand hygiene behavior were knowledge, awareness, action control, and facilitation of behavior (Huis et al. 2012). The less-addressed determinants were social influence, attitude, self-efficacy, and intention. Addressing combinations of different determinants showed better results (Huis et al. 2012).

16.4.5   Delirium Prevention

Delirium is defined as a disturbance in attention, awareness, and cognition with reduced ability to direct, focus, sustain, and shift attention, and reduced orientation to the environment (Herling et al. 2018). Hospitalized

patients frequently, and the most critically ill patients in the ICU, develop delirium with a prevalence rate ranging between 10% and 31% (Martinez et al. 2014). There is strong evidence supporting multicomponent interventions to prevent delirium in hospitalized patients, including multidisciplinary teamwork that included clinical experts, nurses, and physical therapists; staff education and training; and local tailoring of interventions and engagement of frontline clinical staff in the design of the intervention (Siddiqi et al. 2016). Many of the delirium risk factors targeted with multicomponent interventions relate to good basic care, including individualized care, an educational component, systematic cognitive screening, geriatric consultative services, supportive psychotherapy, a scheduled pain protocol, daily reorientation, family involvement in care, and early mobilization. The nature of the interventions that were implemented varied between the studies: some relied on a protocol-driven approach, while others were more pragmatic in the delivery of the intervention (e.g. the family delivered the reorientation intervention; Siddiqi et al. 2016). The evidence is insufficient to identify which elements of multicomponent interventions are most beneficial (Reston and Schoelles 2013).

There is no evidence that pharmacologic interventions (e.g. cholinesterase inhibitors and antipsychotic medications), melatonin, sedation, environmental, and preventive nursing interventions are effective in preventing delirium in hospitalized patients and ICU patients (Siddiqi et al. 2016; Herling et al. 2018). It is unclear why these interventions are not effective in the ICU (Bannon et al. 2019).

16.4.6 Fall Prevention

Falls result in substantial burden for patients and healthcare systems. In hospital settings, the incidence of falls is 5.71–18.0 per 1000 bed days (Cameron et al. 2018). Fall-prevention programs, such as combinations of interventions, including exercise, vision assessment, and treatment (e.g. geriatric assessment), environmental assessment and modification, quality improvement strategies (e.g. case management), multifactorial assessment and treatment, calcium supplementation, and vitamin D supplementation, were associated with a lower risk of injurious falls compared with usual care (Tricco et al. 2017).

Evidence about the successful implementation of multicomponent fall-prevention interventions suggests that the following factors are important: leadership support; engagement of frontline clinical staff in the design of the intervention; guidance by a multidisciplinary committee; pilot testing the intervention; information systems that provide data about falls and facilitate the evaluation of the causes of falls and adherence to the intervention components; and education and training of clinical staff, which are necessary to help ensure that adherence does not diminish (Miake-Lye et al. 2013).

16.4.7 Pressure Ulcers

Pressure ulcers (i.e. bedsores, pressure sores, pressure injuries, decubitus ulcers) are localized damage to the skin and underlying tissue. In the

USA more than one million patients and in Europe one in four patients had a pressure ulcer in acute care settings (Sullivan and Schoelles 2013; McInnes et al. 2015). They are most common in the elderly and immobile, and considered as largely preventable (Sullivan and Schoelles 2013; McInnes et al. 2015). Alternatives to standard hospital foam mattresses reduce the incidence of pressure ulcers in people at risk. The relative merits of alternating and constant low-pressure devices are unclear. Meta-analysis of three trials suggests that Australian standard medical sheepskins prevent pressure ulcers (McInnes et al. 2015).

Evidence for the impact of organizing health services for preventing and treating pressure ulcers, such as transmural care, a care model that provided activities to support patients and their family/partners and activities to promote continuity of care, and multidisciplinary wound care, remains unclear (Joyce et al. 2018). Important components for successful implementation include simplification and standardization of pressure ulcer–specific interventions and documentation, involvement of multidisciplinary teams and leadership, designated skin champions, ongoing staff education, and sustained audit and feedback (Sullivan and Schoelles 2013).

16.4.8 Pain Management

Pain is an unpleasant sensory and emotional experience associated with actual or potential tissue damage, or described in terms of such damage (IASP 1994). Up to 80% of patients experienced post-operative pain (Meissner et al. 2018), with the majority of patients complaining of moderate, severe, or extreme pain. Severe pain after surgery represents a largely unrecognized clinical problem and is associated with an increased incidence of cardiac and pulmonary complications (e.g. pneumonia, deep vein thrombosis, infection, and delayed healing), and in some situations with an increased rate of morbidity and mortality (Meissner et al. 2018).

Poor management of post-operative acute pain can contribute to these medical complications and the development of chronic pain. It is therefore important that all patients undergoing surgery receive adequate pain management, of which assessment of pain is a critical step (Wells et al. 2008). Self-report is the most reliable way to assess pain intensity. Measuring pain intensity in the clinical setting is most often done by using the 0–10 Numerical Rating Scale (NRS; Wells et al. 2008; Meissner et al. 2018). Pain management teams (e.g. an Acute Pain Service team) are an interdisciplinary approach which includes an individualized plan of care for pain control, developed in collaboration with the patient and the family. These teams improve pain assessment and the use of analgesics, but do not clearly affect pain outcomes (Wells et al. 2008; Meissner et al. 2015). Implementation of patient-controlled analgesia, peripheral blocks, and epidural infusions of local anesthetic/opioid mixtures may represent real advances in improving patient well-being and in reducing post-operative morbidity (Meissner et al. 2018). However, post-operative pain is still undertreated in many countries and the quality of nearly half of these teams is questionable (Erlenwein et al. 2016; Meissner et al. 2018). Barriers to achieving patient-satisfactory analgesia include deficient knowledge regarding post-operative pain management among staff, lack of instructions, insufficient pain (re)assessments, and suboptimal treatment. Greater involvement of patients in pain decisions is also seen as a priority area for improving clinical outcomes (Meissner et al. 2018).

16.4.9 Interventions to Prevent Adverse Drug Events

Many hospitalized patients are affected by MEs that can cause discomfort, harm, and even death. Among European Union citizens, 18% claim to have experienced a serious ME during hospital care and 11% to have been prescribed the wrong medication (WHO 2019).

Medication review is a key element in improving the quality of prescribing and in preventing adverse drug events (ADEs; Christensen and Lundh 2016). Although there is no generally accepted definition of medication review, it can be broadly defined as a systematic assessment of pharmacotherapy for an individual patient that aims to optimize patient medication by providing a recommendation or by making a direct change. Christensen and Lundh (2016) in their Cochrane systematic review found no evidence that medication review reduces mortality or hospital readmissions, but they found that medication review may reduce emergency department contacts.

There is a growing focus on *medication reconciliation* at hospital admission and discharge. Medication reconciliation is the formal process in which healthcare professionals partner with patients to ensure an accurate and complete transfer of medication information at interfaces of care (e.g. at hospital admission and hospital discharge; Kwan et al. 2013). It is a major intervention to target and reduce the burden of medication discrepancies and MEs during transitions in care (Kwan et al. 2013). Key aspects of successful intervention components are intensive pharmacy staff involvement and targeting the intervention at a "high-risk" patient population, but the effects of these components on ADEs remains unclear (Kwan et al. 2013). Medication reconciliation alone probably does not reduce MEs. Medication reconciliation supported by an electronic tool was able to minimize the incidence of medications with unintended discrepancy, mainly drug omissions (Mekonnen et al. 2016).

Computerized physician order entry (CPOE) has been defined as an electronic application used by physicians to order drugs, laboratory tests, and requests for consultations, ensuring that all orders are legible and complete. Clinical decision support (CDS) encompasses a wide range of computerized tools directed at improving patient care, including computerized reminders and advice regarding drug selection, dosage, interactions, allergies, and the need for subsequent orders. CPOE linked with CDS has been promoted as having great potential for reducing MEs and ADEs (Prgomet et al. 2017). The percentage of CPOE-related medication prescription errors ranged from 6.1 to 77.7%. "Wrong dose" and "wrong drug" were the most frequent types of errors (Korb-Savoldelli et al. 2018). In hospital-related settings, implementing CPOE is associated with a greater than 50% decline in preventable ADEs. Decreases in MEs are similar and robust to variations in important aspects of intervention design and context (Nuckols et al. 2014). Critical care settings, both adult and pediatric, involve unique complexities, making them vulnerable to MEs and adverse patient outcomes. The currently limited evidence base requires research that has sufficient statistical power to identify the true effect of CPOE implementation. There is also a critical need to understand the nature of errors arising post-CPOE and how the addition of computerized decision-support systems (CDSSs) can be used to provide greater benefit in delivering safe and effective patient care (Prgomet et al. 2017).

Other interventions to prevent ADEs are the participation of a pharmacist in physician rounds and increasing antibiotic guideline compliance. Participation of a pharmacist in physician rounds and timely information exchange and advice to physicians by the pharmacist (i.e. on drug interactions, appropriate dosages, dose intervals, and routes of administration) were associated with a statistically significant reduced ADE rate (Wang et al. 2015). Interventions aimed at increasing antibiotic guideline compliance for pneumonia were associated with a significant reduction in mortality (Davey et al. 2013). Effective intervention components were formal presentations, academic detailing, letters, frequent reminders by pharmaceutical representatives, pre-printed outpatient and admission order sheets, and reporting of outcome data to providers.

Drug treatment is an important clinical process in primary care that is associated with risk of error and adverse events (Lainer et al. 2015). Information technology (IT) can play an important role in preventing ADEs in primary care (see also Chapter 15). Positive results of pharmacist-led IT interventions indicate that IT interventions with interprofessional communication appear to be effective (Lainer et al. 2013). Multifaceted medication safety programs in primary care, including educational training, quality improvement tools, informatics, patient education, and feedback provision, were evaluated. It resulted in a decrease in error rates from 18.6 to 14.6% and in prescription error rates from 0.45 to 0.15% (Khalil and Roughead 2017).

16.5 Strategies to Assure Patient Safety

Besides patient safety strategies focused on specific patient safety problems or patient categories, more general strategies are also necessary to assure patient safety, like leadership, safety culture, and governance. These strategies aim to assure patient safety by optimal prevention and management of adverse events.

16.5.1 Leadership

Struggling healthcare organizations share characteristics that may affect their ability to provide optimal care, which relate to specific organizational culture, infrastructure, mission of the organization, and system shocks (Vaughn et al. 2019). Organizational leaders have an important influence on these issues. There is some research evidence to support the growing recognition that leaders can establish structures, systems, and processes for successful improvement in their organization, which in turn are thought to reduce patient harm. However, the evidence is not strong, especially about how important one or more leaders' actions were compared with other situational factors (Øvretveit 2010). There is also some evidence that hospital managers' time spent and work in quality of care can influence quality and safety clinical outcomes, processes, and performance (Parand et al. 2014).

A common practice for leaders is to engage in walkrounds, where frontline healthcare workers are encouraged by the leadership to identify and resolve issues related to the safe delivery of care. Fundamentally, walkrounds are a form of observable leadership engagement with quality that can be an empowering resource for healthcare professionals, at a time when resources are scarce (Weaver et al. 2013; Sexton et al. 2018). When walkrounds are conducted, acted on, and the results are fed back to those involved, the work setting is a better place to deliver and receive care as assessed across a broad range of metrics, including teamwork, safety, leadership, growth opportunities, participation in decision making, and the emotional exhaustion component of burnout. The effectiveness of walkrounds is unknown, but the link with improved patient safety is demonstrably potent (Sexton et al. 2018). Several studies reported improvement in staff perceptions of safety culture by walkrounds (Weaver et al. 2013).

16.5.2 Safety Culture

Establishing a culture of safety is a cornerstone of efforts to develop high-reliability organizations that ensure patient safety. The Agency for Healthcare Research and Quality's Hospital Survey on Patient Safety Culture (HSOPS) is a validated survey that is widely used to assess safety culture (AHRQ 2019). The survey examines organizational perceptions of 12 domains of culture, ranging from communication about errors to teamwork within and across units (Reis et al. 2018). The set of studies included in the systematic review of Reis et al. (2018) reveals that hospital organizational cultures are often underdeveloped or weak as regards patient safety and comprise dimensions that require strengthening. Strategies to improve patient safety culture should focus on preparing personnel to offer safe, quality healthcare and enhancing a "just culture" approach, which would counter the urge to blame, enhance

professional and institutional accountability, prioritize the identification of systemic failures, and, consequently, proceed to mitigate them (Reis et al. 2018).

To affect the patient safety culture in primary care, two strategies were found: workshops on risk management and significant event audit (Verbakel et al. 2016). These interventions may be effective, but it is not evident which intervention would help practices most to improve their patient safety culture. Ideally, practices choose an intervention close to their momentary needs for improvement and evaluate frequently to assess whether the intervention leads to the desired effect (Zwart et al. 2013).

16.5.3 Governance

Many high-risk industries operate within a strong regulatory context, often with a single or small number of powerful, independent regulators. In the complex healthcare sector with a variety of different players, including national and state governments, public and private providers, insurers, and (representatives of) patients, regulatory mechanisms are necessary to ensure equal and safe healthcare for every citizen. It is, however, unclear which regulatory mechanism, such as self-regulation by health professionals, regulation by government, market forces, or combinations of mechanisms (e.g. enforced self-regulation), drives healthcare providers to improve patient safety most (Devers et al. 2004; Healy and Braithwaite 2006).

Inspection systems are used in healthcare to promote quality improvements (i.e. to achieve changes in organizational structures or processes, healthcare provider behavior, and patient outcomes). These systems are based on the assumption that externally promoted adherence to evidence-based standards (through inspection/assessment) will result in a higher quality of healthcare. Researchers and inspecting bodies should ensure that inspection and data collection are conducted using standardized and validated instruments (Tuijn et al. 2011). A Cochrane review examined whether external inspection of compliance with standards can improve improving healthcare organization behavior, healthcare professional behavior, and patient outcomes (Flodgren et al. 2016). Only two studies were identified, which did not provide conclusive evidence for the effectiveness of such external inspection.

Accreditation is usually a voluntary program in which trained external peer reviewers evaluate a healthcare organization's compliance and compare it with pre-established performance standards (Alkhenizan and Shaw 2011). The increased international focus on improving patient outcomes, safety, and quality of care has led stakeholders, policy makers, and healthcare provider organizations to adopt standardized processes for evaluating healthcare organizations. Accreditation has been proposed as an intervention to support patient safety and high-quality healthcare (Brubakk et al. 2015). However, there is inconsistent evidence that shows that accreditation programs improve the process of care provided by healthcare services and clinical outcomes as mortality. The strategies that hospitals should implement to improve patient safety and organizational outcomes related to accreditation components remain unclear (Alkhenizan and Shaw 2011; Brubakk et al. 2015).

Patient safety governance is (in many countries legally) a responsibility of hospital boards for safe healthcare. They need tools to assist them in their task of governing patient safety (van Gelderen et al. 2017). In the Netherlands, hospitals perform internal audits for detecting patients' risks of adverse events and for encouraging the continuous improvement of patient safety (Hanskamp-Sebregts et al. 2013). Internal audits are systematic evaluations of the quality system of a hospital which aims to improve patient safety by measuring the performance of healthcare providers and preconditions for safe care, and comparing these outcomes with (inter)national standards and guidelines (see Box 16.7). These audits focus

---

Box 16.7   Internal Audit Process in Dutch Hospitals

Phase	Audit activities
Preparation	An audit team prepares the audit, which includes the analysis of quality and policy documents and outcomes of earlier performed audits, observations of care processes, medical record reviews, and self-evaluation forms filled in by the heads of departments or theme leader. The quality of the audited care processes is compared with various prevailing quality and safety standards (e.g. Joint Commission International [JCI], ISO 9000), laws and regulations, and guidelines for healthcare professionals.
Audit visit	During an audit visit, the audit team interviews auditees (e.g. nurses, physicians, and management of the department or working in the audited patient safety area). Specific safety risks will receive additional attention.
Report	Subsequently, the audit team writes an audit report with the audit findings and conclusions based on all collected information. The audit results will be fed back to the audited department heads for quality improvement purposes and to the boards of directors for governance purposes.
Implementation improvement actions	Department heads or team leaders are obligated to develop and implement improvement plans based on the audit results.
Follow-up	Follow-up of the audit findings and recommendations is the responsibility of department heads or team leaders and is monitored by the board of directors or delegated to committees. This audit process should be repeated periodically.

on auditing all departments of the hospital (department-based audits) or specific patient safety areas, for example medication safety, infection prevention, or surgical safety (theme-based audits). These audits are executed on a periodic basis.

For patient safety governance, internal audits are regarded as effective, because they help boards to identify patient safety problems, proactively steer patient safety, and inform boards of supervisors on the status of patient safety (van Gelderen et al. 2017). However, the effectiveness of internal audits on patient outcomes is limited without focus and support (e.g. sufficient time, capacity, management support, information and communication technology support) in the implementation of audit-based improvement actions (Hanskamp-Sebregts et al. 2019).

16.6 Conclusions

Several methods exist to analyze incidents and adverse events, such as medical record review or incident analysis. Healthcare professionals become more aware of unsafe situations by taking part in analysis of incidents and adverse events. Although reporting with feedback to the reporter stimulates notification of incidents, no studies have been found showing a decrease in the number of actual incidents after notification. A lot of time and energy is put into measuring adverse events, and relatively little time is spent on setting up and evaluating interventions to reduce adverse events.

There is some evidence for interventions that have a positive effect on patient safety, such as team training that increases patient safety knowledge and attitude of staff; interventions to improve handovers that reduce the hospital readmission rate; an SSC that reduces postoperative complications, mortality, and infections; and programs preventing falls. To assure patient safety in healthcare and to create a climate to improve patient safety continuously, leadership, safety culture, and governance are indispensable.

References

Agency for Healthcare Research and Policy (2019). *Surveys on patient safety culture (SOPS) hospital survey*. Rockville, MD: AHRQ https://www.ahrq.gov/sops/surveys/hospital/index.html.

Alkhenizan, A. and Shaw, C. (2011). Impact of accreditation on the quality of healthcare services: a systematic review of the literature. *Ann. Saudi Med.* 31: 407.

Aranaz-Andres, J.M., Aibar-Remón, C., Limón-Ramírez, R. et al. (2011). Prevalence of adverse events in the hospitals of five Latin American countries: results of the Iberoamerican study of adverse events (IBEAS). *BMJ Qual. Saf.* 20: 1043–1051.

Aranaz-Andres, J.M., Aibar-Remon, C., Vitaller-Burillo, J., and Ruiz-Lopez, P. (2008). Incidence of adverse events related to health care in Spain: results of the Spanish national study of adverse events. *J. Epidemiol. Community Health* 62: 1022–1029.

Baker, G.R., Norton, P.G., Flintoft, V. et al. (2004). The Canadian Adverse Events Study: the incidence of adverse events among hospital patients in Canada. *CMAJ* 170: 1678–1686.

Bannon, L., McGaughey, J., Verghis, R. et al. (2019). The effectiveness of non-pharmacological interventions in reducing the incidence and duration of delirium in critically ill patients: a systematic review and meta-analysis. *Intensive Care Med.* 45: 1–12.

Battles, J.B. and Lilford, R.J. (2003). Organizing patient safety research to identify risks and hazards. *Qual. Saf. Health Care* 12 (Suppl. sII): ii2–ii7.

Benning, A., Ghaleb, M., Suokas, A. et al. (2011). Large scale organizational intervention to improve patient safety in four UK hospitals: mixed method evaluation. *BMJ* 342: d195.

Bergs, J., Hellings, J., Cleemput, I. et al. (2014). Systematic review and meta-analysis of the effect of the World Health Organization surgical safety checklist on postoperative complications. *Br. J. Surg.* 101: 150–158.

Bergs, J., Lambrechts, F., Simons, P. et al. (2015). Barriers and facilitators related to the implementation of surgical safety checklists: a systematic review of the qualitative evidence. *BMJ Qual. Saf.* 24: 776–786.

Boet, S., Bould, M.D., Fung, L. et al. (2014). Transfer of learning and patient outcome in simulated crisis resource management: a systematic review. *Can. J. Anaesth.* 61: 571–582.

Brennan, T.A., Leape, L.L., Laird, N.M. et al. (1991). Incidence of adverse events and negligence in hospitalized patients: results from the Harvard Medical practice Study I. *N. Engl. J. Med.* 324: 370–376.

Brubakk, K., Vist, G.E., Bukholm, G. et al. (2015). A systematic review of hospital accreditation: the challenges of measuring complex intervention effects. *BMC Health Serv. Res.* 15: 280.

Cameron, I.D., Dyer, S.M., Panagoda, C.E. et al. (2018). Interventions for preventing falls in older people in care facilities and hospitals. *Cochrane Database Syst. Rev.* (9): CD005465. https://doi.org/10.1002/14651858.CD005465.pub4.

Chiozza, M.L. and Ponzetti, C. (2009). FMEA: a model for reducing medical errors. *Clin. Chim. Acta* 404: 75–78.

Christensen, M. and Lundh, A. (2016). Medication review in hospitalised patients to reduce morbidity and mortality. *Cochrane Database Syst. Rev.* (2): CD008986. https://doi.org/10.1002/14651858.CD008986.pub3.

Damiani, E., Donati, A., Serafini, G. et al. (2015). Effect of performance improvement programs on compliance with sepsis bundles and mortality: a systematic review and meta-analysis of observational studies. *PLoS One* 10: e0125827.

Davey, P., Marwick, C.A., Scott, C.L. et al. (2013). Interventions to improve antibiotic prescribing practices for hospital inpatients. *Cochrane Database Syst. Rev.* (4): CD003543. https://doi.org/10.1002/14651858.CD003543.pub4.

Davis, P., Lay-Yee, R., Briant, R. et al. (2002). Adverse events in New Zealand public hospitals I: occurrence and impact. *N. Z. Med. J.* 115: U271.

Deilkås, E.T., Bukholm, G., Lindstrøm, J.C., and Haugen, M. (2015). Monitoring adverse events in Norwegian hospitals from 2010 to 2013. *BMJ Open* 5: e008576.

Deis, J.N., Smith, K.M., Warren, M.D. et al. (2008). Transforming the morbidity and mortality conference into an instrument for systemwide improvement. In: *Advances in Patient Safety: New Directions and Alternative Approaches (Vol. 2: Culture and Redesign)* (eds. K. Henriksen, J.B. Battles, M.A. Keyes and M.L. Grady). Rockville, MD: Agency for Healthcare Research and Quality https://www.ncbi.nlm.nih.gov/books/NBK43710.

Devers, K.J., Pham, H.H., and Liu, G. (2004). What is driving hospitals patient-safety efforts? *Health Aff.* 23: 103–115.

Dy, S.M., Taylor, S.L., Carr, L.H. et al. (2011). A framework for classifying patient safety practices: results from an expert consensus process. *BMJ Qual. Saf.* 20: 618–624.

Erlenwein, J., Koschwitz, R., Pauli-Magnus, D. et al. (2016). A follow-up on Acute Pain Services in Germany compared to international survey data. *Eur. J. Pain* 20: 874–883.

Flodgren, G., Gonçalves-Bradley, D.C., and Pomey, M.P. (2016). External inspection of compliance with standards for improved healthcare outcomes. *Cochrane Database Syst. Rev.* (12): CD008992. https://doi.org/10.1002/14651858.CD008992.pub3.

Fung, L., Boet, S., Bould, M.D. et al. (2015). Impact of crisis resource management simulation-based training for interprofessional and interdisciplinary teams: a systematic review. *J. Interprof. Care* 29: 433–444.

van Gelderen, S.C., Zegers, M., Boeijen, W. et al. (2017). Evaluation of the organisation and effectiveness of internal audits to govern patient safety in hospitals: a mixed-methods study. *BMJ Open* 7: e015506.

Gould, D.J., Moralejo, D., Drey, N. et al. (2017). Interventions to improve hand hygiene compliance in patient care. *Cochrane Database Syst. Rev.* (9): CD005186. https://doi.org/10.1002/14651858.CD005186.pub4.

Grayson, M.L., Stewardson, A.J., Russo, P.L. et al. (2018). Effects of the Australian National Hand Hygiene Initiative after 8 years on infection control practices, health-care worker education, and clinical outcomes: a longitudinal study. *Lancet Infect. Dis.* 18: 1269–1277.

Hansen, L.O., Young, R.S., Hinami, K. et al. (2011). Interventions to reduce 30-day rehospitalization: a systematic review. *Ann. Intern. Med.* 155: 520–528.

Hanskamp-Sebregts, M., Zegers, M., Boeijen, W. et al. (2013). Effects of auditing patient safety in hospital care: design of a mixed-method evaluation. *BMC Health Serv. Res.* 13: 226.

Hanskamp-Sebregts, M., Zegers, M., Boeijen, W. et al. (2019). Process evaluation of the effects of patient safety auditing in hospital care (part 2). *Int. J. Qual. Health Care* 31: 433–441.

Health Foundation (2011). *Evidence: Safer Patient Initiative Phase One: Mixed-Method Evaluation of a Large-Scale Organizational Intervention to Improve Patient Safety in Four UK Hospitals*. London: Health Foundation.

Healy, J. and Braithwaite, J. (2006). Designing safer health care through responsive regulation. *Med. J. Aust.* 184: S56–S59.

Herling, S.F., Greve, I.E., Vasilevskis, E.E. et al. (2018). Interventions for preventing intensive care unit delirium in adults. *Cochrane Database Syst. Rev.* (11): CD00978. https://doi.org/10.1002/14651858.CD009783.pub2.

Hesselink, G., Berben, S., Beune, T., and Schoonhoven, L. (2016). Improving the governance of patient safety in emergency care: a systematic review of interventions. *BMJ Open* 6: e009837.

Hesselink, G., Schoonhoven, L., Barach, P. et al. (2012). Improving patient handovers from hospital to primary care: a systematic review of interventions and effects. *Ann. Intern. Med.* 157: 417–428.

Huis, A., van Achterberg, T., de Bruin, M. et al. (2012). A systematic review of hand hygiene improvement strategies: a behavioural approach. *Implement. Sci.* 7: 92.

Joyce, P., Moore, Z.E., and Christie, J. (2018). Organisation of health services for preventing and treating pressure ulcers. *Cochrane Database Syst. Rev.* (12): CD012132. https://doi.org/10.1002/14651858.CD012132.pub2.

Kemper, P.F., van Dyck, C., Wagner, C., and de Bruijne, M. (2017). Implementation of crew resource management: a qualitative study in 3 intensive care units. *J. Patient Saf.* 13: 223–231.

Khalil, H. and Roughead, L. (2017). Medication safety programs in primary care: a scoping review protocol. *JBI Database System Rev. Implement. Rep.* 15: 1512–1517.

Korb-Savoldelli, V., Boussadi, A., Durieux, P., and Sabatier, B. (2018). Prevalence of computerized physician order entry systems–related medication prescription errors: a systematic review. *Int. J. Med. Inform.* 111: 112–122.

Kripalini, S. (2011). *What Have We Learned about Safe Inpatient Handovers. Perspectives on Safety*. Rockville, MD: Agency for Healthcare Research and Quality.

Kwan, J.L., Lo, L., Sampson, M., and Shojania, K.G. (2013). Medication reconciliation during transitions of care as a patient safety strategy: a systematic review. *Ann. Intern. Med.* 158: 397–403.

Lainer, M., Mann, E., and Sönnichsen, A. (2013). Information technology interventions to improve medication safety in primary care: a systematic review. *Int. J. Qual. Health Care* 25: 590–598.

Lainer, M., Vögele, A., Wensing, M., and Sönnichsen, A. (2015). Improving medication safety in primary care. A review and consensus procedure by the LINNEAUS collaboration on patient safety in primary care. *Eur. J. Gen. Pract.* 21 (Suppl): 14–18.

Leape, L.L. (2002). Reporting of adverse events. *N. Engl. J. Med.* 347: 1633–1638.

Leistikow, I.P., den Ridder, K., de Vries, B., and de Vries, B. (2016). *Patient Safety: Systematic Incident Reconstruction and Evaluation*, 3e. Houten: Bohn Stafleu van Loghum.

Leonard, M., Graham, S., and Bonacum, D. (2004). The human factor: the critical importance of effective teamwork and communication in providing safe care. *BMJ Qual. Saf.* 13 (suppl 1): i85–i90.

Lilford, R.J., Mohammed, M.A., Braunholtz, D., and Hofer, T.P. (2003). The measurement of active errors: methodological issues. *Qual. Saf. Health Care* 12: ii8–ii12.

Lilford, R. and Pronovost, P. (2010). Using hospital mortality rates to judge hospital performance: a bad idea that just don't go away. *BMJ* 340: c2016.

Luangasanatip, N., Hongsuwan, M., Limmathurotsakul, D. et al. (2015). Comparative efficacy of interventions to promote hand hygiene in hospital: systematic review and network meta-analysis. *BMJ* 351: h3728.

Luu, N.P., Pitts, S., Petty, B. et al. (2016). Provider-to-provider communication during transitions of care from outpatient to acute care: a systematic review. *J. Gen. Intern. Med.* 31: 417–425.

MacDonald, R.D. (2016). Articles that may change your practice: crew resource management. *Air Med. J.* 35: 65–66.

Madden, C., Lydon, S., Curran, C. et al. (2018). Potential value of patient record review to assess and improve patient safety in general practice: a systematic review. *Eur. J. Gen. Pract.* 24: 192–201.

Maharaj, R., Raffaele, I., and Wendon, J. (2015). Rapid response systems: a systematic review and meta-analysis. *Crit. Care* 19: 254.

Martinez, F., Tobar, C., and Hill, N. (2014). Preventing delirium: should non-pharmacological, multicomponent interventions be used? A systematic review and

meta-analysis of the literature. *Age Ageing* 44: 196–204.

McGaughey, J., O'Halloran, P., Porter, S., and Blackwood, B. (2017). Early warning systems and rapid response to the deteriorating patient in hospital: a systematic realist review. *J. Adv. Nurs.* 73: 2877–2891.

McInnes, E., Jammali-Blasi, A., Bell-Syer, S.E. et al. (2015). Support surfaces for pressure ulcer prevention. *Cochrane Database Syst. Rev.* (9): CD001735. https://doi.org/10.1002/14651858. CD001735.pub5.

Meddings, J., Rogers, M.A., Krein, S.L. et al. (2014). Reducing unnecessary urinary catheter use and other strategies to prevent catheter-associated urinary tract infection: an integrative review. *BMJ Qual. Saf.* 23: 277–289.

Meissner, W., Coluzzi, F., Fletcher, D. et al. (2015). Improving the management of post-operative acute pain: priorities for change. *Curr. Med. Res. Opin.* 31: 2131–2143.

Meissner, W., Huygen, F., Neugebauer, E.A.M. et al. (2018). Management of acute pain in the postoperative setting: the importance of quality indicators. *Curr. Med. Res. Opin.* 34: 187–196.

Mekonnen, A.B., Abebe, T.B., McLachlan, A.J., and Brien, J.A. (2016). Impact of electronic medication reconciliation interventions on medication discrepancies at hospital transitions: a systematic review and meta-analysis. *BMC Med. Inform. Decis. Mak.* 16: 112.

Mendes, W., Martins, M., Rozenfeld, S., and Travassos, C. (2009). The assessment of adverse events in hospitals in Brazil. *Int. J. Qual. Health Care.* 21: 279–284.

Miake-Lye, I.M., Hempel, S., Ganz, D.A., and Shekelle, P.G. (2013). Inpatient fall prevention programs as a patient safety strategy: a systematic review. *Ann. Intern. Med.* 158: 390–396.

Müller, M., Jürgens, J., Redaèlli, M. et al. (2018). Impact of the communication and patient hand-off tool SBAR on patient safety: a systematic review. *BMJ Open* 8: e022202.

Nuckols, T.K., Smith-Spangler, C., Morton, S.C. et al. (2014). The effectiveness of computerized order entry at reducing preventable adverse drug events and medication errors in hospital settings: a systematic review and meta-analysis. *Syst. Rev.* 3: 56.

OECD (2009). Health quality indicators project: patient safety indicators report 2009. https://doi.org/10.1787/220112312723.

Øvretveit, J. (2010). Improvement leaders: what do they and should they do? A summary of a review of research. *Qual. Saf. Health Care* 19: 490–492.

Øvretveit, J. (2011). *Does Clinical Coordination Improve Quality and Save Money? Volume 1: A Summary Review of the Evidence*. London: Health Foundation.

Parand, A., Dopson, S., Renz, A., and Vincent, C. (2014). The role of hospital managers in quality and patient safety: a systematic review. *BMJ Open* 4: e005055.

Prgomet, M., Li, L., Niazkhani, Z. et al. (2017). Impact of commercial computerized provider order entry (CPOE) and clinical decision support systems (CDSSs) on medication errors, length of stay, and mortality in intensive care units: a systematic review and meta-analysis. *J. Am. Med. Inform. Assoc.* 24: 413–422.

Pronovost, P.J., Nolan, T., Zeger, S. et al. (2004). How can clinicians measure safety and quality in acute care? *Lancet* 363: 1061–1067.

Rafter, N., Hickey, A., Conroy, R.M. et al. (2017). The Irish National Adverse Events Study (INAES): the frequency and nature of adverse events in Irish hospitals—a retrospective record review study. *BMJ Qual. Saf.* 26: 111–119.

Reis, C.T., Paiva, S.G., and Sousa, P. (2018). The patient safety culture: a systematic review by characteristics of hospital survey on patient safety culture dimensions. *Int. J. Qual. Health Care* 30: 660–677.

Rennke, S., Nguyen, O.K., Shoeb, M.H. et al. (2013). Hospital-initiated transitional care interventions as a patient safety strategy: a systematic review. *Ann. Intern. Med.* 158: 433–440.

Reston, J.T. and Schoelles, K.M. (2013). In-facility delirium prevention programs as a patient safety strategy: a systematic review. *Ann. Intern. Med.* 158: 375–380.

Runciman, W., Hibbert, P., Thomson, R. et al. (2009). Towards an international classification for patient safety: key concepts and terms. *Int. J. Qual. Health Care* 21: 18–26.

Schiøler, T., Lipczak, H., Pedersen, B.L. et al. (2001). Incidence of adverse events in hospitals. A retrospective study of medical records. *Ugeskr. Laeger* 163: 5370–5378.

Schmutz, J. and Manser, T. (2013). Do team processes really have an effect on clinical performance? A systematic literature review. *Br. J. Anaesth.* 110: 529–524.

Sexton, J.B., Adair, K.C., Leonard, M.W. et al. (2018). Providing feedback following leadership WalkRounds is associated with better patient safety culture, higher employee engagement and lower burnout. *BMJ Qual. Saf.* 27: 261–270.

Shebl, N.A., Franklin, B.D., and Barber, N. (2009). Is failure mode and effect analysis reliable? *J. Patient Saf.* 5: 86–94.

Shojania, K.G., Burton, E.C., McDonald, K.M., and Goldman, L. (2003). Changes in rates of autopsy-detected diagnostic errors over time: a systematic review. *JAMA* 289: 2849–2856.

Siddiqi, N., Harrison, J.K., Clegg, A. et al. (2016). Interventions for preventing delirium in hospitalised non-ICU patients. *Cochrane Database Syst. Rev.* (3): CD005563. https://doi.org/10.1002/14651858.CD005563.pub3.

SimPatIE (Safety Improvement for Patients in Europe) (2007). *Catalogue of Patient Safety Indicators*. Aarhus: European Society for Quality in Healthcare.

van Sluisveld, N., Hesselink, G., van der Hoeven, J.G. et al. (2015). Improving clinical handover between intensive care unit and general ward professionals at intensive care unit discharge. *Intensive Care Med.* 41: 589–604.

Snijders, C., van der Schaaf, T.W., Klip, H. et al. (2009). Feasibility and reliability of PRISMA-medical for specialty-based incident analysis. *Qual. Saf. Health Care* 18: 486–491.

Soop, M., Fryksmark, U., Koster, M., and Haglund, B. (2009). The incidence of adverse events in Swedish hospitals: a retrospective medical record review study. *Int. J. Qual. Health Care* 21: 285–291.

Sousa, P., Uva, A.S., Serranheira, F. et al. (2018). Patient and hospital characteristics that influence incidence of adverse events in acute public hospitals in Portugal: a retrospective cohort study. *Int. J. Qual. Health Care* 3: 132–137.

Stelfox, H.T., Lane, D., Boyd, J.M. et al. (2015). A scoping review of patient discharge from intensive care: opportunities and tools to improve care. *Chest* 14: 317–327.

Sullivan, N. and Schoelles, K.M. (2013). Preventing in-facility pressure ulcers as a patient safety strategy: a systematic review. *Ann. Intern. Med.* 158: 410–416.

Thomas, E.J. and Petersen, L.A. (2003). Measuring errors and adverse events in health care. *J. Gen. Intern. Med.* 18: 61–67.

Thomas, E.J., Studdert, D.M., Burstin, H.R. et al. (2000). Incidence and types of adverse events and negligent care in Utah and Colorado. *Med. Care* 38: 261–271.

Tricco, A.C., Thomas, S.M., Veroniki, A.A. et al. (2017). Comparisons of interventions for preventing falls in older adults: a systematic review and meta-analysis. *JAMA* 318: 1687–1699.

Tuijn, S.M., Robben, P.B., Janssens, F.J., and van den Bergh, H. (2011). Evaluating instruments for regulation of health care in the Netherlands. *J. Eval. Clin. Pract.* 17: 411–419.

Vaughn, V.M., Saint, S., Krein, S.L. et al. (2019). Characteristics of healthcare organisations struggling to improve quality: results from a systematic review of qualitative studies. *BMJ Qual. Saf.* 28: 74–84.

Verbakel, N.J., Langelaan, M., Verheij, T.J. et al. (2016). Improving patient safety culture in primary care: a systematic review. *J. Patient Saf.* 12: 152–158.

Vincent, C. and Amalberti, R. (2016). *Safer Healthcare. Strategies for the Real World.* Heidelberg: Springer.

Vincent, C., Neale, G., and Woloshynowych, M. (2001). Adverse events in British hospitals: preliminary retrospective record review. *BMJ* 322: 517–519.

Vincent, C., Taylor Adams, S., and Stanhope, N. (1998). A framework for analysing risk and safety in medicine. *BMJ* 316: 1154–1157.

de Vries, E.N., Prins, H.A., Crolla, R.M. et al. (2010). Effect of a comprehensive surgical safety system on patient outcomes. *N. Engl. J. Med.* 363: 1928–1937.

de Vries, E.N., Ramrattan, M.A., Smorenburg, S. M. et al. (2008). The incidence and nature of in hospital adverse events: a systematic review. *Qual. Saf. Health Care* 17: 216–223.

Wang, T., Benedict, N., Olsen, K.M. et al. (2015). Effect of critical care pharmacists intervention on medication errors: a systematic review and meta-analysis of observational studies. *J. Crit. Care* 30: 1101–1106.

Weaver, S.J., Lubomksi, L.H., Wilson, R.F. et al. (2013). Promoting a culture of safety as a patient safety strategy: a systematic review. *Ann. Intern. Med.* 158: 369–374.

Wells, N., Pasero, C., and McCaffery, M. (2008). Improving the quality of care through pain assessment and management. In: *Patient Safety and Quality: An Evidence-Based Handbook for Nurses* (ed. R.G. Hughes). Rockville, MD: Agency for Healthcare Research and Quality, Ch. 17.

Wibrandt, I. and Lippert, A. (2017). Improving patient safety in handover from intensive care unit to general ward: a systematic review. *J. Patient Saf.* https://doi.org/10.1097/PTS.0000000000000266.

Wilson, R.M., Harrison, B.T., Gibberd, R.W. et al. (1999). An analysis of the causes of adverse events from the quality in Australian health care study. *Med. J. Aust.* 170: 411e15.

Winters, B.D., Weaver, S.J., Pfoh, E.R. et al. (2013). Rapid-response systems as a patient safety strategy: a systematic review. *Ann. Intern. Med.* 158: 417–425.

World Health Organization (2009). *WHO Guidelines on Hand Hygiene in Health Care: First*

Global Patient Safety Challenge, Clean Care Is Safer Care. Geneva: World Health Organization.

World Health Organization (2019). Data and statistics. WHO. http://www.euro.who.int/en/health-topics/Health-systems/patient-safety/data-and-statistics (accessed November 7, 2019).

Zegers, M., de Bruijne, M.C., Wagner, C. et al. (2007). Design of a retrospective patient record review study on the occurrence of adverse events among patients in Dutch hospitals. *BMC Health Serv. Res.* 7: 27.

Zegers, M., de Bruijne, M.C., Wagner, C. et al. (2009). Adverse events and potentially preventable deaths in Dutch hospitals: results of a retrospective patient record review study. *Qual. Saf. Health Care* 18: 297–302.

Zegers, M., Geense, W., and Wollersheim, H. (2016a). *Optimal Handover of ICU Patients. Quality Management in Intensive Care: A Practical Guide.* Cambridge: Cambridge University Press.

Zegers, M., Hesselink, G., Geense, W. et al. (2016b). Evidence-based interventions to reduce adverse events in hospitals: a systematic review of systematic reviews. *BMJ Open* 6: e012555.

Zhan, C. and Miller, M.R. (2003). Administrative data based patient safety research: a critical review. *Qual. Saf. Health Care* 12 (Suppl. II): ii58–ii63.

Zingg, W., Holmes, A., Dettenkofer, M. et al. (2015). Hospital organisation, management, and structure for prevention of health-care-associated infection: a systematic review and expert consensus. *Lancet Infect. Dis.* 15: 212–224.

Zwart, D., Lyd, M., and de Bont, A. (2013). Introducing incident reporting in primary care: a translation from safety science into medical practice. *Health, Risk Soc.* 15: 265–278.

17

Health System Strategies for Implementation

Michel Wensing[1,2,3], Holger Pfaff[4], and Richard Grol[5,6]

[1] *Faculty of Medicine, University of Heidelberg, Heidelberg, Germany*
[2] *Department of General Practice and Health Services Research, Heidelberg University Hospital, Heidelberg, Germany*
[3] *Department IQ healthcare, Radboud Institute for Health Sciences, Radboud University Medical Center, Nijmegen, The Netherlands*
[4] *Institute of Medical Sociology, Health Services Research and Rehabilitation Science (IMVR), University of Cologne, Cologne, Germany*
[5] *Radboud University, Nijmegen, The Netherlands*
[6] *Maastricht University, Maastricht, The Netherlands*

SUMMARY

- Policy makers and high-level decision makers in healthcare systems have a broad and non-specific influence on the implementation of innovations in healthcare practice.
- There is a range of strategies to enhance evidence-based policy making, including the presentation of research evidence in ways that support decision makers (knowledge-push strategies) and efforts to increase interest in and understanding of research findings (knowledge-pull strategies).
- Scaling up high-value interventions and practices to broader or other populations and settings often requires policy measures. Many policy strategies imply financial incentives, organizational changes, or directives through regulation.
- The body of empirical research on financial strategies in healthcare is relatively large. Increased financial reimbursement and reduced financial risk for healthcare providers can result in a higher volume of services (and vice versa) which can support the implementation of change in some situations. Pay for performance as a reimbursement method for healthcare providers has, on average, a small positive effect on the implementation of targeted practices.
- Changes in the (macro-level) healthcare system, which may facilitate the implementation of innovations, include changes in the allocation of tasks to health professions or healthcare sectors and changes in the economic structure, such as competition between providers and transparency of performance.

17.1 Introduction

Enhancing the uptake of evidence-based practices and reducing the use of low-value practices (procedures with little added value) are important challenges in healthcare systems which have the attention of many policy makers around the world. Healthcare systems at the national, state, or county level can support or inhibit the implementation of specific healthcare practices in complex ways (Theobald et al. 2018). For instance, laws may inhibit the uptake of advanced professional roles by nurses and pay for performance may focus attention on incentivized aspects of care. Financial incentives, organizational changes, and directives to change a healthcare system may be strategies for the implementation of innovations. In particular, they may influence decisions on whether to take up a new practice (or de-implement an existing practice), whether to sustain implemented innovations over time, and whether to scale up the innovations to larger or different populations and healthcare settings (Aarons et al. 2017). This chapter focuses on implementation strategies in healthcare systems, which may be initiated by policy makers and other high-level decision makers.

The health system approach to the implementation of innovations is heavily influenced by economic perspectives. Indeed, some believe that implementation is largely a matter of the presence or absence of (additional) financial reimbursement of healthcare providers. The underlying assumption is derived from standard economic theory, which predicts that specific activities will be more prevalent if their financial benefits exceed costs in the long run. Transparency of cost and quality is an important component of a well-functioning economic market. Box 17.1 presents an example of a financial incentive and public reporting strategy (Lindenbauer et al. 2007). This chapter will discuss changes in the reimbursement of healthcare providers, changes in the financial risk of patients, and other changes in the economic healthcare system. For instance, economic theory suggests that transparency of performance and price (often labeled "public reporting"), as well as enhanced competition between healthcare providers, overall results in better healthcare outcomes and lower costs (Dixon et al. 2007). As healthcare differs from industry, because it involves collective resource collection and allocation, it remains to be seen whether economic mechanisms function similarly in this context (Gubb et al. 2010).

Health system strategies for implementation tend to influence the implementation of a broad range of innovations, rather than focus on one or a few specific innovations (although such examples exist). Strategies to enhance evidence-based policy making and strategies to scale up specific interventions or practices will be discussed first. Then changes in the financial reimbursement of providers and financial risk of patients will be considered. Finally, changes in the regulations and structure of the healthcare system and their impact on the implementation of innovations are elaborated.

17.2 Strategies to Enhance Evidence-Based Policy Making

Implementation of innovations in health systems may involve policy makers and managers at national, state, and institutional levels. A logical first step in successful implementation is therefore the effective dissemination of knowledge to these individuals in leading positions.

Box 17.1 Pay for Performance and Public Reporting in American Hospitals

This observational study compared 207 hospitals with a pay-for-performance and a public reporting program and 406 hospitals with only a public reporting program (Lindenbauer et al. 2007). These programs were part of two voluntary national programs. Pay for performance is financial reimbursement for a defined quality of healthcare delivery. Public reporting is making the performance of healthcare providers public in terms of scores on performance indicators. These programs were part of two voluntary national programs in the USA. Both programs used performance indicators: 10 of these were used in both programs and concerned aspects of professional performance in myocardial infarction, heart failure, and pneumonia. Hospitals that also participated in the pay-for-performance program made more improvement on the 10 indicators. After controlling for several factors, this led to an additional improvement of 2.6–4.1% on specific indicators. The costs associated with the pay-for-performance program were not reported.

Table 17.1 Overview of reviews on strategies to enhance evidence-based policy making.

Leeman et al. (2015)	Review with 29 studies on strategies to build practitioners' capacity to implement community-based interventions. Capacity-building strategies were found to be effective at increasing practitioners' adoption (n = 10 of 12 studies) and implementation (n = 9 of 10 studies) of evidence-based interventions. Findings were mixed for interventions' effects on practitioners' capacity or intervention-planning behaviors.
Murthy et al. (2012)	Review with 8 studies on strategies to enhance the uptake of systematic review evidence. One of five randomized trials showed effects; these concerned the perceived understanding and usefulness of summary of findings tables in Cochrane reviews. Three other studies showed effects of mailing printed materials.
Petkovic et al. (2016)	Review with 6 studies on evidence summaries, showing that these did not increase the use of systematic review evidence. Specific tables and formats were easier to understand.
Sarkies et al. (2017)	Review with 19 studies on research implementation strategies in health policy and management. Workshops, ongoing technical assistance, and distribution of instructional digital materials may improve knowledge and skills around evidence-informed decision making in US public health departments. Tailored, targeted messages were more effective in increasing public health policies and programs in Canadian public health departments compared to messages and the use of knowledge brokers.

There is a range of strategies to enhance the uptake of evidence-based practices by these decision makers (see Table 17.1). Evidence-based policy making has developed into a special field within implementation science and health systems research (Lavis et al. 2008). Box 17.2 (Lavis et al. 2006) provides an overarching framework for describing implementation policies for knowledge dissemination in a country, state, or county.

Decision makers in healthcare policy and practice are recommended to focus on systematic reviews of knowledge on a topic, because single studies can be highly misleading. A Cochrane review on the subject found few studies of high quality on the impact of various strategies for knowledge dissemination; the few available studies showed an impact of mailing written materials (Murthy et al. 2012). Healthcare managers and policy makers appreciate summaries of evidence (Busert et al. 2018), but it remains uncertain whether these actually increase the uptake of systematic reviews (Petkovic et al. 2016). A review on strategies to develop practitioners' capacity to implement innovations generally, which included a range of study designs, suggested

that various strategies (training, tools, technical assistance, assessment and feedback, peer networking, and incentives) can be effective (Leeman et al. 2015).

Based on experience, Whitty described a number of characteristics of a useful academic paper (Whitty 2015). These include appropriate timing (better fast and 80% correct than 99% correct but too late); interdisciplinary approach of a relevant healthcare topic; reporting with a focus on data and numbers, rather than interpretations and policy recommendations; and reporting on cost implications of changes. He also argues that systematic reviews (rather than reports on single studies) are most useful for decision makers.

A systematic review of studies showed that the knowledge and skills of healthcare policy makers around evidence-based decision making can be improved by education and support (Sarkies et al. 2017). The authors describe a broad set of requirements for achieving actual impact, which include establishing an imperative for practice change, building trust between implementation stakeholders, developing a shared vision, planned use of change mechanisms, the employment of effective communication strategies, and the provision of resources

---

Box 17.2   Framework for Implementation Policy

A report by the World Health Organization (Peters et al. 2013) proposes a framework for describing national implementation policies. It lists seven domains and proposes indicators for each of these domains:

- *Overall climate*: health research funders have the mandate to enhance implementation of knowledge; universities and research organizations stimulate researchers to promote knowledge implementation; potential users appreciate research findings; mediating groups (professional bodies, media) have positive views on research knowledge; there is continuous exchange between researchers and users of research.
- *Knowledge development*: health research funders involve users in priority setting; they commission scoping reviews and systematic reviews of the state of the knowledge in a field; researchers conduct systematic literature reviews before they write a research application.
- *Knowledge dissemination ("push" activities)*: research findings are presented regularly by reliable messengers in an accessible format, customized for different user groups; the impact of these dissemination activities

is regularly evaluated; researchers participate in training programs that help them to improve their knowledge dissemination.

- *Enhance demand for knowledge ("facilitation of user pull")*: health research funders, researchers, and intermediate groups make systematic reviews of relevant knowledge widely accessible; there is a facility to get quick responses to questions; there are training programs to enhance user pull.
- *Knowledge application ("user pull")*: potential users of research knowledge have structures and processes to collect, assess, and apply research findings; they are trained for this; these user pull activities are regularly evaluated.
- *Exchange*: specific individuals maintain relations between researchers and users of research (sometimes named "knowledge brokers"); researchers and users of research maintain partnerships concerning societal or research programs; both participate in programs to enhance skills for exchange.
- *Evaluation*: research funders finance the evaluation of implementation programs in healthcare; all relevant individuals and organizations participate in such evaluations.

Box 17.3   Knowledge Implementation in the US Veterans Administration

The Department of Veterans Affairs (VA) created a comprehensive healthcare system for the about 4.5 million military veterans in the USA. The VA system supports a large research community; for instance, in 2016 it supported 2000 researchers at 83 VA medical centers with US$633 million (Atkins et al. 2017). The VA system adopted comprehensive performance measurements, some of which are related to reimbursement and used for priority setting in QI. In order to address

the gaps between knowledge and practice, the VA initiated the Quality Enhancement Initiative (QUERI) in 1998. The projects in QUERI address important health and social problems, such as mental conditions and homelessness, as well as health system problems, such as physician burnout and waiting times. QUERI may be worldwide the largest and longest-running program of health services research and implementation science in healthcare.

to support change. Specific organizations may act as mediators or brokers between research and practice, aiming to address these requirements of effective knowledge transfer that obviously go far beyond producing scientific publications. These "knowledge brokers" use a wide range of strategies, such as education, planning, and quality improvement (QI; Proctor et al. 2019). Examples of such organizations exist and include, for instance, ZonMW in the Netherlands.

Overall, the body of research on strategies to enhance evidence-based policy making is small. Nevertheless, the scientific literature provides a number of interesting ideas and examples. Some healthcare systems, such as the Veterans Administration, have developed a systematic approach to the implementation of evidence-based practice (see Box 17.3).

17.3 Scaling Up Interventions and Practices

Many strategies to improve an aspect of healthcare have initially been applied in a small number of sites, or only one site. For instance, an innovative QI project may be done in one hospital or in a small number of ambulatory practices. In many of these projects, additional resources for implementation activities are available, which are no longer present after the project ends (Alonge et al. 2019). This is problematic, particularly if resources are scarce, as in low- and middle-income countries. However, most research on scaling up and sustained implementation has been done in high-income countries (Hailemariam et al. 2019) After completion of an initial implementation project, achieving sustained implementation is the next challenge, for which sustained funding, political support, and efficient organization are crucial (Lennox et al. 2018; Shelton et al. 2018). A further challenge is the scaling up of effective interventions and practices to a broader or different population of users.

Sustainability and scaling up are crucial to optimize the impact of innovations for patients and populations. The sustainability and impact of a scale-up innovation are influenced by the financial, regulatory, organizational, and cultural context, which may motivate, facilitate, or enable individuals in the target groups for behavior change. Particularly interaction-based innovations (changes which imply much social interaction) require continuous support of implementation teams to achieve sustained uptake with high fidelity (Fixsen et al. 2017). The ultimate success may be determined by the similarity of the population and healthcare setting of the scale-up setting as compared to the effectiveness research, which provided the evidence of impact (Aarons et al. 2017).

Obviously, there are also examples of interventions, tools, or organizational models which were scaled up in health systems without preceding evaluation research. Examples concern, for instance, the large-scale introduction of an information technology system or healthcare delivery model. This approach may be motivated by commercial or ideological interests, the belief that system change is a prerequisite of clinical effectiveness, difficulties in conducting rigorous evaluation studies, or the absence of resources or time for rigorous evaluation research. It may be possible to examine outcomes after scaling up an intervention, but it can be difficult to de-implement the changes, even if the evaluation shows that these have little benefit. Alternatively, large-scale programs may fail to be sustainable, despite good intentions and substantial investments.

Scaling up interventions has received increasing interest, because it differs from implementation and small-scale improvement projects. A systematic review with 14 studies on scaling up evidence-based practices in primary care (Charif et al. 2017) reported that components of scaling-up strategies were, in order of frequency, components related to human resources (e.g. policy makers/managers, providers, external medical consultants, and community healthcare workers), components related to healthcare infrastructure (e.g. new buildings, linkages between different clinical sites), components related to changes in policy/regulation, and components related to financing (e.g. paying bonuses to healthcare workers). Most of these studies were done in low- or middle-income countries. Box 17.4 provides an example of a successfully scaled-up intervention.

As in small-scale implementation programs, many factors and mechanisms can influence the uptake of interventions in large-scale programs. These include, for instance, cultural factors (e.g. institutionalization of practices), economic factors (e.g. financial benefits and risks), and regulatory factors (e.g. laws). The analysis of contextual factors associated with successful implementation in a small number of sites can provide insight into the likelihood of successful scaling up. For instance, a systematic review on the implementation of structured chronic care suggested that providing support, ensuring resources, and improving the acceptability of interventions for both patients and providers were key factors in its implementation (Davy et al. 2015). A systematic review on QI in hospitals found that a range of contextual factors were associated with their effectiveness, including characteristics of the QI team, QI support and capacity, organization, micro-system, and external environment (Kringos et al. 2015). These findings give clues on factors that need to be addressed in such programs.

17.4 Changes in the Financial Reimbursement of Healthcare Providers

An important set of strategies for implementation of change in health systems comprises changes in the financial reimbursement of healthcare providers. Changes in payment and financial risk are expected to result in changes in professional practice and service delivery. Economic theory suggests that a practice is financially attractive if costs are lower

---

Box 17.4 Scaling Up Maternal and Child Health Care in Ghana

Ghana aimed to achieve two of the country's Millennium Development Goals: reduce child mortality by 60% and maternal mortality by 75%. To reach these goals, a national health systems improvement initiative was introduced in Ghana in 2008 to promote Ghana's existing maternal and child health programs. The approach comprised adding to an existing set of evidence-based maternal and child survival interventions a QI project to improve the transfer of those clinical interventions into daily practice. A consultancy company introduced into the National Catholic Health Service QI methods to implement an evidence-based package of clinical interventions developed by the Ghana Health Service (Step 1: set-up). The scalable unit was the district. Within these districts, there are subdistricts that included a hospital and primary care clinics. The process started with the subdistrict teams. They have been supported by the district management team (Step 2: develop the scalable unit). In the "test of scale-up" phase (Step 3), the project was tested in three provinces of Ghana. During this phase it became apparent that it was necessary to raise local capacity among district and regional supervisors and high-level leaders to use QI methods. The public promotion of the improvements in maternal and child outcomes became an important motivator for regional and national leadership. The project scaled from 35 subdistricts (Step 2) to 265 subdistricts in Step 3, to 554 subdistricts in the "go to full scale" phase over six years (Step 4). The project reached more than 80% of all public and faith-based hospitals in the country (Barker et al. 2016).

than reimbursement (at least in the long run). In healthcare systems, this implies that a higher payment for a specific service ("price") may result in a higher volume of this service. In addition, services with a lower financial risk (e.g. predictable reimbursement) are more attractive for healthcare providers. Prospective reimbursement systems (such as capitation, fixed budgets, and diagnosis-related group systems) imply a higher financial risk for providers, while retrospective reimbursement systems (fee for service, pay for performance) usually imply lower financial risk.

Translating economic theory to healthcare practice is not easy. production costs are not always known; prices of services are often the result of negotiations and politics, rather than a perfect market; demand for healthcare services is partly determined by health professionals rather than patients; and citizens/patients only partly behave as rational consumers. Nevertheless, the available research evidence suggests that

changes in the reimbursement of healthcare providers can be associated with changes in healthcare services, although their impact seems small to moderate (see Table 17.2). Changes in reimbursement are obviously directly associated with costs or savings, which may be substantial. Financial incentives may particularly influence decisions on whether to implement innovations, but they cannot address the educational, organizational, technological, and cultural challenges of implementation.

In many countries financial reimbursement of healthcare providers is an issue for negotiations and contracts with health authorities or health insurers. This implies that contracts can (intentionally or not) influence healthcare organization and delivery. The contract may arrange the maximum volume of specific (expensive) services, the maximum budget for a time period, or the prices of services. Increasingly contracts also address quality of care (performance). For example, since 2004 primary

Table 17.2 Overview of reviews on changes in financial reimbursement of healthcare providers.

Flodgren et al. (2011)	Overview of 4 quantitative reviews covering 32 studies. Payment for working for a specified time period was generally ineffective, improving 3 of 11 outcomes from 1 study reported in 1 review. Payment for each service, episode, or visit was generally effective, improving 7 of 10 outcomes from 5 studies reported in 3 reviews. Payment for providing care for a patient or specific population was generally effective, improving 48 of 69 outcomes from 13 studies reported in 2 reviews. Payment for providing a pre-specified level or providing a change in activity or quality of care was generally effective, improving 17 of 20 reported outcomes from 10 studies reported in 2 reviews. Mixed and other systems were of mixed effectiveness, improving 20 of 31 reported outcomes from 7 studies reported in 3 reviews.
Mathes et al. (2019)	Cochrane review with 27 studies on pay-for-performance schemes for hospitals, focusing on patient outcomes, quality of care, healthcare utilization, and other outcomes. Most studies showed no effect or a very small effect in favor of the pay-for-performance scheme.
Rashidian et al. (2015)	Review with 18 evaluations on financial strategies to influence medication prescribing decisions. Effects on costs, healthcare use, and health outcomes are uncertain or not measured. Pharmaceutical budget caps or targets were found to reduce overall drug use (median relative change −2.8%). Effects of pay for performance and reimbursement rate reduction were uncertain or not measured.
Yuan et al. (2017)	Review with 32 studies on payment of outpatient care facilities. Pay for performance on top of capitation/input-based reimbursement (13 studies) resulted in small improvements of tests and treatments used (relative risk [RR] 1.1), but little or no improvement in quality indicators, healthcare use, and other outcomes.

Box 17.5   Pay for Performance in British Primary Care Practices

In April 2004 new contracts were made between British health authorities and primary care practices. Practice performance was operationalized in terms of about 150 indicators, spread over different domains. Higher scores were associated with higher financial payment, which constituted up to 25% of the total budget of a practice. Physicians were positive about this contract, for which funds had been found in other sectors. In its first year, performance scores were unexpectedly high: on average 91% of the total score. As a baseline measurement had not been done, it remained unclear which improvements had resulted from the new contract. The additional money was spent on administrative staff, practice support, and information technology. Small-scale evaluations showed that physicians had more time for patients with complex medical problems and that nurses were more involved in chronic illness care. Perceived disadvantages were increased costs of coordination and increased bureaucracy. There were also some indications of data manipulation, for instance regarding opening times and discounting or removal of patients who had a negative impact on the performance scores. An evaluation of changes in performance scores for diabetes, asthma, and coronary heart diseases between 1998 and 2007 showed an improvement of about 60–85% of the maximum score (Roland 2004; Campbell et al. 2009). This improvement had started before 2004 (when the contract was introduced). In diabetes and asthma, a significant acceleration of improvement has been found since 2004. This was not found in coronary heart disease. Patient evaluations of communication with physicians and continuity of care remained the same (about 70% gave a positive score). Positive patient evaluations of being able to get an appointment with a specific physician decreased from 40% in 1998 to 30% in 2007.

---

care practices in England have a contract by which they get higher payment when they score higher on performance indicators (see example in Box 17.5). As well as intended effects, there may also be adverse effects. These may include a focus on aspects of care that are incentivized at the expense of other aspects, avoiding specific patients, erosion of intrinsic professional motivation, and manipulation or fraud with data that are used for performance assessments (Mannion and Davies 2008).

17.5   Changes in the Financial Risk for Patients

Strategies to influence the healthcare utilization of patients and citizens may also contribute to the implementation of innovations. Economic theory predicts that the price of a product influences a consumer's decision whether or not to buy the product or service. This implies that the price of medication, nursing care, and other health products and services influences their use. Translation of this economic principle to healthcare is not straightforward, as patients do not necessarily perceive the financial consequences of prices, given the collective reimbursement of healthcare through health insurance or taxes. Various types of financial risk for patients have been introduced (e.g. cost sharing, co-payment) in an attempt to improve the rational use of healthcare. The primary aim is often to reduce (macro-level) costs, but it may be possible to influence the appropriateness of healthcare delivery at the micro level in this way.

Research provides mixed evidence on the impact of various types of co-payment for patients on the use and appropriateness of

---

Box 17.6   Effects of Different Levels of Co-Payment

Between 1970 and 1980 a large randomized study was conducted in the USA on the impact of varying levels of financial risk on healthcare delivery and outcomes (Newhouse 1993). This study was unusual for being a large randomized trial about a health economic intervention (most research in this field is observational). The study was run in six cities and lasted three to five years per city. A total of 7700 individuals (aged below 65 years) were randomly allocated to four health insurance packages: complete coverage of all expenses, 25% co-payment, 50% co-payment, and 95% co-payment. A clear effect on healthcare use and total costs of healthcare services was found: these were highest if all expenses were covered and lowest in the 95% co-payment group. Differences in costs were mainly explained by healthcare-seeking behaviors and not by costs made after the decision to seek help. In study arms with higher co-payment, individuals with a low income reduced their expenses for healthcare more than did individuals with a high income. It appears that individuals did not distinguish between effective and non-effective services: reductions in both were of a similar size in each category of co-payment. Given the differences in the use of healthcare, it was surprising that no effects were found on patient-reported outcomes.

---

healthcare services. A systematic review with 32 publications on studies of cap or co-payment policies for patients who use medication found a large variety of co-payment formats and outcomes, which made it difficult to summarize the results (Luiza et al. 2015). The certainty of evidence was found to be low to very low. Some studies found that co-payment policies reduced overall medication use, including the use of life-sustaining medication. One problem specific to healthcare is that patients may not be able to distinguish between appropriate and inappropriate services and that they may both increase and reduce their use of care as a response to changes in their financial risk (see Box 17.6).

17.6 Changes in the Healthcare System

Health policy makers may change aspects of the healthcare system in order to facilitate the implementation of innovations. Such changes tend to have a generic or "upstream" impact on the implementation of a range of innovations. For instance, policy makers may facilitate the development of specific health professions (e.g. nurses) or reallocate budgets across healthcare sectors or services (e.g. from specialized care to primary care providers). Such changes may contribute to the implementation of recommended practices at a micro level, because they increase the capacity for specific practices. In some situations policy makers can enforce specific measures, for instance when population health is at stake (see Box 17.7 for an example). Such measures are, however, rare in most healthcare systems.

A different category of policy measures is the introduction of economic market mechanisms, based on economic theory, into the healthcare system. The impact of changes in the healthcare system are often ambiguous. For instance, research from the USA found that higher competition initially led to lower costs, but later to amalgamations of healthcare providers and higher prices (Bodemheimer 2005). The example in Box 17.8 illustrates that competition in healthcare can have positive effects on the implementation of innovations. However, competition can be a barrier for collaboration between healthcare providers and thus become a barrier for changes, which depend on this.

Enhanced transparency of healthcare implies that consumers and others get access to

---

Box 17.7   Regulations of Paracetamol

Poisoning by paracetamol overdose is the main cause of acute liver failure. In 1998 the British government introduced regulations to limit the maximum number of paracetamol tablets per box. In an interrupted time- series design, the annual standardized mortality rates from paracetamol poisoning were analyzed (Morgan et al. 2007). This showed that mortality markedly reduced between 1993 and 2004. Similar trends were found for other drugs (aspirin, antidepressants), so it remains unclear what the added impact of specific regulations has been.

Box 17.8   Impact of Competition on Implementation of Case Management in Hospitals

A study from the USA examined whether economic factors were associated with the implementation of case management in hospitals (Roggenkamp et al. 2005). The authors hypothesized that case management was a response of hospital managers to external pressure to reduce costs. It was hypothesized that the implementation of case management was more likely if (1) patients stayed longer in the hospital; (2) costs per admission were higher; (3) patient case mix implied higher costs; (4) local markets included more managed care organizations; and (5) local markets included more hospitals with case management. The study found that hypotheses 2, 3, and 5 were supported. For hypothesis 1, the study found a negative association. Overall, this study suggested that both cost structure and competition were associated with uptake of case management in a hospital.

Box 17.9   Enhanced Transparency in Cardiac Surgery

Public reporting on quality and outcomes of cardiac surgery in New York State was associated with reduced surgical mortality from 3.5 to 2.8% in three years (there was no control group in this evaluation; Chassin et al. 1996). However, there were indications that cardiac surgeons had started to avoid seriously ill patients (Omoigui et al. 1996). The available information on cardiac surgery was not used to select the best surgeons for contracting (Erickson et al. 2000). This example illustrates that negative consequences may result from public reporting.

---

information on services, quality, and costs of healthcare providers. The assumption is that they use this information in a rational decision-making process. For instance, consumers may use information on quality and range of services in their choice of healthcare providers, while healthcare purchasers (such as health insurers) may use information on cost and outcomes in selective contracting with healthcare providers. The reality is that non-conscious decision making, trust, and information in personal networks remain major determinants of such decisions for many individuals. Nevertheless, enhanced transparency implies that market mechanisms in healthcare are strengthened from an economic perspective. Transparency can result in improved patient care because healthcare providers improve specific services as they no longer provide specific low-quality services, or because patients avoid specific care providers. However, risks of harm by enhanced transparency should be taken into account (see Box 17.9 for an example and Chapter 7 for more studies on this topic).

17.7 Conclusions

In many countries, policy makers and high-level decision makers in healthcare systems are expected to represent the interests of citizens. They provide the funding for the healthcare system (through health insurance and taxes) and hold high expectations of its access, performance, outcomes, and financial affordability. Sensible implementation of innovations with proven high value contributes to meeting these expectations. Policy makers have a range of strategies to influence the implementation of innovations in healthcare practice. Some of these are explicitly aimed at enhancing implementation (e.g. strategies for evidence-based policy making); other strategies have multiple aims, of which implementation of innovations is not necessarily the most important (e.g. changes in co-payment by patients). There is a body of research on these strategies, which tends to show that policy strategies tend to have both desired and undesired consequences. Careful evaluation of the benefits and harms of any policy strategy is therefore recommended.

References

Aarons, G.A., Sklar, M., Mustanski, B. et al. (2017). "Scaling-out" evidence-based interventions to new populations or new health care delivery systems. *Implement. Sci.* 12: 111.

Alonge, O., Rodriguez, D.C., Brandes, N. et al. (2019). How is implementation research applied to advance health in low- and middle-income countries. *BMJ Glob. Health* 4: e001257.

Atkins, D., Kilbourne, A.M., and Shulkin, D. (2017). Moving from discovery to system-wide change: the role of research in a learning health care system: experience from three decades of health systems research in the Veterans Health Administration. *Annu. Rev. Public Health* 38: 467–487.

Barker, P.M., Reid, A., and Schall, M.W. (2016). A framework for scaling up health interventions. Lessons from large-scale improvement initiatives in Africa. *Implement. Sci.* 11: 2.

Bodemheimer, T. (2005). High and rising health care costs. Part 1: seeking an explanation. *Ann. Intern. Med.* 142: 847–854.

Busert, L.K., Mütsch, M., Kien, C. et al. (2018). Facilitating evidence uptake: development and user testing of a systematic review summary format to inform public health decision-making in German-speaking countries. *Health Res. Policy Syst.* 16: 59.

Campbell, S.M., Reeves, D., Kontopantelis, E. et al. (2009). Effects of pay for performance on the quality of primary care in England. *N. Engl. J. Med.* 361: 368–378.

Charif, A.L., Zomahoun, H.T.V., LeBlanc, A. et al. (2017). Effective strategies for scaling up evidence-based practices in primary care: a systematic review. *Implement. Sci.* 12: 139.

Chassin, M.R., Hannan, E.L., and DeBuono, B.A. (1996). Benefits and hazards of reporting medical outcomes publicly. *N. Engl. J. Med.* 334: 394–398.

Davy, C., Bleasel, J., Liu, H. et al. (2015). Factors influencing the implementation of chronic care models: a systematic literature review. *BMC Fam. Pract.* 16: 102.

Dixon, J., Chantler, C., and Billings, J. (2007). Competition on outcomes and physician leadership are not enough to reform health care. *JAMA* 298: 1445–1447.

Erickson, L.C., Torchiana, D.F., Schneider, E.C. et al. (2000). The relationship between managed care insurance and the use of lower-mortality hospitals for CABG surgery. *JAMA* 283: 1976–1982.

Fixsen, D.L., Blase, K.A., and Fixsen, A.A.M. (2017). Scaling effective innovations. *Criminol. Public Policy* 16: 487–499.

Flodgren, G., Eccles, M.P., Shepperd, S. et al. (2011). An overview of reviews evaluating the effectiveness of financial incentives in changing healthcare professional behaviours and patient outcomes. *Cochrane Database Syst.*

Rev. (7): CD009255. https://doi.org/10.1002/14651858.CD009255.

Gubb, J., Smith, S., Lawson, N., and Tomlison, J. (2010). Will a market deliver quality and efficiency in health care better than central planning ever could? *BMJ* 340: 568–570.

Hailemariam, M., Bustos, T., Barajas, R. et al. (2019). Evidence-based intervention sustainability strategies: a systematic review. *Implement. Sci.* 14: 57.

Kringos, D.S., Sunol, R., Wagner, C. et al. (2015). The influence of context on the effectiveness of hospital quality improvement strategies: a review of systematic reviews. *BMC Health Serv. Res.* 15: 277.

Lavis, J.N., Lomas, J., Hamid, M., and Sewankambo, N.K. (2006). Assessing country-level efforts to link research to action. *Bull. World Health Organ.* 84: 620–628.

Lavis, J.N., Oxman, A.D., Moyni, R., and Paulsen, E.J. (2008). Evidence-informed health policy I – synthesis of findings from a multi-method study of organizations that support the use of research evidence. *Implement. Sci.* 3: 53.

Leeman, J., Calancie, L., Hartman, M.A. et al. (2015). What strategies are used to build practitioners capacity to implement community-based interventions and are they effective? A systematic review. *Implement. Sci.* 10: 80.

Lennox, L., Maher, R., and Reed, J. (2018). Navigating the sustainability landscape: a systematic review of sustainability approaches in healthcare. *Implement. Sci.* 13: 27.

Lindenbauer, P.K., Remus, D., Roman, S. et al. (2007). Public reporting and pay for performance in hospital quality improvement. *N. Engl. J. Med.* 356: 486–496.

Luiza, V.L., Chaves, L.A., Silva, R.M. et al. (2015). Pharmaceutical policies: effects of caps and co-payment on rational uses of medicines. *Cochrane Database Syst. Rev.* (5): CD007017. https://doi.org/10.1002/14651858.CD007017.pub2.

Mannion, R. and Davies, H.T.O. (2008). Payment for performance in health care. *BMJ* 336: 306–308.

Mathes, T., Pieper, D., Morche, J. et al. (2019). Pay for performance in hospitals. *Cochrane Database Syst. Rev.* (7): CD011156. https://doi.org/10.1002/14651858.CD011156.pub2.

Morgan, O.W., Griffiths, C., and Majeed, A. (2007). Interrupted time-series analysis of regulations to reduce paracetamol (acetaminophen) poisoning. *PLoS Med.* 4: 654–659.

Murthy, L., Shepperd, S., Clarke, M.J. et al. (2012). Interventions to improve the use of systematic reviews in decision-making by health system managers, policy-makers and clinicians. *Cochrane Database Syst. Rev.* (9): CD009401. https://doi.org/10.1002/14651858.CD009401.pub2.

Newhouse, J.P. (1993). *Free for All? Lessons from the Rand Health Insurance Experiment.* Cambridge, MA: Harvard University Press.

Omoigui, N.A., Miller, D.P., Brown, K.J. et al. (1996). Outmigration for coronary bypass surgery in an era of public dissemination of clinical outcomes. *Circulation* 93: 27–33.

Peters, D.H., Tran, N.T., and Adam, T. (2013). *Implementation Research in Health: A Practical Guide.* Geneva: World Health Organization.

Petkovic, J., Welch, V., Jacob, M.H. et al. (2016). The effectiveness of evidence summaries on health policy makers and health system managers use of evidence from systematic reviews: a systematic review. *Implement. Sci.* 11: 162.

Proctor, E., Hooley, C., Morse, A. et al. (2019). Intermediary/purveyor organizations for evidence-based interventions in US child mental health: characteristics and implementation strategies. *Implement. Sci.* 14: 13.

Rashidian, A., Omidvari, A.H., Vali, Y. et al. (2015). Pharmaceutical policies: effects of financial incentives for prescribers. *Cochrane Database Syst Rev* 8: CD006731. https://doi.org/10.1002/14651858.CD006731.pub2.

Roggenkamp, S.D., White, K.R., and Bazzoli, G.J. (2005). Adoption of hospital case management: economic and institutional influence. *Soc. Sci. Med.* 60: 2489–2500.

Roland, M. (2004). Linking physicians pay to the quality of care. A major experiment in the United Kingdom. *N. Engl. J. Med.* 351: 1448–1454.

Sarkies, M.N., Bowles, K.A., Skinner, E.H. et al. (2017). The effectiveness of research implementation strategies for promoting evidence-informed policy and management decisions in healthcare: a systematic review. *Implement. Sci.* 12: 132.

Shelton, R.C., Cooper, B.R., and Wiltsey Stirman, S. (2018). The sustainability of evidence-based interventions and practices in public health and health care. *Annu. Rev. Public Health* 39: 55–76.

Theobald, S., Brandes, N., Gyapong, M. et al. (2018). Implementation research: new imperatives and opportunities in global health. *Lancet* 392: 2214–2228.

Whitty, C.J.M. (2015). What makes an academic paper useful for health policy? *BMC Med.* 13: 308.

Yuan, B., He, L., Meng, Q., and Jia, L. (2017). Payment methods for outpatient care facilities. *Cochrane Database Syst. Rev.* (3): CD011153.

18

Multifaceted Implementation Strategies

Marlies Hulscher[1] and Michel Wensing[1,2,3]

[1] Department IQ healthcare, Radboud Institute for Health Sciences, Radboud University Medical Center, Nijmegen, The Netherlands
[2] Faculty of Medicine, University of Heidelberg, Heidelberg, Germany
[3] Department of General Practice and Health Services Research, Heidelberg University Hospital, Heidelberg, Germany

---

SUMMARY

- Multifaceted implementation strategies can address multiple barriers for implementation, which may enhance their effectiveness. In addition, the interactions between the different components of strategies may increase the total effectiveness.

- Nevertheless, these strategies are not consistently more effective than single strategies. Research does not (yet?) substantiate the assumed effectiveness of multifaceted strategies, probably because only a small proportion of the strategies address key barriers.

- The resource use and costs associated with multifaceted strategies must be considered, as they may be higher than those of single strategies.

18.1 Introduction

The implementation strategies that are described in the previous chapters are often applied in combination with each other in practice. For instance, a large literature overview on the effectiveness of guideline dissemination and implementation strategies, for example, found that 178 of 235 studies (222 of 309 comparisons) relate to combinations of strategies, so-called multifaceted implementation strategies (Grimshaw et al. 2004). This chapter delves more deeply into the subject of combinations of implementation strategies. It describes their effectiveness and the ways to optimize their impact. We summarize key literature published in recent decades

that specifically focuses on the effectiveness of multifaceted implementation strategies (Box 18.1 provides an example).

In describing multifaceted strategies and their effectiveness, it is important to specify what we mean by a "multifaceted implementation strategy." In this book, we employ the Cochrane Effective Practice and Organisation of Care (EPOC) Review Group list, which classifies strategies or implementation activities by mode of delivery. Strategies may also be described in other ways, for example with respect to working mechanisms or goals, which would lead to a different classification of implementation strategies (see Chapter 10). The EPOC list distinguishes various concrete activities, such as "small group conference" or "audit and feedback." We

Improving Patient Care: The Implementation of Change in Health Care, Third Edition. Edited by Michel Wensing, Richard Grol, and Jeremy Grimshaw.
© 2020 John Wiley & Sons Ltd. Published 2020 by John Wiley & Sons Ltd.

Box 18.1 The Effectiveness of Breakthrough Projects

Pre-operative antimicrobial prophylaxis is important in preventing surgical site infection. In one study, 44 hospitals participated in a longitudinal cluster randomized trial to improve the timing, choice, dosage, and duration of prophylaxis in surgical patients. Half the hospitals received a feedback report (with comparison information) and participated in a so-called breakthrough project (short-cycle quality improvement). The other half only received the feedback report. The analysis showed no differences in improvement between the two groups (Kritchevsky et al. 2008).

Quality improvement collaboratives (QICs), or breakthrough projects, are a typical example of a multifaceted implementation strategy. Here, temporary cooperation and learning networks are used to enhance improvement in practice. This multifaceted approach includes teams from multiple healthcare sites coming together to learn, apply, and share improvement methods, best practices, and performance data for a given healthcare topic. An expert group (including medical and improvement experts) is recruited to establish the vision of a new care system and to teach and coach the participating teams. The participating multidisciplinary teams from the various organizations join forces for a specific period and meet during learning sessions. Between meetings, teams are tasked to apply

quality improvement methods and undertake rapid testing (such as Plan–Do–Study–Act cycles) of successful innovations elsewhere in their own work environment to achieve concrete results. They are asked to share data, innovations, and lessons learned from their implementation efforts during the meetings. Making the improvements visible through measurements plays an important role.

QICs have been applied worldwide. Carrying out breakthrough projects involves considerable costs. The first systematic review of the literature (Schouten et al. 2008) identified nine controlled studies, of which seven reported a positive effect on some of the outcome measures. The authors conclude that a moderately positive result emerged from the studies; however, effects could not be predicted with certainty. An update of this review, performed by Wells et al. (2018), identified 64 controlled studies. An improvement was found for one or more of the study's primary effect measures in 83% of the studies. Where reported, absolute differences ranged from modest to substantial. The authors concluded: "However, enthusiasm for these encouraging findings must be tempered by reflection on the limitations in design and reporting of many of these QICs, as well as likely publication bias."

---

speak of a multifaceted implementation strategy as one that combines two or more different single implementation activities from the EPOC list. This approach is obviously debatable. The activities described in the EPOC list are fairly general. Furthermore, some activities in the EPOC classification are labeled single strategies, while in fact they cover various activities. An example of this is the "outreach visits" that are classed as single strategies while they combine multiple activities, such as instruction, feedback, practical help, reminders, and organizational change. It may also be noted that the EPOC list is not

permanently fixed, but revised from time to time on the basis of emerging insights.

18.2 Strategies in Multifaceted Implementation Strategies

What single strategies are included in multifaceted implementation strategies? Looking at the evaluation research (Table 18.1), it can be noted that many multifaceted strategies

Table 18.1 Overview of reviews on multifaceted improvement strategies.

Reviews of reviews	
Ryan et al. (2014)	Patients can contribute to the quality of care and implementation of recommended practices. The authors of this review of reviews about the effectiveness of strategies to encourage healthcare consumers to use medication safely and effectively analyzed 75 systematic reviews (range 1–78 primary studies per systematic review). They conclude that there are many different potential ways to encourage safe and effective medication use. Single strategies can be just as effective for this purpose as complex strategies. None of the strategies improved all the outcomes for all the diseases, medicines, populations, or settings.
Squires et al. (2014)	This review focused on implementation strategies that target healthcare providers and shows, overall, a mixed picture. The authors included 25 systematic reviews published between 1994 and 2012 of their overview of reviews. The reviews included an average of 28 primary studies (range 10–235). The authors conclude that the outcomes of the review supply no compelling evidence for the assumption that multifaceted strategies are more effective than single ones. Of three reviews with a statistical dose–response analysis, two reviews show that increasing the number of strategies does not result in a greater effect; the third review shows that computer reminders as a single-component intervention have an even greater effect than computer reminders as part of a multifaceted intervention. Eight reviews report direct comparisons of the effectiveness of a multifaceted strategy versus a single-component strategy. Four of these reviews provided evidence that combinations are more effective than single interventions – that is to say, each of these reviews shows that more than two-thirds of the primary studies demonstrate the added value of combinations. Three reviews found mixed results – that is to say, each of these reviews demonstrates the added value of combinations in one-third to two-thirds of the primary studies. One review demonstrated the added value in less than one-third of the included primary studies. Twenty-three reviews describe indirect comparisons of multifaceted to single-component interventions by comparing multifaceted interventions to controls and single interventions to controls. Fifteen reviews showed similar overall effectiveness for multifaceted and single strategies when compared to controls. Six of the eight remaining reviews concluded that the single strategies were generally effective, while the multifaceted strategies had mixed results. Only one of the remaining reviews found that multifaceted strategies were generally effective.
Irwin et al. (2015)	This review of 21 reviews aimed at determining the effectiveness of implementation strategies within general practice. Audit and feedback, computerized advice, point-of-care reminders, practice facilitation, educational outreach, and processes for patient review and follow-up all improved quality. Evidence of an improvement effect was higher where baseline performance was low and was particularly demonstrated across process measures and measures related to prescribing. There is not sufficient evidence for the assumption that multifaceted strategies are more effective than single strategies. The authors conclude that evidence exists for a range of quality improvement interventions within general practice.
Johnson and May (2015)	The authors carried out a systematic overview of systematic reviews on the effectiveness of behavior change interventions. In their theory-led analysis of 67 systematic reviews, the authors concentrated on strategies oriented toward professionals. They pay specific attention to the types and combinations of interventions more likely to successfully initiate and sustain professional behavior change. Each strategy type was mapped to the constructs of normalization process theory (NPT), which relate to the mechanisms of change. The authors show that the less effective interventions (e.g. local consensus processes and local opinion leaders) target fewer constructs and only within "coherence" or "cognitive participation." The

(Continued)

Table 18.1 (Continued)

Reviews of reviews	
	most effective strategies (e.g. audit and feedback, reminders, and educational outreach) tend to act across more constructs, but in particular across "collective action" and "reflective monitoring." Interventions based on action (such as audit and feedback, and reminders) and various types of education tend to be more likely to successfully change professional behavior than those based on persuasion, such as local consensus processes and opinion leaders. The authors conclude that combining such effective interventions is most likely to result in behavioral change.
Lau et al. (2015)	The authors included 91 reviews that examined the effectiveness of single or multifaceted implementation strategies performed in predominantly primary care in developed countries. The reviews included between 2 and 235 original studies. The most commonly evaluated strategies targeted individual professionals (e.g. audit and feedback, educational meetings, educational outreach, reminders) rather than organizations (e.g. revising professional roles, facilitation) or context (all focusing on financial strategies). Single strategies targeted at professionals demonstrated a small (that is to say, effect sizes $\leq$5%) to modest (that is to say, effect sizes >5% and $\leq$10%) improvement: median 2–9% improvement in professional practice or behavior compared with no strategy, with considerable variability in the observed effects. The effects of multifaceted strategies targeted at professionals were mixed and not necessarily more effective than single strategies alone. Of the strategies targeting professionals, educational outreach visits, educational meetings, and audit and feedback had the best evidence base. Passive dissemination strategies such as the distribution of educational materials appeared largely ineffective and the effect of local opinion leaders appeared variable. The authors conclude that multifaceted implementation strategies were not necessarily more effective than single implementation strategies and that the effectiveness of multifaceted strategies did not increase incrementally with the number of components. There was relatively little evidence on implementation strategies at the levels of organization and the wider context. Data on the costs of different strategies were scarce or of low quality.
Pantoja et al. (2017)	The authors aimed to provide an overview of the available evidence about the effects of implementation strategies for health systems in low-income countries. They included 39 reviews in their overview of reviews. The reviews included a total of 1332 studies. Most studies in the reviews were from high-income countries; there were no studies from low-income countries in eight reviews. Implementation strategies were categorized based on the level of the healthcare system targeted by the intervention: strategies targeting (i) healthcare organizations (e.g. strategies to change organizational culture; 1 review); (ii) healthcare workers (e.g. printed educational materials; 14 reviews); (iii) healthcare workers to address a specific problem (e.g. unnecessary use of antibiotics; 9 reviews); (iv) healthcare recipients (e.g. medication adherence; 15 reviews). They report that four reviews examined the effects of multifaceted interventions on professional practice and/or patient outcomes, providing mixed and uncertain results on the effectiveness of multifaceted strategies and on the effectiveness of multifaceted strategies compared to single interventions. The authors concluded that most of the available evidence is focused on strategies targeted at healthcare workers and healthcare recipients and relates to process-based outcomes. Evidence of the effects of strategies targeting healthcare organizations is scarce.
Tonkin-Crine et al. (2017)	The authors reviewed the evidence from 33 randomized controlled trials (RCTs) in eight systematic reviews on the effects of interventions aimed at influencing clinician antibiotic prescribing behavior for acute respiratory infections in primary care. They included one systematic review on the effectiveness of multifaceted interventions, of which five RCTs were relevant to this overview: four studies reported that the multifaceted intervention might improve use. Combining these interventions possibly resulted in greater effects, as they influenced different mechanisms of

Table 18.1 (Continued)

Reviews of reviews

	behavior change. For the other interventions, including multifaceted interventions, those centered on clinician education, patient information leaflets, and the use of rapid viral diagnostics, the evidence was of low or very low quality across outcomes; the authors could not confidently draw any conclusions about the effects of these interventions compared to usual care.
Price et al. (2018)	This systematic review of 19 reviews aimed to synthesize the existing evidence base of interventions to improve healthcare worker hand hygiene compliance (HHC). Primary studies in included reviews ranged between 3 and 73 studies; in total 236 unique primary studies were included with overlap between reviews. Eighteen systematic reviews reported the overall effectiveness of interventions in improving HHC: 15 showed positive effects of interventions, whereas 3 reviews evaluating monitoring technology did not. Findings from 10 reviews regarding whether multimodal rather than single interventions are preferable were inconclusive: multimodal interventions were not always effective and not always more effective than single interventions. The authors concluded that several reviewers advocated multimodal interventions, incorporating performance feedback and extending the World Health Organization multimodal strategy for HHC over single interventions to elicit improvements in HHC. Still, this conclusion was not unanimous. Regarding theory, targeting higher numbers of theoretical determinants of behavior (up to five) appears to increase effectiveness, with interventions that address social influence, attitude, self-efficacy, and intention especially effective. There was no clear link between how educational interventions were delivered (demonstration, no demonstration, self-study, video, demonstration and video, an online element) and effectiveness. Although the evidence is sufficient to recommend the implementation of interventions to improve HHC (except for monitoring technology), it is insufficient to make specific recommendations regarding the content or how the content should be delivered.

Reviews

Gagliardi et al. (2016)	This review of 16 studies describes the type and effectiveness of patient-mediated implementation strategies delivered immediately before, during, or after patients with arthritis (osteoarthritis or rheumatoid arthritis) or cancer (breast cancer or prostate cancer) have been seen. Regardless of delivery as a single (10 studies) or multifaceted strategy (6 studies), all interventions had positive effects on at least one of the outcome measures, including satisfaction, knowledge, decision making, communication, and behavior.
Gagnon et al. (2016)	The authors included 92 unique knowledge translation (KT) initiatives for healthcare providers in the area of pediatric pain. KT programs varied in quality and impact. Knowledge-level changes and self-reported increases in comfort or confidence in skills/knowledge were consistently achieved. Practice-level changes were achieved in many areas, with varying success.
Suman et al. (2016)	The authors included 12 papers (9 studies) in this review to assess the effectiveness of multifaceted implementation strategies compared to minimal, single, or no implementation strategy for the implementation of non-specific low back and/or neck pain guidelines in healthcare. Implementation strategies varied between studies. Meta-analyses did not reveal any differences in effect between multifaceted strategies and controls. The authors conclude that multifaceted implementation is not more effective than usual care or minimal implementation.
Alexander et al. (2017)	The aim of the review was to discover what primary care–targeted interventions increased preventive healthcare for pre-school children, excluding vaccinations. The authors included 29 individual studies, of which 24 employed complex, multifaceted interventions.

(Continued)

Table 18.1 (Continued)

Reviews	
Al Aqeel et al. (2018)	This review aimed at assessing the effectiveness of interventions for improving the counseling practice of community pharmacists. The authors included 17 RCTs, of which 15 investigated multifaceted interventions. This did not allow a clear understanding of the effectiveness of individual interventions. Most of the included studies (n = 11) reported some degree of improvement in counseling practices. The authors conclude that their findings of the 17 studies included suggest that educational meetings combined with outreach visits and feedback have a positive effect on community pharmacists' counseling. The use of multifaceted interventions did not allow a clear understanding of the effectiveness of individual interventions.
Desai et al. (2018)	The authors included six before–after studies and one RCT to assess the effectiveness of evidence-based interventions aimed at reducing cervical spine imaging in adults presenting to the Emergency Department with neck trauma. Overall, implementation of interventions aimed at reducing cervical spine image ordering resulted in a statistically significant reduction in imaging; however, heterogeneity was high. Subgroup analysis revealed no differences between studies employing multifaceted versus non-multifaceted interventions.
Kovacs et al. (2018)	The authors evaluated the effect of intervention methods on primary care providers' guideline adherence. They included 36 studies. The review showed a complete range of professional interventions: no example for organizational interventions could be identified. The authors conclude that their review demonstrated that, among a wide span of interventions, single-component interventions were equally effective to complex multifaceted intervention schemes in improving process of care and outcome of care. Multifaceted interventions did not demonstrate a direct relationship between the number of intervention components and effect size.
Phillips et al. (2018)	In this review the authors compared studies describing the impact of interventions on vancomycin dosing, monitoring, and nephrotoxicity. They included six observational studies. In meta-analysis, the overall effect of interventions on outcome measures of vancomycin dosing was OR 2.50 (95% confidence interval [CI] 1.29–4.84). Effect sizes were more likely to be significant for multifaceted interventions. Interventions had no effect on appropriate timing of trough sample, attaining target concentration in patients, or nephrotoxicity.
Rowe et al. (2018)	The effectiveness of strategies to improve healthcare provider practices in low-income and middle-income countries was assessed. The reviewers selected 670 reports from 337 studies of 118 strategies. The majority of strategies were tested by a single study. Contextual and methodological heterogeneity made comparisons difficult. Several multifaceted strategies had large effects, but multifaceted strategies were not always more effective than simpler ones. Two strategy component categories had significant marginal effects: group problem solving and training. Two specific multifaceted strategies targeting infrastructure, supervision, other management techniques, and training (with and without financing), and the combination of group problem solving and training, often had large effects. The authors found that effectiveness was unrelated to the number of components in the strategy. Financial incentives for healthcare providers had modest to moderate effects, as did health system financing and other incentives. Studies of regulation and governance strategies tended to have large effects, but were not studied in isolation. The analyses suggested that certain strategies might be more effective in areas with higher levels of resources than in low-resource settings, and other strategies might be more effective in inpatient settings than in outpatient settings. The authors conclude that – although some approaches were more consistently effective than others – the impact of strategies to improve practices varied substantially.

Table 18.1   (Continued)

Reviews

Stander et al. (2018)	The authors undertook a systematic review to establish the body of evidence regarding KT training programs to improve physiotherapists' use of evidence-based practice (EBP) and clinical practice guidelines (CPG). They included nine studies for review. The KT strategies were all multifaceted, incorporating both passive and active strategies. When KT strategies addressed local barriers to EBP utilization, success rates were better for EBP and CPG uptake. There was no consistency in elements of training programs, but multifaceted programs which included at least five different elements appeared to be more effective in producing significant learning outcomes than programs with fewer elements.
Al Zoubi et al. (2018)	The authors of this systematic review aimed to evaluate the effectiveness of KT interventions to improve the uptake and application of clinical practice guidelines and best practices for a wide range of musculoskeletal disorders and healthcare professionals. They included 11 RCTs. Ten studies assessed effects on professional outcomes: all three studies using single-component interventions had a small effect. Seven studies used multifaceted interventions. Three of these assessed interventions against no intervention; these reported mixed results. The other four studies compared multifaceted interventions against other single or multifaceted interventions; all reported positive findings. The authors conclude that their findings suggest that for professional outcomes, single-component interventions are more effective than no intervention, and multifaceted interventions are more effective than single-component interventions. Four multifaceted studies assessed patient outcomes, and all were ineffective. This suggests that multifaceted interventions delivered to professionals did not improve patient outcomes.

include some form of education for healthcare providers. Education lays the foundation for behavioral change by providing knowledge, skills, and insight, and thus seems to be a logical conditional component of every implementation strategy. In addition, many multifaceted implementation strategies include data-driven performance feedback as well as reminders to healthcare providers. Both strategies address fundamental mechanisms of behavior change and can support the implementation of innovations in many situations.

On the other hand, organizational change and financial incentives seem underrepresented in the multifaceted strategies that have been studied in the context of quality improvement and implementation of innovations in healthcare. This may be related to the logistic difficulties of testing such strategies in designs for rigorous evaluation as well as a focus on different types of outcomes, such as healthcare utilization or health outcomes, in

the available research. Therefore, the body of available research on multifaceted implementation strategies may not completely reflect the types of strategies that are applied in practice across the world.

Focusing on the research literature, it can be observed that the combinations of strategies differ greatly from each other. The literature shows that a unique combination of strategies has been chosen in almost every study. For instance, the review by Grimshaw et al. (2004) identified 68 different combinations of strategies that were tested in 117 studies with a "no intervention" comparison group and 58 different combinations in 61 studies with a control group that received an intervention (Grimshaw et al. 2004). In the first group of studies, the same combination was found a maximum of 11 times; in the second group, a maximum of 6 times. This makes it difficult to draw conclusions about the effectiveness of specific combinations of strategies.

18.3 Effectiveness of Multifaceted Implementation Strategies

Table 18.1 presents a selection of systematic reviews on the effectiveness of multifaceted strategies to improve healthcare and implement innovations. As described in Section 18.2, many studies test almost unique combinations of strategies. This is why literature overviews usually do not differentiate between different combinations; they merely draw conclusions about the effectiveness of the total group of multifaceted strategies. A mixed picture of the effectiveness of multifaceted interventions comes forward from the literature overviews in Table 18.1 – a picture comparable to the conclusions about most of the single strategies. Multifaceted strategies can be effective, but they are not always effective. Furthermore, they are not always more effective than certain single strategies. No combination guarantees success in advance. The subsequent paragraphs will discuss several potential determinants of the effectiveness of multifaceted implementation strategies.

18.4 Tailoring in Multifaceted Strategies

In this book, we recommend tailoring of implementation strategies: a careful analysis of barriers for implementation, matching of strategies to those barriers, followed by application and evaluation. The involvement of stakeholders and the use of relevant theories can enhance the usefulness of this tailoring process. In the published research, the rationale for the choice of most strategies for change is often difficult to deduce (Grimshaw et al. 2004). The designers of the strategies provide little information about the barriers and facilitators (determinants) to implementation, so that it is unclear whether the choice was based upon possible causal mechanisms. A Cochrane

review of the effectiveness of this type of "tailored interventions" provides some support for the assumption that implementation strategies – and therefore also multifaceted implementation strategies – are more effective if they address the identified determinants of practice (Baker et al. 2015). The authors included 32 studies, of which 15 provided enough data to be included in a meta-regression analysis. In general, multifaceted implementation strategies were tested in the included studies. Compared to a control group in which either no intervention took place or a non-tailored intervention was carried out (usually sending educational materials or guidelines), the odds ratio for success was 1.56 (95% confidence interval 1.27–1.93). The authors conclude that tailored implementation strategies can be successful; however, the effect varies and is small to moderate. The best way to design a tailored strategy is still largely unclear. It is not only unknown what method is most likely to identify those determinants of practice that are most important and are most amenable to being addressed through implementation strategies. It is also unclear what method is most appropriate for selecting suitable strategies to address specific determinants of practice (see also Chapter 10).

These uncertainties partially explain why the effect of the investigated tailored strategies varies and is small to moderate. Bosch et al. (2007) carried out a qualitative analysis on a purposeful sample of 20 implementation studies that reported that they had analyzed determinants. She found that there was often a mismatch between the identified determinants and the interventions chosen, suggesting that the tailoring was imperfect (Bosch et al. 2007). Charani et al.'s (2011) review about improving the use of hospital antibiotics comes to similar conclusions: although qualitative research showed the influence of social norms, attitudes, and beliefs on antibiotic prescribing behavior, these determinants were not considered in the choice of implementation strategies.

18.5 Volume and Classification of Strategies

Little research has been done on examining a dose–response relationship between the composition of a multifaceted strategy and its effect. Squires et al. (2014) found – on the basis of two reviews with a statistical analysis of a dose–response relation – no link between the number of strategies and the degree of effectiveness. Thus, increasing the number of strategies does not result in a greater effect. Strategies differ in terms of intensity (e.g. mailing a written flyer versus a comprehensive training program), which might explain the lack of impact of the number of strategies per se. Furthermore, the lack of tailoring in the composition of a multifaceted strategy may explain the lack of such a dose–response relation.

In addition, an explanation can be found in the use of a classification framework that focuses on the mode of delivery of strategies. In answering the question of whether "more" works better, the framework used to classify the implementation strategies appears to be important. An alternative to "modes of delivery" for categorizing implementation strategies could be based on the *targets, ingredients, working mechanisms*, or *content* of the implementation strategy (Colquhoun et al. 2014), as well as specification of *where and how* exactly implementation strategies effect change.

For instance, a classic classification distinguishes predisposing, enabling, and reinforcing factors (Green et al. 1988). Using this model, implementation activities can focus on:

- Predisposing factors, e.g. knowledge, attitudes, opinions, and values, often translated as educational strategies.
- Enabling factors, e.g. skills, the availability of facilities, supportive resources, organizational changes.
- Reinforcing factors, e.g. the attitudes and behavior of others.

In applying this first alternative classification, a multifaceted strategy would consist of implementation activities aiming at factors from two or three groups of factors. Davis et al. (1992) and Solomon et al. (1998) applied Green's classification to explore the effectiveness of continuing education as part of strategies for improving the use of diagnostic tests. After classifying whether the strategies addressed predisposing, enabling, and reinforcing factors, or combinations of these factors, both reviews conclude that there was a direct relation between the number of behavioral factors addressed and the occurrence of positive effects: multifaceted strategies appeared to be effective more often.

A second alternative way of classifying strategies connects to some degree to Green's classification, where implementation activities are classified on the basis of their determinant of or stimulus for change (i.e. behavior change techniques). This method distinguishes nine main categories of determinants for change: knowledge, awareness, social influence, attitude, self-efficacy, intention, action control, maintenance, and facilitation (Abraham and Michie 2008; Bruin et al. 2009). Each category assumes another means of activation or stimulus to arrive at behavioral change. Using this classification, a multifaceted implementation strategy would include activities that provide two or more different determinants for change. The authors of a review of hand hygiene improvement strategies, who applied the behavior change techniques classification, report a dose–response relation between the number of determinants and the degree of effectiveness: median effect size increased substantially in the studies that addressed five rather than fewer determinants (Huis et al. 2012).

A third alternative way that closely connects to a social-constructivist approach to implementation is explored in Johnson and May's (2015) review of reviews. The authors' theory-driven analysis of 67 systematic reviews links each EPOC strategy to the constructs of normalization process theory (NPT). NPT characterizes an implementation process via four mechanisms or constructs (with a total of

16 subconstructs – 4 per construct): (i) coherence (which refers to participants' understanding of the intervention); (ii) cognitive participation (which focuses on enrolment and engagement with the work); (iii) collective action (which focuses on how the work was carried out); and (iv) reflective monitoring (which is about how participants assess their progress). In using this classification, a multifaceted strategy would include activities that work on two or more subconstructs from different constructs. The authors found that the less effective interventions focus on fewer subconstructs and only within "coherence" or "cognitive participation." The most effective strategies work on more subconstructs of more constructs, in particular on "collective action" and "reflective monitoring."

18.6 Combinations of Specific Strategies

The effectiveness of a multifaceted strategy is determined by the effectiveness of the single strategies of which it is composed and the interaction between these strategies. There is yet little understanding of the added value of combining specific strategies. The effect of a multifaceted strategy is not necessarily equal to the sum of the effects of all its individual strategies. On the one hand, largely the same effects may be achieved through different strategies (i.e. through different mechanisms of action). For example, while both feedback and reminders influenced preventive care, the combination of the two produced no greater effect than the separate strategies (Tierney et al. 1986). The same result emerged in a study comparing printed educational materials alone (control) versus printed materials plus other strategies (audit and feedback and educational outreach); the latter did not add to the effectiveness of printed educational materials alone (Cheater et al. 2006). On the other hand, different strategies can enhance

each other's effects, so that the total effect is greater than the sum of the separate effects. For example, what has been learned in an educational meeting can sometimes only be put into practice if organizational barriers have been addressed.

In multifaceted strategies, the coherence and interaction between the different strategies should explicitly be checked. This is yet another subject on which little research has been performed. Ideally, a factorial design would be used to investigate the interaction between the various components of the multifaceted implementation strategy. In such a design, the single strategies are applied both separately and combined, so that the added value of the combination can be directly compared to the single strategy.

An alternative approach is an (observational) analysis of multiple studies that assessed variable multifaceted strategies in a specific clinical domain or with respect to a given outcome. For instance, a systematic review of improving adult immunization and cancer screening services used meta-regression analysis to determine which strategies most influenced the degree of immunization and cancer screening (Stone et al. 2002). It found that organizational strategies were the most relevant; that is, separate office hours for preventive activities, deploying non-doctors for preventive tasks, and improving team functioning and collaboration. The second most influential component concerned patient-oriented strategies such as financial incentives for patients and reminders for their appointments.

Performing a process evaluation is crucial for obtaining insight into the contribution of the different components of a multifaceted strategy (see Chapter 22). While an effect evaluation shows to what extent the multifaceted strategy actually results in observed changes in the study population, a process evaluation provides information about the actual execution of planned strategy components and the factors that play a role in achieving or not achieving the desired outcomes. Effect evaluations often show that a given implementation strategy results in greater improvements for some participants than for others. At the same time, process evaluations may show that not all participants equally participate in the planned implementation activities. By relating the variation in effect to the variation in participation, statements can be made about the relation between the components of the multifaceted strategy and the changes achieved. In this way, insight into the success-determining, crucial components of the strategy can be gained (Boxes 18.2 and 18.3 provide examples). Ideally, linear (additive) as well as non-linear relationships could be explored in quantitative analyses.

In process evaluations, the impact of specific strategies in a multifaceted program group can also be explored qualitatively, using methods such as interviews and (ethnographic)

Box 18.2   Effectiveness of the Subcomponents of a Multifaceted Strategy to Implement Guidelines for Preventing Cervical Cancer

A nationwide program aimed to implement screening for cervical cancer (Hermens et al. 2001). To make sure that as many at-risk women as possible have a Pap smear taken and that the guideline for cervical cancer screening is optimally applied, a national implementation program was set up, combining various strategies at the national, regional, and practice levels:

- *National level*: development and distribution of evidence-based guidelines, special educational materials, a computer module for selecting patients at risk, and financial compensation for extra work.
- *Regional level*: regional coordination of inviting and reminding patients (agreements between municipal health services, comprehensive cancer centers, pathology laboratories, and primary care) and organization of formal continuing medical education for primary care physicians and practice assistants.
- *Practice level*: outreach visits by trained facilitators.

The effect evaluation showed that – after the intervention – adherence to 9 out of the 10 effect parameters or quality indicators had been improved. Large changes had taken place in, among others, the number of practices that invited the patients themselves (from 5 to 30% between 1995 and 1997), sent reminders (from 7 to 44%), or took care of the follow-up (from 35 to 51%). The process evaluation described the degree of participation in each implementation activity in each primary care practice. Regression analysis helped determine which parts of the implementation program contributed to the change. The most important findings were:

- Using the computer module proved essential: it increased the chance of change two- to ten-fold for nine different aspects of the screening (odds ratio [OR] 1.85–10.2 for nine indicators).
- In practices supported by the outreach visitor, more benefits were gained; if there were two or more visits, the chance of change was 1.5–2 times greater (OR 1.46–2.35 for six indicators).
- The continuing medical education of practice assistants had some effect on almost half of the indicators, particularly on tasks that they carried out themselves (OR 1.37–1.90 for four indicators).
- The formal continuing medical education for physicians had no effect.
- Finally, the effect of financial compensation could not be assessed separately because all participants received it, but financial compensation undoubtedly had a supplemental influence.

Box 18.3 Characteristics of Complexity

Characteristics of the intervention itself, e.g.:

- Multiple components (made up of various interconnecting parts).
- Number of groups or organizational levels targeted by the intervention.
- Degree of flexibility or tailoring of the intervention permitted.
- Self-organization, adaptivity, and evolution over time.

Characteristics of the intervention's causal pathway, e.g.:

- Non-linear relationships; phase changes.
- Multiple mediators and moderators of effect.
- Feedback loops.
- Synergy between components.
- Number and variability of outcomes; emergent novel outcomes.
- Connectivity, where individual components of an intervention are linked together in a system, so they influence each other.
- Interaction with context.

Source: Data from Petticrew et al. (2013).

---

observations. The approach may involve specific conceptual frameworks for guidance and interpretation (see Chapter 3). For instance, a complex systems framework emphasizes the dynamic, pluralistic, interconnected, and unpredictable features of social systems (Greenhalgh and Papoutsi 2018). This framework seems particularly relevant for multifaceted implementation strategies, because these comprise a range of activities that are often targeted at multiple goals and aim to address multiple barriers for change. The complex systems approach suggests taking multiple sources of complexity into account, but it remains to be seen whether the resulting strategies are more effective (Brainard and Hunter 2016).

An implementation strategy can be labeled "complex" because of various characteristics. According to Petticrew et al. these fall into two broad categories: characteristics of the intervention itself and characteristics of the hypothesized causal pathway from the intervention to the outcomes (Petticrew et al. 2013; see Box 18.3). Similarly, Shiell et al. distinguish two types of complexity: complexity can arise not only from the intervention itself, but also from important features of the context or system in which the intervention is implemented (Shiell et al. 2008; Tanner-Smith and

Grant 2018). So complexity is a property of the intervention and the context/system into which it is placed; multiple interactions will create non-linear relationships (Hawe 2015). Greenhalgh and Papoutsi (2018) suggested that in this respect "the dancer and the dance are intertwined": the intervention and its context will be inter-related and reciprocally interacting. Complexity increases the unpredictability of effects (Hawe 2015). To understand the effects of interventions, it is therefore important to understand which elements of the complex intervention interacted in what manner with which elements of the context to produce the observed effects (Minary et al. 2018).

18.7 Conclusions

Given the diversity of barriers and facilitators for change in many cases, it is plausible that multifaceted strategies might be more effective than single strategies: combinations of strategies can address more determinants of practice. Multifaceted implementation strategies can indeed effectively improve patient care, but they are not consistently effective, and there is little insight into which combinations of strategies will work best in which situations. As for single implementation strategies, the choice of the most successful combination of strategies needs to be tailored to the experienced barriers and facilitators of change.

The accumulation of knowledge on the effects of multifaceted strategies is difficult, because it involves a high degree of complexity. The resource use and costs of multifaceted implementation strategies tend to be higher than single strategies and should therefore also be considered. A higher likelihood of successful improvement must be weighed against the higher costs of combining a larger number of strategies. The mixed findings on the impact of multifaceted strategies provide a clear rationale for evaluation and research on those strategies.

References

Abraham, C. and Michie, S. (2008). A taxonomy of behaviour change techniques used in interventions. *Health Psychol.* 27: 379–387.

Al Aqeel, S., Abanmy, N., AlShaya, H., and Almeshari, A. (2018). Interventions for improving pharmacist-led patient counselling in the community setting: a systematic review. *Syst. Rev.* 7: 71.

Al Zoubi, F.M., Menon, A., Mayo, N.E., and Bussières, A.E. (2018). The effectiveness of interventions designed to increase the uptake of clinical practice guidelines and best practices among musculoskeletal professionals: a systematic review. *BMC Health Serv. Res.* 18: 435.

Alexander, K.E., Brijnath, B., Biezen, R. et al. (2017). Preventive healthcare for young children: a systematic review of interventions in primary care. *Prev. Med.* 99: 236–250.

Baker, R., Camosso-Stefinovic, J., Gillies, C. et al. (2015). Tailored interventions to address determinants of practice. *Cochrane Database Syst. Rev.* (4): CD005470. https://doi.org/10.1002/14651858.CD005470.pub3.

Bosch, M., Van der Weijden, T., Wensing, M., and Grol, R. (2007). Tailoring quality improvement interventions to identified barriers: a multiple case analysis. *J Eval Clin Pract* 13: 161–168.

Brainard, J. and Hunter, P.R. (2016). Do complexity-informed health interventions work? A scoping review. *Implement. Sci.* 11: 127.

de Bruin, M., Viechtbauer, W., Hospers, H.J. et al. (2009). Standard care quality determines treatment outcomes in control groups of HAART-adherence intervention studies: implications for the interpretation and comparison of intervention effects. *Health Psychol.* 28: 668–674.

Charani, E., Edwards, R., Sevdalis, N. et al. (2011). Behavior change strategies to influence antimicrobial prescribing in acute care: a systematic review. *Clin. Infect. Dis.* 53: 65–62.

Cheater, F.M., Baker, R., Reddish, S. et al. (2006). Cluster randomized controlled trial of the effectiveness of audit and feedback and educational outreach on improving nursing practice and patient outcomes. *Med. Care* 44: 542–551.

Colquhoun, H., Leeman, J., Michie, S. et al. (2014). Towards a common terminology: a simplified framework of interventions to promote and integrate evidence into health practices, systems, and policies. *Implement. Sci.* 9: 51.

Davis, D.A., Thomson, M.A., Oxman, A.D., and Haynes, R.B. (1992). Evidence for the effectiveness of CME. A review of 50 randomized controlled trials. *JAMA* 268: 1111–1117.

Desai, S., Liu, C., Kirkland, S.W. et al. (2018). Effectiveness of implementing evidence-based interventions to reduce C-spine image ordering in the emergency department: a systematic review. *Acad. Emerg. Med.* 25: 672–683.

Gagliardi, A.R., Légaré, F., Brouwers, M.C. et al. (2016). Patient-mediated knowledge translation (PKT) interventions for clinical encounters: a systematic review. *Implement. Sci.* 11: 26.

Gagnon, M.M., Hadjistavropoulos, T., Hampton, A.J., and Stinson, J. (2016). A Systematic

Review of Knowledge Translation (KT) in Pediatric Pain: Focus on Health Care Providers. *Clin J Pain*. 32: 972–990.

Green, L.W., Eriksen, M.P., and Schor, E.L. (1988). Preventive activities by physicians: behavioral determinants and potential interventions. *Am. J. Prev. Med.* 4: S101–S107.

Greenhalgh, T. and Papoutsi, C. (2018). Studying complexity in health services research: desperately seeking an overdue paradigm shift. *BMC Med.* 16: 95.

Grimshaw, J.M., Thomas, R.E., MacLennan, G. et al. (2004). Effectiveness and efficiency of guideline dissemination and implementation strategies. *Health Technol. Assess.* 8 (iii-iv): 1–72.

Hawe, P. (2015). Lessons from complex interventions to improve health. *Annu. Rev. Public Health* 36: 307–323.

Hermens, R.P.M.G., Hak, E., Hulscher, M.E.J.L. et al. (2001). Adherence to guidelines on cervical cancer screening in general practice: programme elements of successful implementation. *Br. J. Gen. Pract.* 51: 897–903.

Huis, A., van Achterberg, T., de Bruin, M. et al. (2012). A systematic review of hand hygiene improvement strategies: a behavioural approach. *Implement. Sci.* 7: 92.

Irwin, R., Stokes, T., and Marshall, T. (2015). Practice-level quality improvement interventions in primary care: a review of systematic reviews. *Prim. Health Care Res. Dev.* 16: 556–577.

Johnson, M.J. and May, C.R. (2015). Promoting professional behaviour change in healthcare: what interventions work, and why? A theory-led overview of systematic reviews. *BMJ Open* 5: e008592.

Kovacs, E., Strobl, R., Phillips, A. et al. (2018). Systematic review and meta-analysis of the effectiveness of implementation strategies for non-communicable disease guidelines in primary health care. *J. Gen. Intern. Med.* 33: 1142–1154.

Kritchevsky, S.B., Braun, B.I., Bush, A.J. et al. (2008). The effect of a quality improvement collaborative to improve antimicrobial prophylaxis in surgical patients: a randomized trial. *Ann. Intern. Med.* 149: 472–480.

Lau, R., Stevenson, F., Ong, B.N. et al. (2015). Achieving change in primary care-—effectiveness of strategies for improving implementation of complex interventions: systematic review of reviews. *BMJ Open* 5: e009993.

Minary, L., Alla, F., Cambon, L. et al. (2018). Addressing complexity in population health intervention research: the context/intervention interface. *J. Epidemiol. Community Health* 72: 319–323.

Pantoja, T., OpiyoN, Lewin, S. et al. (2017). Implementation strategies for health systems in low-income countries: an overview of systematic reviews. *Cochrane Database Syst. Rev.* (9): CD011086. https://doi.org/10.1002/14651858.CD011086.pub2.

Petticrew, M., Anderson, L., Elder, R. et al. (2013). Complex interventions and their implications for systematic reviews: a pragmatic approach. *J. Clin. Epidemiol.* 66: 1209–1214.

Phillips, C.J., Wisdom, A.J., McKinnon, R.A. et al. (2018). Interventions targeting the prescribing and monitoring of vancomycin for hospitalized patients: a systematic review with meta-analysis. *Infect. Drug Resist.* 11: 2081–2094.

Price, L., MacDonald, J., Gozdzielewska, L. et al. (2018). Interventions to improve healthcare workers' hand hygiene compliance: a systematic review of systematic reviews. *Infect. Control Hosp. Epidemiol.* 39: 1449–1456.

Rowe, A.K., Rowe, S.Y., Peters, D.H. et al. (2018). Effectiveness of strategies to improve health-care provider practices in low-income and middle-income countries: a systematic review. *Lancet Glob. Health* 6: e1163–e1175.

Ryan, R., Santesso, N., Lowe, D. et al. (2014). Interventions to improve safe and effective medicines use by consumers: an overview of systematic reviews. *Cochrane Database Syst. Rev.* (4): CD007768. https://doi.org/10.1002/14651858.CD007768.pub3.

Schouten, L.M.T., Hulscher, M.E.J.L., Everdingen, J.J.E.v. et al. (2008). Evidence for the impact of quality improvement collaboratives? A systematic review. *BMJ* 336: 1491–1494.

Shiell, A., Hawe, P., and Gold, L. (2008). Complex interventions or complex systems? Implications for health economic evaluation. *BMJ* 336: 1281–1283.

Solomon, D.H., Hashimoto, H., Daltroy, L., and Liang, M.H. (1998). Techniques to improve physicians' use of diagnostic tests. *JAMA* 280: 2020–2027.

Squires, J.E., Sullivan, K., Eccles, M.P. et al. (2014). Are multifaceted interventions more effective than single-component interventions in changing health-care professionals' behaviours? An overview of systematic reviews. *Implement. Sci.* 9: 152.

Stander, J., Grimmer, K., and Brink, Y. (2018). Training programmes to improve evidence uptake and utilisation by physiotherapists: a systematic scoping review. *BMC Med. Educ.* 18: 14.

Stone, E.G., Morton, S.C., Hulscher, M.E. et al. (2002). Interventions that increase use of adult immunization and cancer screening services: a meta-analysis. *Ann. Intern. Med.* 136: 641–651.

Suman, A., Dikkers, M.F., Schaafsma, F.G. et al. (2016). Effectiveness of multifaceted implementation strategies for the implementation of back and neck pain guidelines in health care: a systematic review. *Implement. Sci.* 11: 126.

Tanner-Smith, E.E. and Grant, S. (2018). Meta-analysis of complex interventions. *Annu. Rev. Public Health* 39: 135–151.

Tierney, W.M., Hui, S.L., and McDonald, C.J. (1986). Delayed feedback of physician performance versus immediate reminders to perform preventive care. Effects on physician compliance. *Med. Care* 24: 659–666.

Tonkin-Crine, S.K.G., Tan, P.S., van Hecke, O. et al. (2017). Clinician-targeted interventions to influence antibiotic prescribing behaviour for acute respiratory infections in primary care: an overview of systematic reviews. *Cochrane Database Syst. Rev.* (9): CD012252. https://doi.org/10.1002/14651858.CD012252.pub2.

Wells, S., Tamir, O., Gray, J. et al. (2018). Are quality improvement collaboratives effective? A systematic review. *BMJ Qual. Saf.* 27: 226–240.

Part VI

Organization and Evaluation

19

Planning of Implementation

Richard Grol[1,2]

[1] Radboud University, Nijmegen, The Netherlands
[2] Maastricht University, Maastricht, The Netherlands

SUMMARY

- Irrespective of the size and ambition of an implementation project, it is a good idea to draw up an explicit plan for the implementation process.
- In the plan, a number of issues will be specified, such as:
  - Development of the plan according to phases in the change process.
  - Planning of activities for different levels of care.
  - Planning of activities over time.
  - Incorporating the implementation plan into existing activities.
  - Testing of the implementation strategies.
  - Setting goals and indicators for the evaluation.
  - Embedding of new practice into routines and organization.

19.1   Introduction

As we have outlined in previous chapters, the first requirement for effective implementation of innovations in patient care is a clear recommendation or proposal for practice. Ideally, it is based on (scientific) knowledge regarding benefits and is relevant for perceived issues in current practice. When it has become clear which innovation professionals would like to introduce, the next steps include analysis of the actual care and the problems encountered, as well as an analysis of the target group and the setting in which the change would need to take place (Figure 19.1). Such an analysis usually identifies a variety of required changes and identifies various ways of introducing effective implementation of new procedures. On the basis of these analyses, implementation strategies and interventions are chosen and elaborated.

A project or program of implementation strategies requires careful preparation (Box 19.1 provides an example). The format of the program depends on whether it is a small-scale project in a single ward or practice, a large-scale implementation program, or a randomized study. Irrespective of this, we recommend elaborating an "implementation plan" for organizing things. In the context of research projects, it may be required to keep specific activities as planned (see Chapter 20). In many

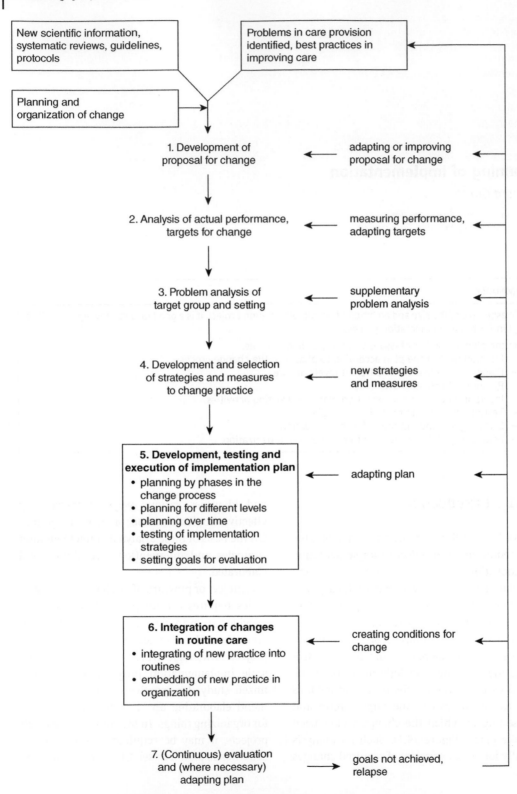

Figure 19.1 The Grol and Wensing implementation of change model.

Box 19.1   Implementation of ParkinsonNet

Parkinson's disease is a complex neurode-generative disorder with increasing prevalence. Several healthcare professionals in primary and hospital healthcare have a long-term involvement in the care of patients with Parkinson's disease. The ParkinsonNet concept was developed in the Netherlands to improve the quality of multidisciplinary community care since 2004 (Nijkrake et al. 2010). ParkinsonNet involves regional networks of healthcare professionals who specialize in Parkinson's disease and who are able to work efficiently together. For the organization of a regional ParkinsonNet, a small number of care professionals who are interested in Parkinson's disease are selected per region. These care providers receive targeted training with respect to evidence-based guidelines and cooperation with other professions. After this training, mutual communication and cooperation within the network are stimulated through a web-based forum and email. Also, the ParkinsonNet facilitates patients with Parkinson's disease being directed specifically to these trained care professionals, resulting in them treating more patients. This will help in keeping their expertise at the required standard and develop a healthy business model. The ultimate aim is to improve the quality of care in the patient's immediate environment.

In subsequent years the added value of the concept has been evaluated scientifically within controlled trials (Munneke et al. 2010). In eight regions the ParkinsonNet concept was introduced, while in eight other regions the usual care was provided. The outcomes showed that the new approach did not change health outcomes for patients, but it did reduce healthcare costs (annual savings of up to about US$100 000). Also, the quality of care improved considerably: in particular, knowledge and use of clinical guidelines improved. Moreover, the number of patients with Parkinson's disease per physiotherapist in the ParkinsonNet areas increased from 6 to 13 patients per therapist. Toward the end of 2010, 80 ParkinsonNet networks were active nationally, resulting in national coverage. Moreover, the number of disciplines participating has been extended, with occupational therapists and speech therapists and more disciplines becoming involved in the national network. How was ParkinsonNet so successfully implemented in the Netherlands? What were its success factors?

- A start was made on a small scale with one network in one region; a lot was learned from this pilot. Upgrading as part of a scientific study led to further experience being gained, which proved to be of importance to the rollout across the country.
- The innovation was connected to the needs of the most important actors. The networks were initially introduced for Professions Allied to Medicine (PAMs) in ambulatory care. There was a perceived need to increase the specific expertise and cooperation among this target group. Therefore, there was a lot of support for this innovation.
- There was a deliberate choice not to attempt to solve all problems immediately within the project. The project was initially aimed at physiotherapy care for Parkinson patients. Other disciplines became involved later.
- Financial support for the innovation was gradually raised and secured; this proved essential to realize the development nationally. One of the key selling arguments was that ParkinsonNet provided an exemplary model for modern healthcare for patients with complex chronic diseases who need multiprofessional care.
- Two "champions" (a neurologist and a physiotherapist) led ParkinsonNet and promoted it over many years by raising attention in the national and international media,

(Continued)

> **Box 19.1 (Continued)**
>
> presentations at conferences, and a continuous flow of scientific publications and doctoral theses.
> - The way the project team had been set up: the personal effort of all those involved in the project and the shared ambition to improve care for patients with Parkinson's
>
> disease contributed to the success of the project.
> - Over the whole course of the project, research and evaluation had been incorporated into it; this yielded important information to shape the project and it kept all involved alert to the possibilities.

situations, however, such a plan can be handled flexibly; it can be adjusted on the basis of experiences gained during the course of the implementation.

19.1.1 Planning of the Implementation Process

In general, the following issues are addressed in the implementation plan:

- Development of the plan according to phases in the change process:
  - The plan takes into account the phases in the change process: orientation, understanding, acceptance, change, and maintenance.
- Planning of activities for different organizational levels:
  - The plan takes into account different levels of healthcare (central, institution, department/team/practice, individual professional, patient) on which the implementation can be focused.
- Planning of activities over time:
  - Activities are not all offered at the same time.
  - Activities can be subdivided into manageable units.
  - Activities are presented in a logical order.
  - Evaluation points are incorporated into the time schedule.
- Incorporating the implementation plan into existing activities:
  - Implementation activities are, if possible, incorporated into existing programs for training and improvement.

- Testing of the implementation strategies:
  - Testing the strategy on a small scale prior to large-scale implementation of the innovation.
  - Adjusting the strategy where necessary.
- Setting goals for evaluation:
  - Formulating targets for change at the start of the implementation process.
  - Goals, while suitably ambitious, are also concrete and measurable.
  - Monitoring, using indicators, will be a permanent feature.
- Integration and embedding:
  - Support permanent change through the attention of leaders, involvement of the target group, adequate staff and budget, visibility of the outcomes, proper coordination, etc.

The recommendations given in this chapter have been predominantly based on knowledge gained through experience, since scientific research into the planning of implementation processes is relatively scarce.

19.2 Development of the Plan According to Phases in the Change Process

In Chapter 3 we showed that there is broad consensus that implementation requires a process in which change for care providers and teams occurs in different steps. We have summarized that "ideal" process of five steps in Chapters 3 and 10:

- Orientation
  - Awareness of the innovation
  - Interest and involvement
- Insight
  - Understanding
  - Insight into own routines
- Acceptance
  - Positive attitude, motivation to change
  - Positive intention or decision to change
- Change
  - Actual adoption in practice
  - Confirmation of benefit or value of change
- Maintenance
  - Integration of new practice into routines
  - Embedding of new practice in the organization

A plan to disseminate and implement a new procedure or improvement in care must, in principle, give adequate attention to each of these steps, allowing for the scale and dimension of the implementation activity, the nature of the innovation, and any implementation problems encountered (see Chapter 10 for examples of strategies per phase). For instance, in the implementation of a new multidisciplinary guideline for stroke with recommendations for treatment involving a large number of disciplines, initial attention must be given to developing a good dissemination plan to inform all stakeholders. If, however, the percentage of post-operative wound infections on a ward is seen as unacceptably high, much more emphasis must be placed on a thorough analysis of the problem and the development of a good implementation plan with continuous monitoring and feedback on wound infections.

It matters a great deal whether a group has much experience with working on quality improvement and a positive attitude with regard to change, or whether a group is completely new to the idea of working on improvement. In the latter case a lot of attention will have to be paid to creating a "context or a culture of change" (see Box 19.2). It is therefore recommended that the plan deals with the intended implementation of the innovation and the target group, as well as the setting in which the implementation is to take place. This procedure will determine which steps in the change process will need to be given most attention.

The steps in the process of changing do not all require the same attention, and the planned sequence will not always be followed. However, different steps do, to some degree, necessitate other actions.

Box 19.2 Model for Change through Persuasion

On the basis of experiences with the introduction of changes in a hospital, Garvin and Roberto (2005) developed a model for change, in which the emphasis lies on making the target group ready for change. Prior to announcing a plan for a different procedure and executing it, a lot of preparatory work is needed to create a receptive environment. In their model, the following steps are distinguished:

1) Convince employees that radical change is imperative: demonstrate why the new direction is the right one.
2) Position and frame a preliminary plan: gather feedback, announce final plan.

3) Manage employee mood through constant communication.
4) Reinforce behavioral guidelines to avoid backsliding.

Central to the model is that, initially, sufficient time should be given to persuade the target group that change is unavoidable and to involve the target group in what the change is going to look like. Only then will the plan be implemented and monitored definitively and in a very strict way. This will form the basis for a permanent change.

19.3 Planning of Activities for Different Levels of Care

Assuming that a combination of strategies, adapted to the target group, is most effective in the majority of cases, the question is which strategies should be targeted and carried out at what level of care provision. Mittman et al. (1992) distinguished three types of situations, each of which requires a different strategy:

- *Small groups* (two or three people): strategies include, particularly, face-to-face instruction by trained personnel, individual consultation by "expert," and personal contact between colleagues.
- *Medium-sized groups* (e.g. members of a hospital department, care team, health center, or local groups of physicians or paramedics): strategies here are the use of opinion leaders and key figures, interactive study groups, preparing consensus agreements, clinical audit and quality circles, but also monitoring and financial incentives.
- *Large groups* (e.g. all leaders of a professional group, all care providers in a region, or all hospitals in a country): an important strategy here will be the use of mass media, public reporting, or national development of guidelines.

For the effective introduction of an innovation, it is sometimes necessary to work on multiple levels at the same time, especially when it concerns programs on a national or regional scale or all employees in an institution or home-care organization. The activities on different levels (central, local, department/practice, or individual) then have different goals and contents (Table 19.1):

- *Central*: on a central level, professional organizations, policy makers, and payers can provide support by creating good preconditions for the implementation of the innovation and by providing the necessary infrastructure, provisions, and regulations. By contributing a definite, positive point of view about the change, they can make their influence felt across the system.
- *Local/institution*: local organizations of care providers or an institution can help with introducing a successful change by making local agreements among all of those involved to support a new procedure and include it in their policies, to clearly communicate this to the target group, and to assist in and support the achievement of the necessary organizational and structural conditions.

Table 19.1 Introducing changes on multiple levels.

Level	Possible methods
Central	Publication in journals and online platforms Written or email mailings Development of information and educational materials Financial incentives Regulation and support to facilitate infrastructure
Local/ institution	Local courses Local consensus and protocol development Use of key people/opinion leaders Quality projects in institutions Leaders support improvement
Department, team, practice	Setting goals for department or practice Developing a protocol or work agreements Setting up quality projects with data collection Improve information technology infrastructure Outreach visits for instruction and help Introduction of checklists in routine care
Individual professional	Self-study, courses Audit and feedback Reminders Skill training

- *Department, team, or practice*: at the level of a department of an institution, a team, or a practice, there is usually a multidisciplinary group of care providers who must accept and apply the change or innovation. Various methods discussed in previous chapters can facilitate the change.
- *Individual professional*: finally, the individual care provider must become informed and motivated, and for this they must participate in education, audit and feedback programs, and similar activities.

19.4 Planning of Activities over Time

The different elements of the implementation must also be scheduled. Among the important considerations are:

- The *activities* should not all be offered at the same time, as this could overwhelm the target group and overtax the organization. A *logical order* must be decided upon: What is the most important thing to do first, and what can be done later?
- The plan should be *divided* into a number of well-organized and manageable components that can be introduced and evaluated separately.
- The *sequence* of these components can be determined by the different *steps in the change process* that the care providers and teams undergo (see Chapter 10). It is advisable to make both a *dissemination plan* and an *implementation plan*.
- The *most important problems*, as identified by an analysis of the target group and setting, should receive the greatest attention.
- *Evaluation and feedback* at regular intervals should be incorporated into the plan. This is necessary to identify problems in the introduction, to respond to new priorities and the needs of the target group, and to identify any slowdown in the process. Therefore, a plan

for evaluation is made at the outset. The methods for this are described in the following chapters.

- It should be recognized and accepted that the full course of many implementation and change processes *requires time* (sometimes years). Experiences across many projects have shown that the time required often was a disappointment: "Progress is not linear, but three steps forward and two steps back" (Wye and McClenahan 2000). However, while changes usually proceed slowly, at the same time a certain speed and boldness are necessary to prevent the loss of momentum. Those in the target group generally want quick success, once they have committed themselves to a new way of working.

19.5 Incorporating the Implementation Plan into Existing Activities

Experience in numerous implementation projects has shown the great importance of *integrating the implementation plan into existing structures and channels* for contact with, training of, and improving the quality of the target group. It is advisable to make use of what is already available (Wye and McClenahan 2000): regular team or educational meetings, existing audit and visiting procedures, and familiar communication channels. In other words, use the media with which the target group is already familiar, which they trust and can use without extra effort. Across the various levels, this will look slightly different:

- *Central*: scientific and professional journals for professionals, as well as newsletters from professional organizations.
- *Institute*: existing quality programs, quality and safety committee meetings, accreditation programs, and monitoring systems.
- *Local groups*: for example, for primary care this may include local study groups, care

---

Box 19.3   Evaluation of National Quality Improvement Programs

The Netherlands Organization for Health Research and Development (ZonMw) initiated 10 national quality and safety improvement programs in healthcare in the Netherlands. Øvretveit and Klazinga (2010) conducted a meta-evaluation on these 10 programs, which yielded the following results:

- In order to start a program successfully, an explicit division of roles and clear coordination are necessary.
- Make sure the data are correct – at the start, as well as during and after the project has finished – so that the targets aimed at can be evaluated.

- Make sure the program has been sufficiently embedded in the policy and arrange for clear agreements on the follow-up.
- Make sure the activities are embedded in existing improvement programs and geared to specific target groups and levels.

The most important recommendation of the authors is to spend more time and energy in arranging for "sustainable change." This can be done by studying how best practices in different countries have been sustained and distributed, by fitting in with existing structures and activities in a better way, and by learning from each other across sectors and disorders.

---

team meetings, continuing medical education courses, and local professional group meetings, and for medical specialists their clinical discussions and team meetings.

- *Partnership, team*: visiting programs, clinical audit, and department-related quality improvement projects.
- *Practice*: practice meetings, clinical audit projects.
- *Individual*: re-registration programs, educational initiatives.

Box 19.3 provides a summary of lessons learned from a large improvement program.

19.6   Testing of the Implementation Strategies

An important question is what will constitute the set strategies for improvement and implementation of innovations into practice. Differing considerations may shape the choices of implementation strategies to be incorporated into the plan: for example, the question of which strategies have a *proven value* within the setting and target group of interest. Previous chapters can provide leads on this. The transferability of findings from published research needs to be considered by representatives or experts of the target group and setting.

The choice is also influenced by the *available budget* and the effort required by staff and volunteers, as well as by considerations of *cost-effectiveness*. There is most likely an optimum beyond which considerably more resources are required to achieve a small additional effect or beyond which the effect may even decrease. The latter can occur, for example, because the plan evokes a negative reaction in the target group, which does not want to be continually faced with initiatives for change. A study of the effectiveness of the effort of trained outreach visitors to improve prevention in primary care showed that a greater number of visits was not associated with more changes (Hulscher et al. 1997). A review by Grimshaw et al. (2004) of 235 studies in the field of the implementation of new knowledge in care also showed that more interventions do not by definition lead to more effect. Data on the cost-effectiveness of diverse improvement activities are still scarce (see Chapter 23).

The conclusion will sometimes be that the scientific literature offers little assistance to the specific situation in which changes are introduced, making it necessary to elaborate strategies substantially. In this situation, it is important to *begin small*: choose a few changes that you want to introduce and test these in a small, motivated group. The small-scale *testing of the implementation strategy* and its components can thereby be seen as a crucial element in preparing the implementation (Green et al. 1989; Cretin 1998). What has been developed at the desk, or by a group of experts, usually turns out differently when it is put into practice. We know, for example, that the use of outreach visitors is an effective way to make changes in some aspects of care delivery, but who should best fill this role, how often the visits should be made, what materials the visitor should use, and what position he or she should have in the team cannot be determined in advance for specific innovations. This should be tried out on a small scale and then gradually built up on the basis of the first experiences (see Box 19.4). The *triability* of an innovation is, according to Rogers (2003), one of the characteristics of a successful implementation. However, not everything can be planned in advance. The plan should often be *flexible* and amenable to repeated readjustment and adaptation (*tailoring*) to the requirements or other attributes of the target group. This means that the plan must be able to offer help with concrete introduction problems in specific care settings, and in seeking alternatives when a given approach does not appear to work well.

19.7 Setting Goals for Evaluation

A component of the planning and performance of the procedure of implementation, continuing on to the next step in the implementation cycle, is the formulation of *concrete goals* and measurable indicators, with which the progress and success of the activities can be measured. Evaluation activities are ideally integrated into the change process from the very beginning. For this purpose, it is necessary to formulate specific goals. These should be ambitious, while also being very concrete and attainable within the setting of implementation (Schellekens 2000). A goal such as "lowering the number of cesarean sections" is too loosely defined. "Reducing the number of cesarean sections by 15% within 1 year" contains points against which success can be evaluated. The goals should be sufficiently ambitious to get real changes started, such as 25% fewer post-operative wound infections, 80% shorter time to perform certain procedures, or 40% fewer amputations in patients with diabetes (Schellekens 2000). There should also be clear time deadlines for achieving the goals. It is clear that when ambitious goals are set, evaluation of progress toward them cannot be delayed to the end of the project. The implementation plan must be regularly and repeatedly reviewed: Is it still suitable for stimulating the

---

Box 19.4 Testing and Introduction of a Plan for Change

Changing is a cyclic process, in which a number of steps are taken time and again. The PDSA cycle (Plsek 1999) is a practical model, having the following as steps:

- *Plan*: set goals and generate ideas about how the goals can best be achieved.
- *Do*: carry out the plan and record what has been done.
- *Study*: analyze data, reflect on the lessons that can be learned.
- *Act*: continue, adapt, or change the activities, formulate new ideas for the plan.

The starting point is always to test the changes on a small scale and repeatedly go through the cycle, adding or sharpening ideas. Multiple cycles are planned to test the changes before the real implementation begins. Begin on a small scale and gradually expand. In each cycle data are collected on the principle that ideas can be added. Ideally, the test is carried out in different surroundings, under different conditions.

Box 19.5   Success Factors in Improving Mental Healthcare

In a Breakthrough Collaborative program in mental healthcare, 26 teams from 29 mental health hospitals worked on the implementation of three multidisciplinary guidelines. The effects and success factors were collected through monitoring data and questionnaires. Teams with an active and inspiring leader, that received support from the management in their improvement actions and had sufficient time, resources, and staff support, achieved more improvements.

---

intended changes or does it need adaptation? Begin small, check to be sure things are on the right track, improve the plan, and expand to other segments of the target group: a cyclic process (see Box 19.5). The evaluation requires carefully developed indicators and measuring methods. Chapter 7 presents an elaborate explanation on how indicators can be developed and the actual care be monitored.

19.8   Integration and Embedding of New Practice into Routines and Organization

Even when the improvements aimed at have been implemented into daily healthcare routines, experience has taught us that as soon as the official implementation project has finished, the risk of reverting to old routines is high. After an initial period in which everyone has a supportive attitude toward the change, attention often wanes or the circumstances in an institution of practice are such that the new procedure cannot be successfully continued. A loss of the improvement of care is expensive, and it could undermine the confidence and support of the target group for future programs. Therefore, arranging for permanent and sustainable improvements, through integration of the new procedure into existing routines and facilitating it with the right organizational measures, is very important. This is something that needs to be thought through during the implementation plan.

The literature on sustainability of change in healthcare is growing and comes up with many different terms for sustainable change, such as *sustainability*, *resilience*, *viability*, *stability*, *maintenance*, *institutionalization*, *continuation*, *scaling out*, and *normalization* (May et al. 2007; Gruen et al. 2008; Tricco et al. 2016; Aarons et al. 2017; Reed et al. 2018; Shelton et al. 2018). These terms can apply to maintaining certain outcomes of care with patients, successfully continuing an improvement program, embedding a continuous improvement in a care system, or maintaining the possibility of introducing a new procedure. Box 19.6 describes a review of sustainability approaches.

Box 19.6   A Systematic Review of Sustainability Approaches in Healthcare

A systematic review of publications on sustainability of change approaches, models, and frameworks included 62 publications describing 32 frameworks, 16 models, 8 tools, and 4 strategies (Lennox et al. 2018). Constructs across approaches were compared and 40 individual constructs for sustainability were found, with 6 constructs included in 75% of the approaches:

• General resources available

• Demonstration of effectiveness
• Monitoring progress over time
• Stakeholder participation
• Integration of change in existing programs and policies
• Training and capacity building.

Also organizational readiness, belief in the initiative, and leadership and champions proved to be important in many approaches.

Different authors reviewed the research on sustainability in healthcare. For instance, Stirman et al. (2012) reviewed the research methods used in knowledge translation studies and identified 125 studies, of which almost half relied on self-reports. Few studies employed rigorous methods of evaluation. Tricco et al. (2016) aimed to characterize the interventions used in sustainability studies to manage chronic diseases and included 62 studies in their review. More than half were randomized controlled trials, but few studies focused on the sustainability of the interventions.

Gruen et al. (2008) checked 84 studies on sustainability and came up with a list of conditions for successful sustainable change, such as:

- The *continuous attention* of managers.
- The *involvement* of the target group and local managers.

- An *improvement* that fits the more general aim of the organization.
- *Sufficient staff and budget* for a long-term continuation of the new procedure or the project.
- An enthusiastic pioneer (*champion*).
- *Positive outcomes* of the project being visible.
- The improvement project will be *well directed and well coordinated*.

The conditions for success presented are similar to those found in other reviews (e.g. Scheirer 2005; Shelton et al. 2018), which also pointed at the importance of resources, staffing and support within the organization, leadership, adaptability of the interventions, training and supervision, and perceived benefits of the new procedure. Box 19.7 presents a structured approach to assessment of sustainability from the UK.

Box 19.7   National Health Service Sustainability Model

In the UK, the National Health Service (NHS) developed an instrument to be used in the planning and evaluation of the "sustainability" of a proposal for change or an implementation project (Maher et al. 2007). The following aspects of implementation are dealt with in this model.

Procedure That Needs to Be Improved

- Does this procedure have extra advantages, apart from better patient care (more efficient, easier)?
- Is the basis of the new procedure credible for the staff?
- Can the new procedure be adapted to the organization's demands?
- To what extent does continuation of the procedure depend on specific persons, money, or technology?
- Is there a system to monitor if and how the procedure is applied, are data available, is feedback given on the outcomes?

Professionals

- Involvement and training of professionals: Are professionals involved in the implementation plan and do they receive training?
- Professionals' attitude: Are they motivated, sufficiently involved, and sufficiently able to implement the quality project or the improvement?
- Leadership: Are formal and clinical leaders involved in the project and do they assume their responsibility for the project, also in the longer run?

Organization

- Does the new procedure have links to the strategic goals and culture of the organization, is there a change culture, has the organization successfully implemented improvements in the past?
- Is there an infrastructure (equipment, training, logistics, staff, etc.) for sustainable change?

19.9 Conclusions

The successful implementation of innovations in the practice of patient care requires good preparation and planning. Although the scientific literature in the field of planning of implementation and improvement projects is limited, there is now extensive experience in setting up such projects in many different sectors of healthcare. Ideally, a small-scale start with testing the plan on motivated persons, groups, or institutions leads on to the activities being gradually expanded. A realistic time schedule is planned (usually more time is required than anticipated). The plan is incorporated into the normal activities of the target group and provides sufficient attention to the embedding of the changes in existing, set work routines. Continuing evaluation is carried out to add to the plan where necessary. The way in which the evaluation can be designed will be explained in the following chapters. Box 19.8 provides a checklist for implementation activities.

Box 19.8   Checklist for Implementation Activities

1) **Goals of the implementation**
   - Is there a clear description of what exactly is being implemented (guideline, care pathway, protocol, best practice, technique)?
   - Is there a clear description of the target group(s) on which the implementation is focused?
   - Has the target group been involved in formulating the targets for improvement?
2) **Toolkit**
   Have specific tools been developed that assist in the implementation process?
   - Tools for professionals (summaries, decision trees, decision-support systems)?
   - Tools for patients (leaflets, internet applications, videos)?
   - Tools for organizations (care pathways, protocols, models for cooperation)?
3) **Dissemination plan**
   Have specific plans been made to inform the target group about change proposals?
   - Is there a clear description of the target groups?
   - Has a different approach to the various sections in the target groups been planned?
   - Is there an actual description of the channels through which information is spread (written, personal)?
   - Is there an actual description detailing who is responsible for spreading information?
4) **Indicators and measurement**
   Has a systematic approach of the development of indicators, measurement, and feedback been used?
   - Has a limited set of core recommendations or core goals been selected that need to be measured?
   - Have valid and reliable indicators been developed for these core recommendations?
   - Has the actual care been measured, in order to determine the most important problems?
   - Have the measurement outcomes been used to select a number of very concrete goals for improvement?

(Continued)

Box 19.8   (Continued)

---

5) **Problem analysis**

Has a systematic analysis of factors that influence implementation positively or negatively been conducted?

- Has an analysis been made of all those involved in the implementation process (who is important, who has what role)?
- Have factors that hinder or promote change been mapped (preferably per planned change goal):
  - With professionals?
  - With patients?
  - With teams, in care processes?
  - In an organizational context (staff, resources, culture, leaders, etc.)?
  - In a political, economic, legal context?
- Have factors that will play a part in the implementation plan been prioritized?

6) **Implementation of the plan**

Has a systematic approach to the change in practice been used?

- Have interventions and measurements, related to the outcomes of the problem analysis, been selected?
- Has a plan been made for when which part of the intervention will take place?
- Is there an allocation of tasks (who does what)?
- Has the target group been involved in the change plan?
- Have measures been anticipated to sustain and embed the desired new procedure, also when the project has finished?

7) **Evaluation of the outcome**

- Have the methods of collecting, analyzing, and feedback of (indicator) data been determined?
- Has a plan been made when and which evaluations will take place in the course of time?

8) **Organization of the plan**

- Is there a project team with a suitable leader and sufficient expertise?
- Have a budget and other means/staff been determined?
- Has there been support from (senior) management, also in the long run?
- Has the target group been sufficiently involved in the project at all important moments?
- Has a concrete, clearly described plan with all steps for the implementation project been made?

References

Aarons, G., Sklar, M., Mustanski, B. et al. (2017). "Scaling-out" evidence-based interventions to new populations or new healthcare delivery systems. *Implement. Sci.* 12: 11.

Cretin, S. (1998). *Implementing Guidelines: An Overview*. Santa Monica, CA: RAND.

Garvin, D.A. and Roberto, M.A. (2005). Change through persuasion. *Harv. Bus. Rev.* 83: 104–112.

Green, L., Gottlieb, N., and Parcell, G. (1989). Diffusion theory extended and applied. In: *Advances in Health Education and Promotion* (eds. B. Ward and F.M. Lewis), 3. Greenwich, CT: JAI Press.

Grimshaw, J.M., Thomas, R.E., MacLennan, G. et al. (2004). Effectiveness and efficiency of guideline dissemination and implementation strategies. *Health Technol. Assess.* 8 (iii–iv): 1–72.

Gruen, R.L., Elliott, J.H., Nolan, M.L. et al. (2008). Sustainability science: an integrated approach for health-programme planning. *Lancet* 372: 1579–1589.

Hulscher, M.E.J.L., van Drenth, B.B., van der Wouden, J.C. et al. (1997). Changing preventive practice: a controlled trial on the effects of outreach visits to organize prevention of cardiovascular disease. *Qual. Health Care* 6: 19–24.

Lennox, L., Maher, L., and Reed, J. (2018). Navigating the sustainabily landscape: a systematic review of sustainability approaches in healthcare. *Implement. Sci.* 13: 27.

Maher, L., Gustafson, D., and Evans, A. (2007). *Sustainability Model and Guide.* NHS Institute for Innovation and Improvement: Coventry.

May, C., Finch, T., Mair, F. et al. (2007). Understanding the implementation of complex interventions in health care: the normalization process model. *BMC Health Serv. Res.* 7: 148.

Mittman, B.S., Tonesk, X., and Jacobson, P.D. (1992). Implementing clinical practice guidelines: social influence strategies and practitioner behaviour change. *QRB Qual. Rev. Bull.* 18: 413–422.

Munneke, M., Nijkrake, M.J., Keus, S.H. et al. (2010). Efficacy of community-based physiotherapy networks for patients with Parkinson's disease: a cluster-randomised trial. *Lancet Neurol.* 9: 46–54.

Nijkrake, M.J., Keus, S.H.J., Overeem, S. et al. (2010). The Parkinson-net concept:

development, implementation and initial experience. *Mov. Disord.* 25: 823–829.

Øvretveit, J. and Klazinga, N. (2010). *Meta-Evaluation of Ten National Quality Improvement Programmes in the Netherlands 2004–2009.* The Hague: ZonMw.

Plsek, P.E. (1999). Section 1: evidence-based quality improvement, principles, and perspectives. Quality improvement methods in clinical practice. *Pediatrics* 103: 203–214.

Reed, J., Howe, C., Doyle, C. et al. (2018). Simple rules for evidence translation in complex systems: a qualitative study. *BMC Med.* 16 (92).

Rogers, E.M. (2003). *Diffusion of Innovations.* New York: Simon and Schuster.

Scheirer, M.A. (2005). Is sustainability possible? A review and commentary on empirical studies of program sustainability. *Am. J. Eval.* 26: 320–347.

Schellekens, W. (2000). Een passie voor patiënten [A passion for patients]. *Med. Contact* 55: 412–414.

Shelton, R., Cooper, B., and Stirman, S. (2018). The sustainability of evidence-based interventions and practices in public health and healthcare. *Annu. Rev. Public Health* 39: 55–78.

Stirman, S., Kimberly, J., Cook, N. et al. (2012). The sustainability of new programs and innovations: a review of the empirical literature and recommendations for future research. *Implement. Sci.* 7: 17.

Tricco, A., Ashoor, H., Cardoso, R. et al. (2016). Sustainability of knowledge translation interventions in healthcare decision-making: a scoping review. *Implement. Sci.* 11: 15.

Wye, L. and McClenahan, J. (2000). *Getting Better with Evidence.* London: King's Fund.

20

Experimental Designs for Evaluation of Implementation Strategies

Michel Wensing[1,2,3] and Jeremy Grimshaw[4,5]

[1] *Faculty of Medicine, University of Heidelberg, Heidelberg, Germany*
[2] *Department of General Practice and Health Services Research, Heidelberg University Hospital, Heidelberg, Germany*
[3] *Department IQ healthcare, Radboud Institute for Health Sciences, Radboud University Medical Center, Nijmegen, The Netherlands*
[4] *Clinical Epidemiology Program, Ottawa Hospital Research Institute, Ottawa, Ontario, Canada*
[5] *Department of Medicine, University of Ottawa, Ottawa, Ontario, Canada*

SUMMARY

- Experimental designs aim to attribute outcomes to interventions, thus going beyond description of outcomes or goal attainment after intervention.

- They are characterized by comparison of outcomes in two or more purposefully created study groups, of which at least one is exposed to an intervention (e.g. a program for improving healthcare practice).

- Experimental evaluations can be designed in different ways. In the field of quality improvement and knowledge implementation, most are cluster randomized and pragmatic (i.e. close to routine practice).

- Many aspects of study procedures (e.g. data collection, measurement, regulations for research) need to be considered for the successful running of experimental evaluations.

- Experimental designs have an important role in quality improvement and knowledge implementation, alongside other study designs and methods.

20.1 Introduction

Evaluation is a crucial component of a structured approach to the implementation of change in healthcare (Figure 20.1). While evaluation may take various forms, we refer here to data-driven assessment: reflection guided by systematically collected empirical data. Evaluation can be used in various phases of the design, piloting, implementation, sustaining, and scaling-up of programs. Evaluation may address outcomes (e.g. patients' health), processes (e.g. quality of care), and costs (e.g. time investment by healthcare providers). Experimental designs are crucially important for the accumulation of scientific knowledge (Baldasarri and Abascal 2017). As resources are usually limited, not every question can be answered through evaluation research. Evaluation is practically important, if the stakes are high and the effects of an intervention are uncertain. This may be the case, for instance, if a program requires many resources, affects many individuals, involves risks for targeted individuals, or if the program's feasibility is uncertain. In such situations, it is important to assess the benefits, risks, feasibility, and costs

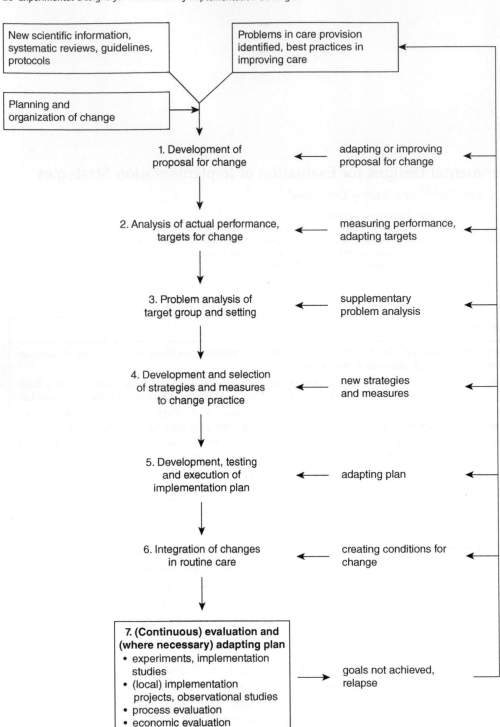

Figure 20.1   The Grol and Wensing implementation of change model.

Box 20.1   Audit and Feedback to Reduce Cesarean Section Rates

Cesarean section is associated with risk of harm and should be only be conducted if medically indicated. To reduce the rising rates of cesarean section in Canada, a multifaceted program, which included audit and feedback to providers and other interventions, was conducted over 1.5 years (Chaillet et al. 2015). In a cluster-randomized trial, 32 hospitals were allocated to either an intervention group or a control group. The program had a small, statistically significant effect on cesarean section rate (the primary outcome in this trial). This rate decreased from 22.5 to 21.8% in the intervention group, while it increased from 23.2 to 23.5% in the control group. The effect size, adjusted for hospital and patient characteristics (odds ratio [OR] 0.90, 95% confidence interval [CI] 0.80–0.99), was statistically significant. The effect estimate was based on data concerning 105 351 deliveries.

---

as rigorously as possible, preferably before sustaining and scaling-up of interventions.

This chapter will focus on experimental designs for evaluation, while subsequent chapters will focus on observational designs, process evaluation, and economic evaluation. Box 20.1 provided an example of an evaluation study that was designed as an experiment or randomized trial. It is beyond the scope of this chapter to provide a comprehensive elaboration of experimental designs and methods, because the literature on the topic is very large. After describing several options for study design, this chapter will discuss some aspects of conducting experimental evaluations in research on quality improvement and knowledge implementation. The design, conduct, and analysis of experimental evaluations of interventions for quality improvement and knowledge implementation can be complex, but in some situations these are relatively straightforward, highly feasible, and relatively cheap.

20.2 Experimental Study Designs

Like many other methodological concepts, the term "experimental" is not consistently used across scientific domains. In epidemiology and the behavioral and social sciences, it usually refers to a specific type of study design for the evaluation of intervention outcomes, which aims to minimize the risk of bias in the estimation of effectiveness (that is, a causal relationship between intervention and outcome). The interventions are not necessarily "experimental" in the sense of "innovative" or "first in humans." If an intervention, or its use in a target group, is innovative, it is recommended to start with theory-based analysis and observational research in order to explore and optimize the intervention, before it is tested in experimental research (Craig et al. 2008).

Experimental designs are characterized by the application of one or more interventions, measurement of pre-specified outcomes, and comparison between two or more study groups (one of which does not get the interventions of interest). Many experimental designs are prospective studies, but some use routinely collected data, which may be captured retrospectively after the intervention period has been completed. The primary reason for having a non-intervention ("control") group in experimental designs is that it controls for change due to natural trends, concurrent initiatives, and non-specific intervention effects. In many studies of improvement in healthcare practice, control groups' performance improves in the same direction as the intervention groups (Chen et al. 2016). This may be positive for the quality and outcomes of healthcare, but it needs to be taken into account in the interpretation of change and attribution of outcomes to interventions.

Ideally, the allocation of participants (e.g. patients or healthcare providers) is randomly done, using a valid procedure, because this balances known and unknown confounders (factors which distort causal interpretation) between study groups across all experimental studies in a field. It may be noted that most single experimental studies do not achieve balanced study groups, but the methods for analysis do not assume such balance. The procedure for random allocation (e.g. a computerized generator of random numbers) should be concealed from the healthcare providers and patients involved. For instance, in many cluster-randomized trials, participants are randomized at the start of the study by an independent statistician. Ideally, study participants (e.g. physicians and their patients) are unaware of their treatment status ("blinding") and the researcher sticks to the planned intervention. In quality improvement and knowledge implementation, however, blinding of study participants is hardly ever possible.

While randomized trials have theoretically the lowest risk of bias when estimating intervention effectiveness, various aspects can still induce substantial bias, such as the use of an inadequate randomization procedure, lack of concealment of randomization, absence of blinding for study arms for participants, high drop-out of participants, and suboptimal outcome measures or incomplete reporting (Schünemann et al. 2013). Attribution of changes in outcomes to interventions is problematic, if such aspects emerge. Regardless of the allocation method, trials can be designed in different ways. For instance, there may be more than two study groups if multiple interventions are being tested. The allocation of individuals to study groups may be based on individual patients, healthcare providers, or healthcare organizations. Trials may use sequential or one-off recruitment and allocation of interventions. The follow-up period after intervention delivery may be short (e.g. days) or long (e.g. months). Interventions vary from

completely standardized to somewhat flexible and adaptable with pre-specified boundaries. Some options for experimental designs will be provided in this section. Rather than presenting a few ideal-type designs (e.g. patient-randomized trial, cluster-randomized trial, etc.), a number of key aspects of study design are discussed.

20.2.1 Pragmatic versus Explanatory Trials

Explanatory trials focus on the effects of an intervention under ideal circumstances, while pragmatic trials test whether an intervention will work under real-world circumstances (Schwartz and Lellouch 2009). Pragmatic and explanatory are two extremes on a continuum rather than a dichotomy (Dal-Re et al. 2018). The degree of pragmatism influences the eligibility and recruitment of participants, the setting and organization where the trial is done, flexibility in intervention delivery and adherence, intensity of follow-up monitoring, choice of primary outcome, and data-analysis approach (Loudon et al. 2015). PRECIS-2 is a structured instrument to assess the degree of pragmatism of a trial (see http://rethinkingclinicaltrials. org). The generalizability of findings to real-world populations and settings is better in pragmatic trials, thus these are most frequently applied in quality improvement and knowledge implementation. Box 20.2 provides an example of a pragmatic randomized trial.

20.2.2 Cluster Randomization

In many randomized trials of clinical interventions, patients are randomly allocated to intervention or control groups. This design is often problematic in the evaluation of quality improvement and implementation programs, because healthcare providers (who are usually not blinded for these programs) tend to change their routines in both intervention and control patients (Eccles et al. 2003). Such contamination can result in a dilution of intervention effects, because the contrast between intervention and control groups is lowered. A common

---

Box 20.2   Improvement Plans in the Context of Practice Accreditation

Improvement plans were part of a comprehensive, data-based accreditation program for primary care practices in the Netherlands. To examine the effects of making improvement plans in the context of a multifaceted improvement program, a pragmatic cluster-randomized trial was designed (Nouwens et al. 2014). Forty-five practices were randomly allocated to one of two groups. In block A, practices were requested to make improvements in cardiovascular risk management in their practices. In block B, practices were requested to focus their improvement plans on other clinical or organizational domains. In both blocks, performance indicators for cardiovascular risk management were measured on the basis of chart audit in samples of cardiovascular patients. For practical reasons, no measurements of other conditions were done. The trial showed no effect on the primary outcome, which concerned controlled systolic blood pressure (achieved in 40% of patients), controlled cholesterol level (achieved in 39%), and prescription of antiplatelet medication (achieved in 83%) in eligible patients. Six of 17 secondary outcomes showed effects and physicians reported high levels of goal attainment (scores of about 8 on a 10-point scale). Making elaborated, written improvement plans had no observable value in the context of practice accreditation.

---

way to address this problem is to allocate healthcare providers (with all their patients) to intervention or control groups. This is called cluster randomization. Cluster-randomized trials need larger sample sizes than patient-randomized trials, because the statistical clustering needs to be taken into account in the power calculation (Eldridge and Kerry 2012). In a few cases, it may be more attractive to design a patient-randomized trial of larger size and adjust for clustering in the analysis (Torgerson 2001). This may be the case if the intervention of interest largely focuses on individual patients (e.g. home visits by nurses), but also includes some components targeted at care providers, which could induce contamination (e.g. the education of physicians).

20.2.3   Options for Choice of Study Groups

The classic two-arm randomized trial allocates participants to either an intervention group or a control group. The latter group may receive a placebo, a minimal intervention, a different intervention, or no intervention. In many studies of quality improvement and knowledge implementation, control groups receive either no intervention (which may be labeled "usual care") or minimal intervention, such as paper-based guidelines (which is assumed to have little impact on professional practice). Control groups may show a large variation in outcomes (e.g. professional behaviors), which complicates the interpretation of differences with intervention groups. There is a range of advanced study designs (e.g. factorial designs, see Box 20.3), which aim to determine the added value of intervention components combined, compared to their effectiveness as single intervention components.

20.2.4   Block Designs

A specific category of trials randomizes not only participants to study groups, but also blocks of activities to these groups. Within these blocks of activities (e.g. types of diagnostic tests ordered), participants receive the same interventions (e.g. feedback). Thus, all participants receive interventions, which is often attractive to both participants and policy makers. This approach may also enhance the recruitment and retention of participants in the study.

Box 20.3   Reducing Prescribing of Antibiotics

The aim of this randomized trial with a 2 × 2 factorial design (Cals et al. 2009) was to evaluate the effect of testing for C-reactive protein (CRP) in the consultation room and specific training in communication skills. The primary outcome was prescribing antibiotics at the index consultation. Forty physicians included 431 patients with symptoms of lower respiratory tract infections. Four groups of practices were formed: (i) physicians who were given a desktop CRP test device; (ii) physicians who had been trained in communication; (iii) physicians who had been exposed to both interventions; and (iv) physicians without any intervention

(usual care). Physicians in the CRP test group prescribed antibiotics to 31% of the patients compared to 53% in the no-test group. In the communication training group antibiotics were prescribed to 27% of the patients compared to 54% in the no-training group. Both differences were statistically significant. Physicians in the combined intervention arm (iii) prescribed antibiotics to 23% of the patients (the interaction term was not-significant). A combination of the illness- and disease-focused approaches may be necessary to achieve the greatest reduction in antibiotic prescribing for this common condition in primary care.

The analysis and interpretation of these trials are based on the assumption that an intervention in block A (e.g. feedback on laboratory tests ordered) does not influence behaviors in block B (e.g. ordering imaging tests), and vice versa. The advantage is that all participants receive the same level of attention (intervention and data-collection procedures), which theoretically balances non-specific effects. However, appropriate analysis of trials with block designs is complex (Steen et al. 2014). Boxes 20.4 and 20.5 provide examples.

20.2.5   Allocation of Participants to Study Arms

The approach to allocation of participants to study arms is an important aspect of study design, which has direct implications for the logistics of the study. Allocation of participants (patients or clusters) can theoretically be done at different times within a trial: before recruitment of participants (pre-randomization), after recruitment and informed consent of participants, or after baseline measurement.

Box 20.4   Nurse Practitioners in Out-of-Hours Care

There is increasing demand for out-of-hours care (care during evenings, nights, and weekends) and shortages of physicians to provide this care. Substitution of physicians with nurses may help to reduce these problems, but outcomes such as patient safety and costs were uncertain. In one primary out-of-hours care organization in the Netherlands, teams of four physicians were compared with teams of three physicians and one nurse practitioner (Van der Biezen et al. 2016). The nurse

practitioner was trained to care for patients with a wide range of symptoms, with the exception of a few categories of symptoms. The effects were examined in a cluster-randomized design, in which weekend days were randomly rotated between the two types of teams. Analysis of data on a total of 12 089 patients showed no difference in resource use, including X-rays, medication prescription, and referrals to hospital emergency care.

Box 20.5   Computerized Decision Support in Primary Care

The effects of a computerized decision-support system in primary care were examined in a pragmatic cluster-randomized trial in 60 general practices in the north of England (Eccles et al. 2002). In a block design, the practices received support for decisions in either asthma or angina, while they contributed data on both conditions before and after the intervention. No effects were found on adherence to guidelines, based on review of case notes. The authors explain the absence of effects by the low levels of use of the software. Examples of outcome measures for angina care were percentage of patients with blood pressure recorded (80% adherence in the intervention arm), body weight recorded or advised (26%), and smoking education given (4%). Examples of outcome measure for asthma care were percentage of patients with lung function assessed (43%), inhaler technique assessed (19%), and asthma education or action plan (5%).

Pre-randomization (also known as Zelen design) is a logical possibility, but it is associated with practical problems (e.g. low participation rates among pre-randomized individuals). In many cluster-randomized trials, participants are allocated all at once at the start of the study. Cluster trials raise specific ethical issues, such as who are research participants, or when and how to seek consent from participants (Weijer et al. 2012). If participants are recruited over a long period, they may be allocated sequentially over time, like in many patient-randomized trials. In case of sequential allocation, small numbers of participants (e.g. four or six) are allocated to study arms shortly after enrollment into the trial (block randomization). The allocation may be restricted by specific requirements, for instance that study groups have equal size or similar composition (e.g. regarding hospital size). Adaption of the allocation to study groups while the trial is running is an innovative approach in patient-randomized trials, but its usefulness for research on improving healthcare is not known.

Furthermore, participants in the intervention group may receive the intervention (e.g. quality improvement or implementation program) at the same point in time or sequentially. The cross-over trial is a classic example: in this design, each of the groups receives the intervention, but at different phases, while measurements are done in all phases. An important risk, however, is the possibility of carry-over effects: effects of a preceding intervention which continues to have impact. The stepped-wedge trial, another design which involves a sequential intervention start, has been proposed and elaborated in recent years (Barker et al. 2016; Copas et al. 2015). In this design, participants are allocated to four or more study groups (ideally at random). All study groups eventually receive the intervention, but they are randomly allocated to different moments in time for the start of the intervention. Outcomes are measured throughout all phases. Box 20.6 provides an example of a cluster-randomized trial with a stepped-wedge design. While the design has attractive features (e.g. all participants receive the intervention), an appropriate analysis is complex and requires substantial statistical expertise (Barker et al. 2016).

20.3   Outcome Measures and Data-Collection Methods

Outcome evaluations can use a variety of measures, such as measures of patients' health and health utilization, providers' decisions and activities, and their perceptions and views on aspects of healthcare practice. In many situations, it is wise to include a variety of measures

---

Box 20.6   Improving Safety of Prescribing in Primary Care

In a cluster-randomized trial with two arms and a stepped-wedge design, 34 practices were allocated to various start dates for a multifaceted program to enhance safety of prescribing during a 48-month period (Dreischulte et al. 2016). Recruited practices were stratified by list size tertile and randomly allocated within strata to one of 10 starting dates. Due to the nature of the study, allocation concealment of practices was only possible until the time they switched over to a different intervention status. The program comprised professional education, informatics to facilitate review of medical records, and financial incentives. The primary outcome was a composite measure of prescribing of non-steroidal anti-inflammatory drugs or selected anti-platelets in nine high-risk patients (e.g. patients with chronic kidney disease). High-risk prescribing was on average reduced from 3.7% of patients immediately before the start of the intervention to 2.2% of patients at the end of the intervention (a statistically significant difference).

---

in different domains (e.g. patient outcome and provider behaviors), because change often involves different domains and research users may be interested in different outcomes. Ideally, outcomes are organized in a causal chain, based on theory or previous research (Glasgow et al. 1999). For instance, if clinical research showed the effects of a treatment on a patient outcome, application of that treatment can be expected to result (on average) in a change of outcome. The linkages between provider and patient perceptions, such as their intention to perform specific behaviors, and actual behavior or health outcomes tend to be complex. Therefore, it is recommended to measure actual behavior, rather than self-reported behavior, whenever possible. In the context of outcomes evaluations, it is particularly important that measures are responsive to change in professional behavior and healthcare delivery.

Proctor et al. (2009) proposed a set of implementation outcomes, including acceptability, adoption, appropriateness, cost, feasibility, fidelity, penetration, and sustainability. Lewis et al. (2015) identified 104 instruments across these 8 constructs, of which 50 related to acceptability. In the context of this book, we relate these constructs largely to process evaluation rather than to outcome evaluation of implementation strategies. The exception would be adoption, if it is measured in terms of behaviors of health professionals, managers, or policy makers.

In randomized trials, and ideally in all other study designs, primary outcomes need to be defined a priori, so that the study can be adequately powered to detect relevant change on those outcomes and the risk of switching primary outcomes during analysis is reduced. Strictly, a trial is only hypothesis-testing research with respect to this primary outcome. Various considerations influence the choice of primary outcome, such as the importance to stakeholders, the body of knowledge on the intervention of interest, and the availability of validated measures. The primary outcome measure may reflect health outcomes, but more likely aspects of provider behaviors or healthcare delivery in research of quality improvement and knowledge implementation. Randomized trials of clinical interventions which also include measures of intervention implementation have been labeled hybrid effectiveness–implementation trials (Curran et al. 2012). In many of these trials, the emphasis remains on answering a research question concerning clinical effectiveness.

The type of data in many studies of quality improvement and knowledge implementation comprises data from clinical or administrative databases and questionnaires, which are completed by providers or patients. Other types of data include (videotaped) consultations of patients and providers, tracking on mobile devices, and independent clinical measurements (e.g. a psychiatric interview). We refer to Chapter 7 for a discussion of the feasibility and validity of various types of measures of professional behaviors and quality of healthcare. The use of routinely collected data (e.g. for administrative or clinical purposes) in the context of trials may have benefits, but a key issue is whether the available routine data map onto the outcomes of interest. Also, in some jurisdictions there may be legal hurdles to using routine data (McCord et al. 2018). For instance, it may be difficult to use data for other than their original purposes, if these data include individual identifiers.

Recruitment and retainment of participants in evaluations can be a challenge, which is not limited to experimental designs but is often perceived to be highest in such designs. There is high variation in the rates of recruitment and retainment. While participation rates of 5–20% may be typical for recruitment in unselected healthcare providers, these rates can be much higher (e.g. 60–100%) in existing networks or programs (personal experiences of the authors). Likewise, drop-out rates of healthcare providers in the course of the research vary between studies, with a rate of 5–20% as an experienced estimate. A systematic review of 45 studies suggested that telephone reminders, financial incentives, opt-out designs, and open trial designs were promising in patient-randomized trials (Treweek et al. 2013). It seems plausible that these findings can be generalized to evaluations in quality improvement and implementation science.

20.4 Statistical Power and Data Analysis

We refer to books and papers on statistics for a detailed discussion of the design and analysis of randomized trials and related designs (e.g. Donner and Klar 2000; Eldridge and Kerry 2012; Friedman et al. 2015). In this section only some key aspects are highlighted. The sample size in an evaluation should be sufficiently large to detect meaningful change over and above random error ("noise") in the primary outcome. This can be enhanced by high fidelity of intervention delivery, accurate outcome measurement, and higher numbers of measurements. A statistical power calculation focuses on the latter: the sample size. It is required by most funders of research, although the assumptions are often (at least partly) tentative in quality improvement and knowledge implementation. Based on a range of assumptions, such as distribution of the primary outcome and the expected effect size, it predicts the required sample size. Many studies of quality improvement and implementation have a complex data structure, which needs to be taken into account in the statistical power calculation and data analysis. These complexities include, for instance, clustering in the data and repeated measurements. It is often most efficient to have many clusters of small size (e.g. many primary care practices, each with a few patients) but this is not always feasible.

The primary data analysis in a randomized trial and related designs is focused on between-groups comparison of follow-up measurements (after completion of the intervention). Looking at changes within groups only is misleading (Bland and Altman 2015) and comparison of changes between groups reduces the statistical power unnecessarily (Egbewale et al. 2014). Baseline data may be included in the analysis, for instance in a regression model, to adjust for the remaining differences between groups. The primary analysis in explanatory trials should be based on intention to treat, meaning that all participants allocated to study groups should remain included in the study. If there is a substantial number of missing values, imputing missing values may be considered. Multiple imputation of missing values has been recommended in patient-randomized trials. Ideally, the plan for data analysis is elaborated before analyzing the data begins (Gamble et al. 2017).

20.5 Regulatory and Ethical Considerations

From a scientific and ethical perspective, any trial is only justified if there is honest uncertainty ("equipoise") about the benefit and risk of the intervention. For instance, it may be difficult to justify a non-intervention control group in a trial of audit and feedback to providers, an intervention of proven effectiveness (Ivers et al. 2014). In reality, the added value of a study is often based on professional judgment, which may be suboptimal or inadequate. Furthermore, replication of previous research findings can be scientifically highly relevant, but it is often difficult to judge how many replications are useful.

An important ethical as well as methodological requirement, which is reinforced by many research funders and scientific journals, is that randomized trials should be registered in a recognized trial register (DeAngelis et al. 2004). This is no different for trials of strategies for quality improvement and knowledge implementation. Ideally, registration occurs before recruitment and data collection start. The registration documents, among other things, the intervention, study population, and primary outcomes. It is also good practice to develop and publish a study protocol for a randomized trial, in fact for all rigorous studies.

The regulations for research on quality improvement and knowledge implementation in healthcare differ between jurisdictions (Goldstein et al. 2018). In some jurisdictions it is completely exempted from regulations for research. In others it falls under regulations for research, but is exempted from research ethics review. This may be the typical situation for research in university hospitals and medical faculties. A third possibility (which might emerge in the coming years) is

that it is considered part of the learning healthcare system and dealt with through a set of regulations which differ from those for research. It may be noted that many scientific journals require a statement by an independent ethics committee for any empirical study they publish.

Regardless of the need for ethics approval, improvement interventions and research should obviously adhere to all prevailing law and regulations. For instance, the European law on data protection (active since 2018) has specified strict regulations for collecting and handling non-anonymous data on individuals. This often implies that written informed consent is required from all patients and providers in a study. Other regulations specify how long data have to be stored, and whether data can be used for other purposes than those for which they were primarily collected.

20.6 Conclusion

This chapter provided an introduction and overview of designs and methods of experimental evaluation of improvement and implementation programs. Experimental evaluation has an important role, alongside other study designs and methods, particularly if the stakes are high and the uncertainty on intervention effectiveness is substantial. Ideally, experimental studies are preceded by systematic intervention development and accompanied by rigorous process evaluation (which is the topic of Chapter 22). The quality and relevance of clinical trials are less than what may be achievable (Ioannidis 2014). This likely also applies to trials in the field of quality improvement and knowledge implementation. For instance, a methodological assessment found that most trials of quality improvement in diabetes care have a high risk of bias (Ivers et al. 2013). Experimental evaluation is not always possible and affordable. A range of observational designs and methods for evaluation is available, which is the topic of Chapter 21.

References

Baldasarri, D. and Abascal, M. (2017). Field experiments across the social sciences. *Annu. Rev. Sociol.* 43: 41–73.

Barker, D., McElduff, P., D'Este, C., and Campbell, M.J. (2016). Stepped wedge cluster randomized trials: a review of the statistical methodology used and available. *BMC Med. Res. Methodol.* 16: 69.

Bland, J.M. and Altman, D.G. (2015). Best (but often forgotten) practices: testing for treatment effects in randomized trials by separate analyses of changes from baseline in each group is a misleading approach. *Am. J. Clin. Nutr.* 102: 991–994.

Cals, J.W., Butler, C.C., Hopstaken, R.M. et al. (2009). Effect of point of care testing for C reactive protein and training in communication skills on antibiotic use in lower respiratory tract infections: cluster randomised trial. *BMJ* 338: b1374.

Chaillet, N., Dumont, A., Abrahamovic, M. et al. (2015). A cluster-randomized trial to reduce cesarean delivery rates in Quebec. *N. Engl. J. Med.* 372: 1710–1721.

Chen, Y.F., Hemming, K., Stevens, A.J., and Lilford, R.J. (2016). Secular trends and evaluation of complex interventions: the rising tide phenomenon. *BMJ Qual. Saf.* 25: 303–310.

Copas, A.J., Lewis, J.J., Thompson, J.A. et al. (2015). Designing a stepped-wedge trial: three main designs, carry-over effects and randomisation approaches. *Trials* 16: 252.

Craig, P., Dieppe, P., Mcintyre, S. et al. (2008). *Developing and Evaluating Complex Interventions. New Guidance.* London: Medical Research Council.

Curran, G.M., Bauer, M., Mittman, B. et al. (2012). Effectiveness–implementation hybrid designs. Combining elements of clinical effectiveness and implementation research to enhance public health impact. *Med. Care* 50: 217–2226.

Dal-Re, R., Janiaud, P., and Ioannidis, J.P.A. (2018). Real-world evidence: how pragmatic are randomized controlled trials labelled as pragmatic? *BMC Med.* 16: 49.

DeAngelis, C.D., Drazen, J.M., Frizelle, F.A. et al. (2004). Clinical trial registration: a statement from the International Committee of Medical Journal Editors. *JAMA* 292 (11): 1363–1364.

Donner, A. and Klar, N. (2000). *Design and Analysis of Cluster Randomization Trials in Health Research.* London: Arnold.

Dreischulte, T., Donnan, P., Grant, A. et al. (2016). Safer prescribing – a trial of education, informatics, and financial incentives. *N. Engl. J. Med.* 374: 1053–1064.

Eccles, M., Grimshaw, J., Campbell, M., and Ramsay, C. (2003). Research designs for studies evaluating the effectiveness of change and improvement strategies. *Qual. Saf. Health Care* 12: 47–52.

Eccles, M., McColl, E., Steen, N. et al. (2002). Effect of computerised evidence based guidelines on management of asthma and angina in adults in primary care: cluster randomised controlled trial. *BMJ* 325: 941.

Egbewale, B.E., Lewis, M., and Sim, J. (2014). Bias, precision and statistical power of analysis of covariance in the analysis of randomized trials with baseline imbalance: a simulation study. *BMC Med. Res. Methodol.* 14: 49.

Eldridge, S. and Kerry, S. (eds.) (2012). *A Practical Guide to Cluster Randomized Trials in Health Services Research.* Hoboken, NJ: Wiley.

Friedman, L., Furberg, C., DeMets, D. et al. (2015). *Fundamentals of Clinical Trials*, 5e. Heidelberg: Springer.

Gamble, C., Krishan, A., Stocken, D. et al. (2017). Guidelines for the content of statistical analysis plans in clinical trials. *JAMA* 318: 2337–2343.

Glasgow, R.E., Vogt, T.M., and Boles, S.M. (1999). Evaluating the public health impact of health promotion interventions: the RE-AIM Framework. *Am. J. Public Health* 89: 1322–1327.

Goldstein, C.E., Weijer, C., Brehaut, J.C. et al. (2018). Accomodating quality and service improvement research within existing ethical principles. *BMC Med Ethics* 19: 334.

Ioannidis, J.P.A. (2014). Clinical trials: what a waste. Trials that are unregistered, unfinished, unpublished, unreachable, or simply irrelevant. *BMJ* 349: g7089.

Ivers, N.M., Grimshaw, J.M., Jamvedt, G. et al. (2014). Growing literature, stagnant science? Systematic review, meta-regression and cumulative meta-analysis of audit and feedback interventions in health care. *J. Gen. Intern. Med.* 29: 1534–1541.

Ivers, N.M., Tricco, A.C., Taljaard, M. et al. (2013). Quality improvement needed in quality improvement randomized trials: systematic review of interventions to improve care in diabetes. *BMJ Open* 3: e002727.

Lewis, C.C., Fischer, S., Weiner, B.J. et al. (2015). Outcomes for implementation science: an enhanced systematic review of instruments using evidence-based rating criteria. *Implement. Sci* 10: 155.

Loudon, K., Treweek, S., Sullivan, F. et al. (2015). The PRECIS-2 tool: designing trials that are fit for purpose. *BMJ* 350: h2147.

McCord, K.A., Salman, R.A., Treweek, S. et al. (2018). Routinely collected data for randomized trials: promises, barriers, and implications. *Trials* 19: 29.

Nouwens, E., Van Lieshout, J., Bouma, M. et al. (2014). Effectiveness of improvement plans in primary care practice accreditation: a clustered randomized trial. *PLoS One* 9: e114045.

Proctor, E.K., Landsverk, J., Aarons, G. et al. (2009). Implementation research in mental health services: an emerging science with conceptual, methodological, and training challenges. *Admin. Policy Mental Health Serv. Res.* 36: 24–34.

Schünemann, H., Brozek, J., Guyatt, G., and Oxman, A. (eds.) (2013). *Handbook for Grading the Quality of Evidence and the Strength of Recommendations Using the GRADE Approach.* Version of October 2013. GRADE Working Group. http://gdt.guidelinedevelopment.org/central_prod/_design/client/handbook/handbook.html.

Schwartz, D. and Lellouch, J. (2009). Explanatory and pragmatic attitudes in therapeutical trials. *J. Clin. Epidemiol.* 62: 499–505.

Steen, I.N., Campbell, M.K., Eccles, M.P. et al. (2014). The use of Latin squares and related block designs in implementation research. *J. Clin. Epidemiol.* 67: 1299–1301.

Torgerson, D.J. (2001). Contamination in trials: is cluster randomization the answer? *Br. Med. J.* 322: 355–357.

Treweek, S., Lockhart, P., Pithethly, M. et al. (2013). Methods to improve recruitment to randomized controlled trials: Cochrane systematic review and meta-analysis. *BMJ Open* 3: e002360.

Van der Biezen, M., Adang, E., Van de Burgt, R. et al. (2016). The impact of substituting general practitioners with nurse practitioners on resource use, production and healthcare costs during out-of-hours: a quasi-experimental study. *BMC Health Serv. Res.* 17: 132.

Weijer, C., Grimshaw, J.M., Eccles, M.P. et al. (2012). The Ottawa statement on the ethical design and conduct of cluster randomized trials. *PLoS Med.* 9: e1001346.

21

Observational Evaluation of Implementation Strategies

Michel Wensing[1,2,3] *and Jeremy Grimshaw*[4,5]

[1] *Faculty of Medicine, University of Heidelberg, Heidelberg, Germany*
[2] *Department of General Practice and Health Services Research, Heidelberg University Hospital, Heidelberg, Germany*
[3] *Department IQ healthcare, Radboud Institute for Health Sciences, Radboud University Medical Center, Nijmegen, The Netherlands*
[4] *Clinical Epidemiology Program, Ottawa Hospital Research Institute, Ottawa, Ontario, Canada*
[5] *Department of Medicine, University of Ottawa, Ottawa, Ontario, Canada*

SUMMARY

- Randomized trials have, in principle, the lowest risk of bias in estimating the effectiveness of interventions, including implementation strategies. However, they are not always feasible and affordable. Also, the generalizability of their results to routine practice is a topic of debate.

- Observational designs provide an alternative approach to the evaluation of the effectiveness of implementation strategies. These designs include cross-sectional or post-intervention study, before–after study, and controlled before–after study. The integration of repeated measurements can reduce the risk of bias in these designs.

- Multiple case studies and developmental research (e.g. using "embedded researchers") are alternative designs which can provide tentative insights into the effects of implementation strategies.

- Data analysis in observational evaluations often requires the use of advanced statistical methods. Systematic consideration of relevant theory, previous research, and common sense can further enhance the plausibility of observed effects.

21.1 Introduction

In Chapter 20 we argued that a well-performed randomized trial is the best study design for providing estimates of intervention effectiveness with a low risk of bias. Randomized trials are crucial for major decisions which have important consequences for outcomes, risks, and costs of healthcare. They can also provide an important contribution to the scientific body of knowledge, if they address scientifically relevant questions. However, randomized trials can be expensive and time consuming, and the procedures involved in trials can influence the natural course of events (Black 1996). Furthermore, randomized trials are not the most efficient design for all research questions on interventions (Claxton et al. 2001). For instance, before an intervention is put up to evaluation in a randomized trial, it is often efficient to test it in an observational design. Also, observational designs may be applied to evaluate interventions that are targeted at all healthcare providers in a setting and a control group cannot be established.

Improving Patient Care: The Implementation of Change in Health Care, Third Edition. Edited by Michel Wensing, Richard Grol, and Jeremy Grimshaw.
© 2020 John Wiley & Sons Ltd. Published 2020 by John Wiley & Sons Ltd.

Compared to experimental designs, observational evaluation designs are characterized by a lower degree of control by the research team, and in particular by the absence of random allocation of participants to intervention and control arms. Observational evaluation designs have been widely used in health research for many decades (Bärnighausen et al. 2017; Craig et al. 2017; Handley et al. 2018; Hendricks Brown et al. 2017). Risk of bias in the causal attribution of outcomes to interventions is generally higher in observational designs than in a well-conducted randomized trial (Deeks et al. 2003; Portela et al. 2015). Nevertheless, a comparative observational evaluation can be convincing, particularly if estimates of effectiveness are appropriately adjusted for confounders, if it shows substantial effect size, and if it presents evidence of a dose–response relationship (Schünemann et al. 2013). Compared to randomized trials, observational designs tend to interfere less with the natural course of activities, which enhances both their generalizability to routine practice and the feasibility of the study. Box 21.1 (Horwitz et al. 2007) provides an example of an observational evaluation.

This chapter describes a number of designs and methods for observational evaluation of the effectiveness of implementation and improvement strategies. After a brief elaboration of concepts, we will discuss a number of "epidemiological" designs followed by two alternative observational designs, which are close to process evaluation (the topic of Chapter 22). Finally, we discuss some key aspects of data analysis in observational designs.

21.2 Designs for Observational Evaluations

There is a range of non-randomized evaluation designs, some of which are close to randomized trials and others quite different. Confusingly, varying terms are used to describe observational evaluations, which is the consequence of different methodological traditions in applied health research (Box 21.2). Most observational evaluations of intervention effects examine naturally occurring variations between or within study participants (such as healthcare providers), with the aim of assessing outcomes of an intervention.

Box 21.1 Regulation of Working Times of Medical Residents

It is difficult to set up a randomized trial to study the effects of regulating working times for medical residents on medical errors. Therefore, an observational study with before–after comparison was conducted in an academic hospital in the USA comparing baseline error rates before regulations were implemented with a follow-up period after implementation (Horwitz et al. 2007). Hospital administrators adapted the working schedules as a response to the regulations, so that medical residents worked fewer hours per week. On the basis of experience elsewhere, fewer errors due to fatigue but more errors due to patient transfer were expected. Multivariate regression modeling was used, taking relevant patient characteristics into account and trends in departments that did not have medical residents. After testing several options, an appropriate distribution and link function for each outcome measure was chosen (e.g. a Poisson distribution). Bootstrapping was applied to determine confidence intervals. The study found improvement in three outcome measures: reduction in use of intensive care, increased discharge of patients to home or revalidation centers, and reduced use of interventions by pharmacists to avoid medication errors. No differences were found in other measures such as admission time, readmissions to hospital within 30 days, medication interactions, or mortality in hospital.

Box 21.2   Terminology for Observational Designs

- *Epidemiology*: observational designs include controlled before-and-after study, concurrent cohort study, historical cohort study, case–control study, before-and-after study, cross-sectional study, and analysis of case series (Deeks et al. 2003).
- *Public health*: quasi-experimental studies include the difference-in-difference design, instrumental variables design, and regression discontinuity design (Bärnighausen et al. 2017)
- *Psychology*: non-equivalent group designs include untreated control group, with pre-test and post-test; non-equivalent depend-

ent variables; removal of treatment, with pre-test and post-test; repeated treatment; reversed treatment; non-equivalent control group with pre-test and post-test; cohort in institutions with cyclic turnover; post-test-only design with predicted higher-order interactions; and regression-discontinuity design (Cook and Campbell 1979).
- *Quality improvement*: observational designs include audit and monitoring studies, developmental studies, descriptive case studies, comparative studies, impact evaluations, and community intervention studies (Harvey and Wensing 2003).

The researcher has or takes little control over this variation (Deeks et al. 2003). In observational designs with two or more study arms, a crucial aspect is how subjects are allocated to study groups, because this influences the risk of bias in the attribution of outcomes to interventions (Deeks et al. 2003). Besides random allocation there is a range of options, varying from actively choosing a non-exposed group for comparison (e.g. healthcare providers in a different region) to using non-participants from the same setting as a reference group (e.g. in programs with voluntary enrollment).

21.3   Cross-Sectional Studies

In this observational design, measurements are conducted at one point in time. In the context of outcome evaluation, the measurement is done after intervention has been introduced, and often after intervention completion. "Post-design" is therefore an alternative name for this observational evaluation design. It can show to what extent the desired performance or outcome is present, or to what extent goals have been achieved in the perception of participants ("goal attainment"). As a baseline

measurement is not available in this design, it is also uncertain whether there has in fact been a change due to the intervention in professional performance or healthcare processes. Nevertheless, cross-sectional studies can provide quick and helpful information to clinicians, managers, and other decision makers. The design is widely used in quality improvement projects in local settings. The analysis is often straightforward and descriptive, but more advanced statistical methods can be applied to enhance the interpretation of data. Box 21.3 provides an example.

21.4   Before–After Comparisons

Before–after comparisons are observational studies in a study population or cohort (e.g. healthcare providers) in which outcomes are measured before and after an intervention (e.g. a quality improvement program) is introduced into a setting. They are among the most applied evaluation designs. In quality improvement and knowledge implementation, the follow-up measurement is often several months

---

Box 21.3 Evaluation of Bundles of Care to Reduce Mortality in Hospitals

Care bundles are concise clinical guidelines, which recommend interventions of proven effectiveness. In a London hospital clinicians were trained to use care bundles with the aim of reducing mortality in hospital. Eight care bundles were selected, which addressed catheters and line sepsis, diarrhea, stroke, ventilator-related pneumonia, resistant staphylococcal infections, heart failure, infections after surgery, and chronic obstructive pulmonary disease. An inventory study in 2008 was performed to examine whether the recommended procedures were implemented and which outcomes were achieved (Robb et al. 2010). Given the largely cross-sectional design, the effect needs to be interpreted carefully: it remained uncertain whether the care bundles had caused reduced hospital mortality or whether other factors contributed to the success.

---

after the baseline measurement. The design potentially allows the detection of change (e.g. in care providers' behavior) within the examined groups following the introduction of an intervention. The number of participants may be small (e.g. in pilots of interventions), but may also be substantial or very high (e.g. in nationwide evaluations). The generalizability of the study is influenced by the methods used for sampling of participants into the study, and thus varies substantially. For instance, a study in one hospital department is often not generalizable, but a study in a random sample of all providers in a geographical area may have good representativeness. The key threats to validity in simple before-and-after comparisons are secular changes (underlying trends in performance, or "maturation") or concurrent initiatives occurring around the same time as an intervention is introduced ("history").

Before–after comparisons can be strengthened by including multiple measurements before and after the intervention and applying advanced methods for quantitative analysis. In this design, the pre-intervention measurements are used to determine the usual variation and trend, which may be, for instance, gradual improvement of professional performance over time. The assumption is that the observed variation and trend reflect the natural course of

professional behaviors and healthcare processes. This information can be used as a reference for further analyses. In statistical process control, the measurements are analyzed with respect to the boundaries of "usual variation" (Benneyan et al. 2003). Statistical control designs protect against misinterpretation of fluctuations over time, which are in fact due to secular trends, natural random fluctuation, and measurement error. In an interrupted time-series approach, segmented regression analysis is done to determine if there is a step change or change in trend of performance after the introduction of the intervention. Interrupted time series protect against secular trends, but not against concurrent initiatives occurring around the same time as an intervention is introduced. While these methods of analysis are complex, the interpretation of findings is straightforward and intuitively understandable. Box 21.4 provides an example of statistical process control and Box 21.5 an example of interrupted time-series analysis.

Figure 21.1 presents a hypothetical interrupted times-series study in one cohort, in which an intervention started in month 12. The difference between observed scores after month 12 is compared with the projected trend, using the observed trend before month 12. In this hypothetical example, both an absolute difference and a gradual change can be observed.

Box 21.4   Statistical Monitoring of Adverse Events

Cumulative monitoring of adverse events can be used to examine trends in quality and outcomes of healthcare services, but the challenge is to distinguish "real" trends from random variation. For this purpose several statistical methods can be used (Spiegelhalter et al. 2003). A retrospective study tested one method, the classic sequential probability ratio test, which was developed in World War II. Different datasets were analyzed, including the annual mortality rates for open heart surgery on children under one year of age from the Bristol Royal Infirmary Inquiry (1985–1995) and the mortality rates for male and female patients aged 65 years or over on the practice list of Dr. Harold Shipman (1977–1998). Comparative data referring to similar sites were sought for statistical testing. The analysis of the Bristol case suggested that mortality has been higher than comparative data since 1991 ($p < 0.001$) or 1994 ($p < 0.001$), depending on the comparative data used. The analysis of the Shipman case suggested that mortality in women has been higher than national data since 1997 ($p < 0.000001$); the low p-value is chosen because the national data are based on 27 000 doctors. In both cases, statistical analysis of cumulative data on mortality could have detected the divergent performance earlier than it actually happened.

Box 21.5   Evaluation of a Performance Dashboard in Maternal Newborn Care

An online registry for data on quality and outcomes of maternal newborn care was launched in 2012 in Ontario, Canada. The registry was used to provide feedback on performance to providers, targeting specific performance indicators. As all hospitals participated, a control group in the same province could not be established. The effects were assessed in a before–after study which used monthly figures over a period of about five years (Weiss et al. 2018). Data were analyzed for six selected indicators, using a linear segmented regression model. Two and a half years after introduction, the feedback program showed improvements on five of six indicators. For instance, cesarean section in low-risk women before 39 weeks decreased to 10.4 per 100 women (95% confidence interval [CI] 9.3–11.5). Six non-targeted indicators and outcomes were not changed. The authors concluded that the audit and feedback program was associated with improvements in the majority of targeted indicators.

21.5 Controlled Before–After Comparisons

A different method for strengthening before–after comparisons is to add one or more control study populations or cohorts, which allows comparison between study arms as in randomized trials. While allocation of participants to study arms is non-random by definition in this observational design, there is a spectrum of alternative methods for allocation. The key challenge in designing controlled before–after designs is to minimize selection bias by identifying a control group that is highly similar to the intervention group at baseline. Convincing control groups can occasionally be found. This may be the case, for instance, if groups of rotating medical residents are compared, as it seems plausible that group composition is largely based on chance. In many other situations,

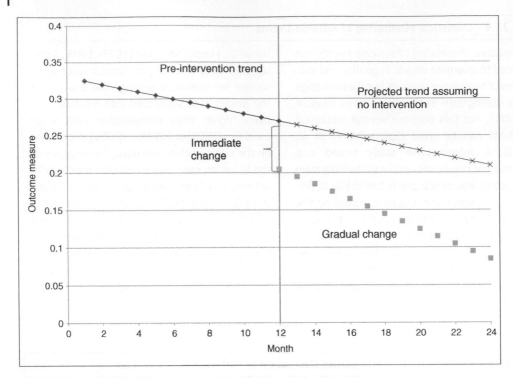

Figure 21.1 Hypothetical example of an interrupted time-series study.

Box 21.6   Evaluation of a Program to Strengthen Primary Care

In 2008 a program for strengthening primary care was introduced in Baden-Wuerttemberg, a German state with about 10 million inhabitants. Physicians and patients were offered the possibility to voluntarily join a program, involving case management of patients with chronic diseases in disease management programs, coordination of access to medical specialists, and physician participation in quality improvement activities. The evaluation design comprised cross-sectional and longitudinal comparisons between cohorts of enrolled patients and cohorts of other patients in the same region, adjusted for (many) patient and physician characteristics (Wensing et al. 2017). Compared to the control patients, enrolled patients had more visits in primary care, fewer non-coordinated contacts with medical specialists, lowered costs of pharmaceutical treatment, and fewer hospital admissions. In addition, patients' five-year survival was slightly higher in the enrolled patients. Despite the large numbers (1.7 million patients in the year 2016) and the advanced statistical analysis, bias in effect estimations cannot be ruled out, given the observational evaluation design.

---

finding an appropriate comparison group may be difficult. For instance, a comparison group may be composed of individuals who did not volunteer to join an intervention. This may be feasible, if data from non-participants are easily available (Box 21.6 provides an example). This design is relatively weak, because the motivation to participate in an intervention is likely to be a confounder of effectiveness estimations. The latter design can also be described as a "comparative cohort study," because the phrase "controlled" suggests more control of confounders than is actually achieved.

21.6 Multiple Case Studies

So far, we focused on "epidemiological" observational study designs, which are (under different names) used across a range of scientific disciplines that conduct quantitative studies in populations (e.g. in the behavioral and social sciences). Case studies come from a different scientific tradition, which may be described as constructivist social science. They are somewhat similar to case series in the clinical sciences: elaborated descriptions and thorough analyses of a small number of patients with specific features. In the context of the implementation of changes in patient care, a case may be, for instance, a hospital department, ambulatory practice, or participants in a quality improvement program. Box 21.7 provides an example. In many case studies, the focus is on how individuals and their interactions influence behaviors and institutions; this reflects the constructivist stance.

From a methodological perspective, case studies are characterized by a large number of measures compared with the number of cases, which tends to be low (often fewer than 10). Ideally cases are selected to reflect sufficient variation concerning relevant factors (purposeful sampling), for instance both high and low performers. Case studies are not defined by any specific method of data collection. A range of sources of data may be used, which are analyzed quantitatively (e.g. questionnaires or routinely collected clinical data) or qualitatively (e.g. interviews or direct observation). Triangulation of data from different sources is recommended to strengthen the validity of the findings. Case studies have low generalizability of their results from a statistical perspective (Deeks et al. 2003), but a purposeful sample of cases can nevertheless show the range of possible outcomes of an

---

Box 21.7   Comparative Case Study of a Quality Improvement Program in Hospitals

A large program to improve various organizational and clinical procedures in 24 hospitals in the Netherlands was carried out in the years 2004–2008 (Vos et al. 2010). It was mainly aimed at improving patient safety and the efficiency of work processes. A subprogram aimed to reduce time between first visit to an outpatient department and start of treatment or hospital admission by at least 30% in targeted patients. The core of the improvement method was repeated use of Plan–Do–Study–Act (PDSA) quality circles. An external advisor was involved to enhance a focus on delivery processes. Seventeen improvement teams in eight hospitals participated in the evaluation, which used mixed methods. Participants (n = 17) and project leaders (n = 17) were interviewed and surveyed on factors associated with the improvement process, partly on the basis of validated measures. The external advisor was observed. Performance data collected by the participants were copied. These different data sources were combined in the analysis for each improvement project. Most of these projects were related to elective procedures, but two projects concerned acute care. Eleven projects found improvement in logistics, but in six other projects no such improvements were found. The PDSA quality circle was well applied in five projects, but not in the other twelve projects. The interviews showed that this quality circle was perceived as time consuming and that assessing goal attainment was viewed as non-relevant when preconditions for improvement were not met. The improvement teams had the feeling that the necessary conditions of meaningful use for the method were not met.

intervention and suggest patterns in exposure to interventions and outcomes.

The results of a single case study are tentative by definition and perhaps most convincing as process evaluation. However, multiple or comparative case studies can explore whether interventions, or other factors in cases, are associated with outcomes by systematic comparison between cases (Yin 1989). This approach is similar to "realist evaluation" (Pawson and Tilley 1997), which aims to identify patterns or stable combinations of contextual factors, intervention components, and types of outcomes. While the number of cases is usually too low for statistical testing, the use of a priori defined hypotheses provides some protection against spurious effects.

21.7 Developmental Research

An observational evaluation may aim to support an implementation or improvement program while it is running, which may lead to adaptations of the program before the research is completed (see Box 21.8). Developmental research (also called participatory or action research) is research that involves study participants actively participating in the study, not only to evaluate the changes but also to (co-)create and optimize the improvement program (Waterman et al. 2001). The design matches well with the idea that stakeholders (e.g. patients, providers, payers) should be involved in the design and conduct of interventions to improve healthcare practice. Another related concept is "integrated knowledge translation," which refers to collaboration between researchers and decision makers during the research. It uses a range of methods, such as interviews and advisory boards, which have yet to prove their added value (Gagliardi et al. 2016). Embedding researchers in teams of practitioners in routine practice may be another type of developmental evaluation research (Marshall et al. 2014), although embedded research is not necessarily restricted to action research models.

All these approaches differ from "traditional" evaluation designs (whether experimental or observational), which typically restrict actions by researchers during program delivery. Developmental research may be one component of a flexible intervention program, in which activities are planned and adapted on the basis of developing insight into goal attainment and barriers for change (Harvey and

---

Box 21.8 Step-wise Approach to Reduce Catheter-Related Infections

Catheter-related bloodstream infections are among the most prevalent hospital-related infections in children in intensive care units. An improvement project aimed to reduce the number of catheter-related infections by 25% in 24 months (Bhutta et al. 2007). A step-wise approach was followed, with continuous monitoring and quarterly reports to the medical and nursing staff. Activities included preventive interventions relating to intubation of catheters (November 1998), impregnation of catheters with antibiotics (July 1999), yearly campaigns to promote hand washing (March 2000), creating a separate room for catheter procedures instead of open wards for patients (April 2003), and use of chlorhexidine as the recommended disinfecting agent (May 2003). All physicians and nurses were obliged to participate in educational sessions on the prevention of infections. The number of catheters used increased from 242 in 1998 to 481 in 2005. The number of hospital admissions and hospital days also increased in this period. The number of blood infections with a central venous catheter decreased from 9 to 3 per 1000 days. This study showed that a long-term effort by a multidisciplinary team, which collects data for monitoring, can result in substantial improvement.

Wensing 2003). It has also been debated whether developmental research can provide valid assessment of intervention effectiveness, although some authors believe that it can (Burke and Shojania 2018). We would suggest that the type of evidence from developmental studies is tentative and practical (Harvey and Wensing 2003).

21.8 Data Analysis in Observational Evaluation Designs

Many principles and methods for data analysis in experimental studies (see Chapter 20) also apply to the data analysis in observational evaluation of interventions. This applies to quantitative population science designs in particular. From an "epidemiological" perspective, important biases for internal validity include (Handley et al. 2018):

- *History bias*: development, policies, or events outside the interventions influence outcomes in ways that differ between study arms.
- *Maturation bias*: individuals with study arms develop independently of the interventions in ways that differ between study arms.
- *Selection bias*: individuals in different study arms differ in ways that relate to outcomes (this would be addressed by random allocation in experimental designs).
- *Lack of blinding* (this also applies to most experimental studies of implementation and improvement): individuals are aware of interventions in ways that relate to outcomes, a mechanism that has been described as the Hawthorne effect or nocebo effect.
- *Drop-out*: individuals drop out of the study, or do not contribute to outcome measurements, in ways that differ between study arms.
- *Variable exposure to interventions*: individuals are variably exposed to interventions in ways that influence outcomes.

Given the higher risk of bias in attribution of outcomes to interventions, it is essential to take a careful approach to data analysis in observational designs. Ideally, potential interpretations of findings are systematically identified and considered in relation to the data. While data analysis in a two-arm, randomized trial is relatively straightforward, the analysis and interpretation can be rather complex in observational designs. Craig et al. (2017) distinguish a number of approaches to data analysis in what they call "natural experiments," which they describe as study designs in which the allocation or the assignment of participants to interventions is not under the control of the research team. These approaches are:

- *Pre–post*: outcomes of interest are compared in a population pre- and post-exposure to an intervention.
- *Regression adjustment*: outcomes are compared in exposed and unexposed units, and a statistical model fitted to take account of differences between groups in characteristics thought to be associated with variation in outcomes.
- *Propensity scores*: likelihood of exposure to the intervention calculated from a regression model and either used to match exposed and unexposed units or fitted in a model to predict the outcome of interest.
- *Difference-in-differences*: likelihood of exposure to the intervention calculated from a regression model and either used to match exposed and unexposed units or fitted in a model to predict the outcome of interest.
- *Interrupted time series*: trend in the outcome of interest compared pre- and post-intervention, using a model that accounts for serial correlation in the data and can identify changes associated with introduction of the intervention. Change also compared in exposed and unexposed populations in controlled time-series analyses.
- *Synthetic controls*: trend in the outcome of interest compared in an intervention area and a synthetic control area, representing a weighted composite of real areas that mimics the pre-intervention trend.

- *Regression discontinuity:* outcomes compared in units defined by scores just above and below a cut-off in a continuous forcing variable that determines exposure to an intervention.
- *Instrumental variables:* a variable associated with exposure to the intervention, but not with other factors associated with the outcome of interest, is used to model the effect of the intervention.

Besides the use of advanced quantitative methods of data analysis, it is important to consider the plausibility of observed effects in observational designs. As the allocation of interventions is not under the control of the research team, it is crucial to document exposure to interventions among the targeted individuals and use this information in the analysis of intervention effects. Also, available theory, previous research, and common sense can help to assess the plausibility of observed effects. For these reasons, process evaluation is essential to strengthen the conclusions on intervention effects (Chapter 22 elaborates on this).

21.9 Conclusions

This chapter describes a number of observational designs. Observational studies have higher risk for biased effect estimations than trials, but may have the advantage that they are less disruptive to the natural flow of activities. We recommend using a comparative design when possible, using measurements before the intervention starts and a control arm without the intervention of interest. If the aim of the evaluation is to assess whether goals have been reached, it may be sufficient to use a before–after comparison or a cross-sectional study. In our experience, appropriate data analysis in observational designs is often complex and this complexity is frequently underestimated. Not only may advanced quantitative data analysis be required, a convincing interpretation of data from observational designs also depends on deep knowledge of relevant theory, previous research, and routine practice. We recommend using prevailing methodological recommendations and reporting guidelines for all types of observational studies.

References

Bärnighausen, T., Rottingen, J.A., Rockers, P. et al. (2017). Quasi-experimental study designs: 1. Introduction: two historical lineages. *J. Clin. Epidemiol.* 89: 4–11.

Benneyan, J.C., Lloyd, R.C., and Plesk, P.E. (2003). Statistical process control as a tool for research and health care improvement. In: *Quality Improvement Research. Understanding the Science of Change in Health Care* (eds. R. Grol, R. Baker and F. Moss). London: BMJ Books.

Bhutta, A., Gilliam, C., Honeycutt, M. et al. (2007). Reduction of bloodstream infections associated with catheters in paediatric intensive care unit: stepwise approach. *BMJ* 334: 362–365.

Black, N. (1996). Why we need observational studies to evaluate the effectiveness of health care. *BMJ* 312: 1215–1218.

Burke, R.E. and Shojania, K.G. (2018). Rigorous evaluations of evolving interventions: can we have our cake and eat it too? *BMC Qual. Saf.* 27: 251–254.

Claxton, K., Neuman, P.J., Araki, S.S., and Weinstein, M.C. (2001). The value of information: an application to a policy model of Alzheimer's disease. *Int. J. Technol. Assess. Health Care* 17: 38–55.

Cook, T.D. and Campbell, D.T. (1979). *Quasi-Experimentation: Design and Analysis Issues for Field Settings*. Chicago, IL: Rand McNally.

Craig, P., Kattikiredi, S.V., Leyland, A., and Popham, F. (2017). Natural experiments: an overview of methods, approaches, and contributions to public health intervention research. *Annu. Rev. Public Health* 38: 20.1–20.13.

Deeks, J.J., Dinnes, J., D'Amico, R. et al. (2003). Evaluating non-randomised intervention studies. *Health Technol. Assess.* 7 (iii–x): 1–173.

Gagliardi, A.R., Berta, W., Kothari, A. et al. (2016). Integrated knowledge translation (IKT) in health care: a scoping review. *Implement. Sci.* 11: 38.

Handley, M.A., Lyles, C.R., McCulloch, C., and Cattamanchi, A. (2018). Selecting and improving quasi-experimental designs in effectiveness and implementation research. *Ann. Rev. Public Health* 39: 5–25.

Harvey, G. and Wensing, M. (2003). Methods for evaluation of small-scale improvement projects. *Qual. Saf. Health Care* 12: 210–214.

Hendricks Brown, C., Curran, G., Palinkas, L.A. et al. (2017). An overview of research and evaluation designs for dissemination and implementation. *Annu. Rev. Public Health* 38: 1–22.

Horwitz, L.L., Kosiborod, M., Lin, Z., and Krumholz, H.M. (2007). Changes in outcomes for internal medicine inpatients after work-hour regulations. *Ann. Intern. Med.* 147: 97–103.

Marshall, M., Pagel, C., French, C. et al. (2014). Moving improvement research closer to practice: the researcher-in-residence model. *BMJ Qual. Saf.* 23: 801–804.

Pawson, R. and Tilley, N. (1997). *Realistic Evaluation*. London: Sage.

Portela, M.C., Pronovost, P.J., Woodstock, T. et al. (2015). How to study improvement interventions: a brief overview of possible study designs. *BMJ Qual. Saf.* 24: 325–336.

Robb, E., Jarman, J., Suntharalingam, G. et al. (2010). Using care bundles to reduce in-hospital mortality: quantitative survey. *BMJ* 340: 861–863.

Schünemann, H., Brozek, J., Guyatt, G., and Oxman, A. (eds.) (2013). *Handbook for Grading the Quality of Evidence and the Strength of Recommendations Using the GRADE Approach*. Version of October 2013. GRADE Working Group. http://gdt.guidelinedevelopment.org/central_prod/_design/client/handbook/handbook.html.

Spiegelhalter, D., Grigg, O., Kinsman, R., and Treasure, T. (2003). Risk-adjusted sequential probability ratio tests: applications to Bristol, Shipman and adult cardiac surgery. *Int. J. Qual. Health Care* 15: 7–13.

Vos, L., Dückers, M.L.A., Wagner, C., and van Merode, G.G. (2010). Applying the quality improvement collaborative method to process redesign: a multiple case study. *Implement. Sci.* 5: 19.

Waterman, H., Tillen, D., Dickson, R. et al. (2001). Action research: a systematic review and guidance for assessment. *Health Technol. Assess.* 5: 111–157.

Weiss, D., Dunn, S.I., Sprague, A.E. et al. (2018). Effect of a population-level performance dashboard intervention on maternal-newborn outcomes: an interrupted time series study. *BMJ Qual. Saf.* 27: 425–436.

Wensing, M., Szecsenyi, J., Stock, C. et al. (2017). Evaluation of a program to strengthen general practice care for patients with chronic disease in Germany. *BMC Health Serv. Res.* 17: 62.

Yin, R.K. (1989). *Case Study Research: Design and Methods*. London: Sage.

22

Process Evaluation of Implementation Strategies

Marlies Hulscher[1] and Michel Wensing[1,2,3]

[1] Department IQ healthcare, Radboud Institute for Health Sciences, Radboud University Medical Center, Nijmegen, The Netherlands
[2] Faculty of Medicine, University of Heidelberg, Heidelberg, Germany
[3] Department of General Practice and Health Services Research, Heidelberg University Hospital, Heidelberg, Germany

SUMMARY

- To understand why some implementation strategies and some participants successfully bring about improvement while others fail to change practice, it is necessary to look into the "black box" of strategies and into the context in which the strategies are applied.

- Important aims of process evaluation are to describe the implementation strategy as planned, the strategy as delivered, the actual exposure of the target population to the strategy, factors that influence the intervention outcomes, as well as the target populations' experiences and opinions about the strategy.

- Many process evaluations are based on surveys and interviews with participants and other stakeholders. In addition, other sources of data may be involved, such as direct observations and routinely collected data for administrative or clinical purposes.

- Process evaluation is crucial for the optimization of implementation strategies as well as the accumulation of scientific knowledge on the implementation of innovations in healthcare.

22.1   Introduction

A wide variety of implementation strategies can be used to improve healthcare and implement innovations in practice. Research has shown that most of these strategies are effective in some individuals and organizations, but not in others (see Chapters 11–18). The effectiveness of a given implementation strategy not only varies from study to study, but we usually see differences within studies as well – some recipients of the strategy are more successful in improving patient care than others. To understand in more detail why some strategies and some participants are successful while others fail to change practice, it is necessary to look inside the "black box" of interventions (as in Box 22.1) and the context in which they are applied. For instance, activities that are part of the implementation strategy, the actual delivery of these activities, the participants' exposure to or actual participation in these activities, their experience of these activities, and various factors in the participants' contexts may have influenced the final result (success or failure). A "process evaluation" can illuminate the factors and processes responsible for the outcomes and their variation within target groups. Process evaluation can relate to both the implementation strategies as well as to the interventions or practices which are implemented.

Box 22.1 Head-to-Head Comparison of Two Strategies to Improve Antibiotic Use for Complicated Urinary Tract Infections

Complicated urinary tract infections (UTIs) are among the most prevalent infectious diseases, substantially contributing to antibiotic use in the hospital setting. In a cluster-randomized trial (Spoorenberg et al. 2015) to improve antibiotic use in patients with a complicated UTI, 38 departments of internal medicine and urology were allocated to one of two implementation strategies: a multifaceted strategy and a competitive feedback strategy. Appropriate antibiotic use was measured using nine quality indicators at baseline and post-intervention. The multifaceted implementation strategy included feedback, educational sessions, reminders, and help with additional/optional improvement actions, and was based on a tailored strategy that previously effectively improved antibiotic use in patients with lower respiratory tract infections. Departments allocated to

the second strategy received a one-time feedback report providing professionals with comparative feedback on the appropriateness of the ward's antibiotic use, by non-anonymously ranking the various departments. These competitive feedback reports contained, for each quality indicator, a list of all 38 departments' performance scores, in which the names of the departments were blinded but the others were visible. Contrary to expectations, the multifaceted strategy was just as (limitedly) effective as the feedback strategy. Process evaluation data on participation of the target population in the planned activities showed that participation by both groups was generally low and varied strongly between the departments. Compliance with the strategies was, therefore, suboptimal, and better compliance was associated with more improvement.

Understanding mechanisms is important for optimization of interventions and accumulation of scientific knowledge, but process evaluation is not a substitute for evaluation of outcomes (Craig et al. 2008). If the effects of a strategy are not known, the practical and scientific value of a process evaluation is limited, because its findings cannot be contextualized. In pilot studies, it may only be possible to get a first impression of outcomes, and the emphasis may be largely on exploration of the feasibility, acceptability, and attractiveness of strategies.

This chapter starts with a definition of the concept of "process evaluation" and an overview of the type of questions in process evaluations. Subsequently, specific attention is paid to determining the fidelity of implementation strategies, which is the core component of process evaluation. Finally, a practical approach to the performance of a process evaluation is presented.

22.2 Frameworks for Process Evaluation

Many frameworks for process evaluation have been published (e.g. Dusenbury et al. 2003; Hulscher et al. 2003; Bellg et al. 2004; Carroll et al. 2007; Grant et al. 2013; Masterson-Algar et al. 2018; Moore et al. 2015; Pérez et al. 2016). They tend to converge into a similar set of questions and domains (Box 22.2). According to these frameworks, process evaluation aims to (meticulously) document the implementation strategy as developed and planned, the strategy as delivered, the actual exposure of participants to the implementation activities as part of the strategy, the experience of the people exposed (participants), and the contextual factors or circumstances that also might play a role. In this chapter, we first focus on a framework by Grant et al. (2013; Box 22.2). It distinguishes between clusters

Box 22.2 Key Questions and Framework for Process Evaluation

The key questions for process evaluation can be summarized as follows:

- To describe the strategy as planned, for example:
  - What is the exact nature of the implementation activities as part of the strategy?
  - What material investments, time investments, etc. are required?
  - What factors and circumstances does the strategy aim to influence?
- To check the actual performance of and exposure to the implementation strategy, for example:
  - Were all activities performed as planned?
  - To what degree did the target population actually participate in the planned activities?
  - Did end-users (patients, citizens) notice any changes?
- To describe the experiences of those exposed to the strategy, for example:
  - How did the target group experience the strategy and the activities that were part of it?
  - How did the target group experience the resulting change?
- To check whether changes occurred in factors and circumstances that influence study outcomes, for example:

  - Were there any changes in the factors and circumstances that the strategy aimed to influence?
  - Were there any changes in other factors and circumstances that might positively or negatively influence study outcomes?

Grant et al. (2013) developed a framework for process evaluations of cluster-randomized controlled trials. The framework emphasizes the importance of considering two levels of intervention delivery and response. The first level is the strategy that is delivered to clusters of professionals; the second level is the change in care which the cluster professionals deliver to individual patients. The framework distinguishes between clusters – where the cluster is the unit of randomization – and individuals on whom outcome data are collected. On both levels, process evaluation can focus on several key questions to describe processes that help explain variation in outcomes:

- Clusters that receive the intervention (areas, institutions, individual professionals):
  - How are clusters sampled and recruited? Who agrees to participate?
  - What intervention is actually delivered to each cluster? Is it the intended intervention?
  - How is the work of the intervention and trial implemented in and adopted by clusters?
- Individuals in the target population:

  - Who actually receives the work of the intervention in each setting? Are they representative?
  - What intervention is delivered in each cluster? Or what behavior change has occurred because of the intervention?
  - How does the target population respond?

Besides delivery and response, the framework also emphasizes the role of:

- Theory:
  - What theory has been used to develop the intervention?
  - Can a theory be considered to interpret the effects of the intervention?
- Context:

  - What is the wider context in which the trial is being conducted and it is affecting the processes being examined?

(e.g. healthcare providers) and target groups (e.g. patients) and emphasizes the role of context.

A process evaluation serves a number of different, related purposes. First, a process evaluation provides a detailed description of the "strategy as planned." Such a description acts as a blueprint to help change agents to apply the implementation strategy as intended in a uniform way within the target population. A clear description of the planned strategy also provides a point of reference for other components of process evaluation.

Second, a process evaluation provides a description of the "strategy as delivered" or the "strategy as received." A process evaluation provides information on the actually provided activities as part of the implementation strategy and/or on the exposure to and participation of the target population in these activities. A comparison of the actual activities with the planned activities reveals any gaps in the performance of the implementation strategy. Researchers or evaluators can use this information to detect gaps in exposure in a timely manner and revise the strategy during the course of the study. However, this makes it more difficult to interpret the findings of an outcomes evaluation. In many cases, it is recommended "to sit on your hands" and not interfere (substantially) with the implementation strategy after its launch. In such situations, researchers or evaluators can use the information afterward to explain success or lack of effect (see also Section 22.5).

Third, a process evaluation provides information on the experiences of the participants. This includes their view on the quality of delivery and on the unique and essential features of the strategy that determined success. This information can be used to improve the implementation strategy either during its application (the developmental approach) or afterward (the experimental approach).

Finally, this evaluation can provide insight into factors and processes that influence study outcomes and in which changes occurred.

Factors that mediate or moderate effects can be analyzed. On the one hand, this concerns changes in the factors and circumstances that the strategy aimed to influence, which makes it possible to check whether the assumed explanatory model behind the strategy and the impact of the context is correct. On the other hand, this concerns changes in other factors and circumstances that might have influenced the outcomes in a positive or negative way. For example, changes in the characteristics of the target group, the healthcare institution, or the health system can help explain the effects, or lack thereof.

Process evaluation not only provides information that aids in optimization of the implementation strategy and the interpretation of its outcomes. Information from a process evaluation also provides estimates of implementation costs in terms of time and money, contributing valuable data for an economic evaluation of the improvement strategy (see Chapter 23). Process evaluation also helps interpret the generalizability of findings to other contexts by describing the targeted group and context in detail. Finally, process evaluation supports the analysis and interpretations of implementation strategies in systematic literature reviews by facilitating comparisons between studies. Thus, process evaluation contributes in many important ways to the accumulation of scientific knowledge on how to improve healthcare.

22.3 Process Evaluation and Implementation Strategies

Process evaluation can be applied to implementation strategies at any stage of their development. We distinguish between strategies at three stages of development:

- Evaluation of pilot studies and small improvement projects.
- Evaluation of strategies in experimental designs.

Box 22.3   Improving CT Scan Use in Adults with Head Injuries

After researchers had succeeded in implementing a clinical decision rule that successfully reduced the number of cervical spine scans, they performed the same intervention – in the same emergency department – to reduce the number of computerized tomography (CT) scans in adults with head injuries (Curran et al. 2013). The strategy to implement these clinical decision rules consisted of achieving local consensus, an educational meeting (one hour), and a mandatory reminder at the point of requisition. The second study was not effective; the number of scans even increased. The reason behind the variation in effect across the two studies was unclear. To find out the underlying reasons for these results, the researchers used – as a proof-of-concept study – the theoretical domains framework (a framework in which 128 explanatory constructs from 33 behavioral theories are grouped in 12 theoretical domains to explain behavioral change; Michie et al. 2005) to design a retrospective theory-based process evaluation. They conducted a number of semi-structured telephone interviews using an interview guide that was based on the theoretical domains framework. The interviews showed that the explanations could be found within six of the explored domains. Examples of barriers that may have prevented physicians from consistently applying the rule – or not – included beliefs about the consequences of the use of the decision rule, their belief in their own capabilities, and the social influence of patients and family members.

- Evaluation of improvement programs in observational designs.

22.3.1   Evaluation of Pilots and Small Improvement Projects

An evaluation of the effects of a newly developed implementation strategy that is being tested in a pilot study, or used within a small-scale improvement project, gives an estimate of the potential degree of improvement in patient care. The process evaluation can provide answers to questions on the feasibility and acceptability of performing the implementation strategy: "Who actually participated in the implementation activities?" and "How did the target group experience the implementation strategy and the implementation activities that were part of it?" The answers to these kinds of questions might prompt revision of the implementation strategy. Thus, researchers and implementers of this type of implementation strategy can use process information to investigate whether they are on the right track

or whether their approach needs adjustment (see Box 22.3).

22.3.2   Evaluation of Strategies in Experimental Designs

In an experimental study of the effectiveness of a specific implementation strategy, the central issue is to test the effectiveness of the strategy under conditions that reduce the risk of bias in effect estimations (see Chapter 20). The process evaluation can provide answers to questions like "Were the planned improvement activities indeed delivered in a uniform way?" and "Has the target population actually been exposed to the implementation activities as planned?" In this case, process evaluation yields information that can help explain the heterogeneity in or absence of effects: researchers and implementers of these strategies can use process information to detect gaps in exposure to the implementation activities that might be responsible for failure or for disappointing outcomes of a strategy (Box 22.4 provides an example). This requires careful

---

Box 22.4   Examination of Variation between Practices in the Effectiveness of a Multicomponent Implementation Strategy to Reduce High-Risk Primary Care Prescribing

A large proportion of emergency hospital admissions are caused by high-risk prescribing of commonly prescribed drugs, with non-steroidal anti-inflammatory drugs and anti-platelets being among the main drugs implicated. As described in Box 20.6, a multi-faceted implementation strategy was evaluated in a pragmatic cluster-randomized controlled stepped-wedge trial in 33 Scottish general practices (Dreischulte et al. 2018). The strategy combined professional education (an educational outreach visit by a pharmacist, written educational material, and regular newsletters which also provided regular feedback on progress) with financial incentives and access to a web-based information technology (IT) tool. The strategy turned out to be effective: across all practices, the targeted high-risk prescribing fell from 3.7 to 2.2% (primary outcome). Reductions were sustained in the year after financial incentives stopped. In addition, there were reductions in emergency hospital admissions.

High-risk prescribing was reduced by 37%. Effectiveness ranged from a relative increase in high-risk prescribing of 24.1% to a relative reduction of 77.2%. A quantitative process evaluation was performed to understand what influenced review activity (extent and nature of documented reviews) and effectiveness at practice level (relative reductions in the primary end-point). The evaluation was based on the 2013 framework for process evaluations of cluster-randomized controlled trials of Grant et al. (2013). Associations were assessed between documented review activity and practice characteristics and "adoption" (self-reported implementation work done by practices), and between effectiveness and practice characteristics, adoption, and review activity. Not being an approved general practitioner training practice and higher adoption were significantly associated with higher review activity. Higher baseline high-risk prescribing and adoption (but not documented review activity) were significantly associated with greater effectiveness in the final multivariate model, explaining 64.0% of variation in effectiveness.

---

specification of mediating and moderating factors in a conceptual framework, followed by well-designed quantitative analyses of data. Advanced knowledge of methodology and statistical methods is required for such analyses. In addition, factors may be explored in a qualitative study.

and experience of the implementation activities. In a situation where a control group is lacking, the results of process evaluations can provide some information about the relationship between the strategy and the changes achieved. Boxes 22.5 and 22.6 provide examples.

22.3.3   Evaluation of Improvement Programs in Observational Designs

In large-scale programs for improving patient care, analyses of the effects show the extent to which the goals of the implementation strategy have been achieved, whereas process evaluation can provide information about the "strategy as delivered" and about exposure to

22.4   Assessing the Fidelity of Implementation Strategies

An implementation strategy can only have its theoretically optimal impact *if* its plan is consistent with the underlying theory (fidelity of design) and *if* it is performed as intended by its developers (fidelity of conduct, subsequently

Box 22.5   Improving Cervical Cancer Screening

In a national prevention program (Hermens et al. 2001), physicians and practice assistants were exposed, over a period of 2.5 years, to a comprehensive strategy aimed at introducing national guidelines for cervical cancer screening. The strategy comprised, on a national level, formulating and distributing guidelines, supplying educational materials and a software program, and providing financial support. On a regional level, agreements were made between the relevant parties (primary care, municipal health services, comprehensive cancer centers, and pathology laboratories), and continuing medical education (CME) meetings were organized for physicians and practice assistants. On a local level, trained outreach visitors called at practices and helped them to improve the organization of preventive services and to use the software. The evaluation (in a random, one in three sample of 988 practices) showed considerable improvements at the practice level: after the intervention, adherence to nine out of the ten key indicators had been improved (Hermens et al. 2001).

Information on actual exposure to program elements was collected by postal questionnaire after intervention. Almost all practices in the study population (94%) had been informed about the national prevention program. For practices that had had contact with an outreach visitor through a practice visit (40%), the median number of practice visits was two (range 1–13). The software program to select eligible women was used by 474 practices (48%), either in full or in part. CME meetings for physicians were used by 30% of the practices; 30% also participated in CME meetings for practice assistants. CME meetings for doctors were not related to change. Crucial elements for the successful implementation of the guidelines were:

- Making use of the software program (odds ratio [OR] 1.85–10.2 for nine indicators).
- Having received two or more outreach visits (OR 1.46–2.35 for six indicators).
- Practice assistants having attended the CME meeting (OR 1.37–1.90 for four indicators).

Box 22.6   Process Evaluation of a Routine Vaccination Program in General Practice

In England, general practitioners (GPs) perform the routine childhood and adult vaccination program based on government guidance. Data show that there have been multiyear decreases in coverage across many vaccines. The guidance leaves autonomy to practices as to how they organize the program. For one study (Crocker-Buque et al. 2018), nine geographically and demographically diverse general practices were recruited and demonstrated varying vaccination coverage. In total, 52 staff members participated in 26 interviews. These data were used to develop a care delivery value chain (CDVC): a visual representation of the main activities involved in providing routine vaccinations at general practices. Next, staff involved in *vaccination* were asked to provide information on vaccination appointments by using activity logs. Interview data were supplemented with the activity log

data on 372 vaccination appointments to confirm details from the interviews. The resulting CDVC described 14 core activities. Variation between practices in performance of the 14 core activities was demonstrated. The areas of greatest variation included the method of reminder and recall activities, the structure of vaccination appointments, and task allocation between staff groups. Mean appointment length varied considerably. Non-clinical administrative activities comprised about 60% total activity (range 48.4–67.0%). The authors concluded that the introduction of organized reminder and recall activities for adults could improve coverage. Appointment length and time spent on vaccination did not appear to be related to coverage; however, capacity in terms of availability of appointments per patient could be related and requires further investigation.

Box 22.7   Evaluating the Fidelity of the Implementation Strategy

To evaluate the fidelity of an implementation strategy, several concepts have proposed (Dusenbury et al. 2003; Carroll et al. 2007):

1) *Adherence to the blueprint*: the extent to which the specified implementation activities were delivered as planned by the strategy developers.
2) *Dose/exposure*: the "amount" of strategy received by the participants, or the extent to which the participants actually participated in – or were exposed to – the specified implementation activities as planned by the strategy developers (number, duration).

3) *Quality of delivery*: qualitative aspects of the manner in which the deliverer performed the specified implementation activities.
4) *Participant responsiveness or experiences*: participant response to the specified implementation activities, or participants' experiences with these activities.
5) *Differentiation*: identification of unique and essential features of different implementation activities, or identification of determinants of success.

---

described as strategy fidelity). Process evaluation can help determine whether a lack of impact derives from a poorly conceptualized strategy or from a failure to deliver it as planned. Particularly the latter – assessing the degree to which the "strategy as performed" is in line with the "strategy as planned" – is an important part of most process evaluations. In the literature, the degree to which strategies are performed as intended by the strategy developers is termed the *fidelity* or *integrity* of the implementation strategy (see Box 22.7). If the actually performed implementation strategy differs significantly from the original blueprint, then this can be described as an *implementation error* (Swanborn 1999). Failing to detect implementation error has been characterized in terms of type III error, by analogy with statistical type I and type II errors (Dusenbury et al. 2003; Carroll et al. 2007).

Strategy fidelity influences how far the strategy has the opportunity to change outcomes: high fidelity is assumed to result in more opportunity and poor fidelity in less. Fidelity constitutes a source of potential effect mediation – influencing the relationship between strategies and their intended effects – and should therefore always be measured and included in the

evaluation of an implementation strategy (Carroll et al. 2007). This is especially necessary in multisite studies, where the same strategy may be implemented and received in different ways. Fidelity is, however, not straightforward in relation to strategies that are designed to be adapted to local circumstances. Adaptations may enhance the effectiveness of strategies, but they may also reduce their effectiveness. One of the research questions for process evaluation may relate to this issue. In that case, process evaluation is important to record variations in strategy performance, so that fidelity can be assessed in relation to the degree of standardization required by the study protocol (Craig et al. 2008).

Bellg et al. proposed that researchers or evaluators develop plans – adapted to the needs of a specific study – for enhancing and monitoring fidelity at the outset of the study (see later Box 22.12). In addition, they should put consistent efforts into adhering to this fidelity plan throughout the study period to counter threats to the study's internal and external validity. Such a plan could, for example, comprise the following aspects:

- Dose (number, frequency, and length of contact) is adequately described and is the same for each subject within a particular treatment condition. There is a plan for setbacks (e.g. providers dropping out).

- Training is conducted similarly for different providers using well-defined performance criteria.
- Potential differences between providers are monitored and controlled for. Contamination across conditions is minimized.
- Participants understanding of the information provided in the intervention and their ability to use skills taught in the intervention are ensured.
- Participants' enactment of skills provided in the intervention in daily practice is ensured.

In this chapter, we focus largely on the fidelity of strategies for quality improvement and knowledge implementation, but equally relevant is the fidelity of the clinical or prevention interventions that are implemented. Both fidelity of the clinical or prevention intervention that is being implemented and fidelity of strategies to implement these interventions may impact outcomes. Clarification of this distinction is relevant in all evaluations which include both patient health and professional behaviors as outcomes, as they simultaneously evaluate the effects of an implementation strategy on professionals' behavior (e.g. the use of an evidence-based intervention) and of that intervention on change in patient behavior and health outcomes (Slaughter et al. 2015). The framework for process evaluations of cluster-randomized controlled trials developed by Grant et al. (2013) can be used to specify these two levels of fidelity. The first level addresses the implementation strategy that is delivered to clusters of professionals; the second level addresses the change in evidence-based care interventions which the cluster-level professionals deliver to individual patients. On both levels, process evaluation can focus on several key questions to describe processes that help explain variation in outcomes (see Box 22.3).

Most literature on process evaluation and intervention fidelity addresses clinical or prevention interventions rather than fidelity of implementation and improvement strategies. Such adaptations of clinical or prevention interventions are common. For example, Wiltsey Stirman et al. performed a review that explored whether evidence-based interventions are frequently modified or adapted in daily practice; the authors identified 258 modifications in 32 published articles (Wiltsey Stirman et al. 2013). The authors proposed a framework for systematic description of adaptations of interventions, which specifies the following dimensions: (i) when and how in the implementation process the modification was made; (ii) whether the modification was planned/proactive (i.e. an adaptation) or unplanned/reactive; (iii) who determined that the modification should be made; (iv) what is modified; (v) at what level of delivery the modification is made; (vi) type or nature of context- or content-level modifications; (vii) the extent to which the modification is fidelity consistent; and (viii) the reasons for the modification, including the intent or goal of the modification (e.g. to reduce costs) and contextual factors that influenced the decision (Wiltsey Stirman et al. 2019).

Focusing on the fidelity of implementation strategies, Slaughter et al. (2015) identified 25 systematic reviews that measured the fidelity of the implementation strategies. The review identified 72 research reports, but many studies lacked details and none of them included a conceptual framework or a fidelity definition. A review on hand hygiene implementation strategies confirmed this (Musuuza et al. 2016). For instance, only 8 out of 100 studies reported on five fidelity domains; reporting *adherence* and *dose/exposure* were uncommon.

Hulscher et al. (2003) developed a process evaluation framework that specifically aims to evaluate implementation strategies aimed at professionals (see Box 22.8). This framework can be used for evaluation of the fidelity of implementation strategies. The framework points to the importance of fidelity of the envisioned features of (i) the target group; (ii) the

---

Box 22.8   A Process Evaluation Framework to Evaluate Implementation Strategies Aimed at Professionals

Hulscher et al. (2003) developed a framework that contains features of implementation strategies that might influence their success or failure. The authors advise the users of the framework to measure – for each single implementation strategy (see Chapter 10 for the various taxonomies describing single implementation strategies), which may or may not be part of a multifaceted strategy – the following features:

- *Features of the target group/participants*: strategy aimed at groups (homogeneous or heterogeneous?) or individuals, number of individuals and/or groups, profession, motivation for participation (e.g. voluntary, obligatory, incentive for participation?).

- *Features of the implementers or change agents*: profession, opinion leadership, authority, embedded in participating organizational unit.
- *Intensity of the implementation strategy*: frequency of performing/repeating the selected implementation strategy for the same participants, time intervals between them, duration.
- *Features of the information imparted on the innovation/guideline*: type of information, presentation form, medium.
- *Features of the information imparted on professional performance of the innovation/guideline*: type of information, presentation form, medium, feasibility of comparing information about performance.

---

implementers or change agents; (iii) the intensity of the implementation activity; and (iv) the information imparted. Deviation from the planned features may impact effectiveness. Applying, for example, external change agents instead of the envisioned "implementers in residence" (i.e. change agents who are embedded in the participating organizational units) will influence the impact of the implementation strategy (Vindrola-Padros et al. 2017; Wolfenden et al. 2017).

22.5   Framing Process Evaluations

The specific research questions that underlie a process evaluation obviously determine which data should be collected. There is no validated, widely applicable set of measures for process evaluation. The available frameworks for process evaluation specify a range of concepts, components, and domains which should be considered. So far, we have used

the framework by Grant et al. (2013) as a guidance. An alternative is the guidance on process evaluation of complex interventions by the British Medical Research Council (MRC), which is widely used in the UK and beyond (see Box 22.9). Among other things, this framework provides practical guidance by specification of a series of steps, which should be followed in process evaluation. It does not, however, explicitly distinguish between clinical or prevention interventions, and the strategies to implement these.

Depending on the body of available research and theory, it is possible to take a hypothesis-generating approach (inductive) or a hypothesis-testing approach (deductive) to evaluation. A mix of both is also possible. Regardless of the chosen approach, it is recommended to specify the intervention components and theory underlying the intervention at all times. This can be done in advance of a program, using program descriptions and consultation of program developers, and then adapted and extended on the basis of the findings in

---

Box 22.9   MRC Guidance for Process Evaluation of Complex Interventions

In 2015, the MRC guidance for process evaluation of complex interventions was published (Moore et al. 2015). This framework provides guidance to "assess fidelity and quality of implementation, clarify causal mechanisms, and identify contextual factors associated with variation in outcomes." The framework offers key recommendations for process evaluation within four domains: planning, design and conduct, analysis, and reporting of process evaluation.

Planning of process evaluation:

- Define relationships of evaluators with intervention developers or implementers.
- Ensure that the research team has the correct expertise.
- Decide the degree of separation or integration between process and effect evaluation teams.

Design and conduct of process evaluation:

- Describe the intervention and clarify causal assumptions.
- Identify key uncertainties and select the most important questions to address.
- Select methods appropriate to the research questions.

Process evaluation analysis:

- Provide descriptive quantitative information on fidelity, dose, and reach.

- Consider modeling of variations between participants or sites.
- Examine whether effects differ by implementation or pre-specified contextual moderators, and test hypothesized mediators.
- Collect and analyze qualitative data iteratively.
- Ensure that quantitative and qualitative analyses build upon one another.
- Initially analyze and report process data before trial outcomes are known to avoid biased interpretation.
- Transparently report whether process data are being used to generate hypotheses or for post hoc explanation.

Process evaluation reporting:

- Identify existing reporting guidance specific to the methods adopted.
- Report the logic model/intervention theory and how it was used to guide selection of research questions and methods.
- Disseminate findings to policy and practice stakeholders.
- Clarify, if multiple journal articles are published from the same process evaluation, the context of each article within the evaluation as a whole.

---

the process evaluation (e.g. Dixon-Woods et al. 2013).

Data for process evaluation can be both qualitative and quantitative. Many studies utilize a combination of qualitative and quantitative approaches to process evaluation; they perform so-called mixed-method process evaluation to integrate findings and draw inferences from both types of data (Bryman 1998; Tashakkori and Creswell 2007; O'Cathain et al. 2008; Odendaal et al. 2016). The use of such

combinations requires careful planning, because such an approach may overstretch the logistic and analytical resources of an evaluation. Some other studies utilize the "realist evaluation method" to understand "what works, for whom and under what circumstances" by theorizing and empirically examining underlying mechanisms (Bonell et al. 2012). This method of process evaluation uses qualitative methods and theoretical analysis to look for patterns in the relationships between context, intervention components, and outcomes.

In most studies, process evaluation data are collected by:

- On-site observation, either on the spot using an observer (direct observation) or using audio or video recordings (indirect observation).
- Self-report, using interviews or questionnaires among change agents (providers of the implementation strategy), targeted individuals and organizations, and other stakeholders, such as payers and regulators.
- Pre-existing data sources or records (secondary sources), with the aim of systematically extracting process data from them.

On-site observation is feasible whenever the presence of an observer (person, camera, or audio tape) is not obtrusive and may not alter the behavior of those observed. Observation appears attractive and simple, but can pose several problems. The method is not easily taught or quickly learned, it is time consuming, and sometimes it produces information that is hard to analyze or summarize. The less structured the observation or the more complex the implementation strategy performed, the more problematic the method becomes. It is therefore very important to train observers and to assess reliability.

Self-report (interviews and questionnaires) can be used either through periodic reports throughout the intervention period or through retrospective reports after the intervention has ended. Periodic reports probably provide more accurate data. The number of measurements during an intervention period depends on the homogeneity of the activities (the more homogeneous the activities, the less often data have to be gathered), the amount of time available for scoring and interpreting information, and the assessment of people's tolerance for interruptions. Reports gathered after an intervention has ended are most reliable when done as soon as possible after the event.

Pre-existing data sources or records can also be used for extracting process data. This means that information is used that is already routinely recorded, independent of the process evaluation, in administrative and service records (e.g. the pocket diary in which the outreach visitor records appointments with practices). This is a relatively inexpensive method, providing data that are often easy and cheap to obtain and analyze. Records may vary from narrative reports to highly structured data forms used by staff to check what activities have been performed. Examples of such secondary sources include minutes of meetings, bills, purchase orders, invoices, certificates upon completion of activities, attendance logs, signing in and signing out sheets, checklists, referral letters, diaries, news releases, and so on. Using pre-existing records has some limitations. They will seldom cover all the information needed, so it will usually be necessary to collect additional information. Given the possible problems of using existing records, it is sometimes necessary to set up a project-specific recording system. Checklists are, for example, feasible and efficient to use; no narrative information has to be provided – checking off relevant items is sufficient. They are also usable as a mnemonic device, reminding the user of what activities should be performed.

Whatever measurement method (or group of methods) is chosen, a number of issues need to be considered: for instance, the circumstances (e.g. the amount of time available for gathering and interpreting data), practical issues, the homogeneity of the data, privacy and confidentiality, and the estimated tolerance levels of the respondents who will be asked to provide data. In addition, the instruments selected should ideally be simple and user friendly so that they are not burdensome for the user. On the other hand, they must be detailed enough to answer the evaluation questions. Where possible, existing, validated instruments should be used. When selecting the instruments, it is necessary to consider whether the method of data collection will have an undesirable influence on the ongoing evaluation or on the actual use of the implementation activities as part of the implementation strategy. It is also important that data are gathered in a valid and reliable manner from the target population or a sample thereof.

Irrespective of the chosen measurement method (or combination of methods), it is crucial that a clear and coherent plan is established in the early phases of a study to account for how the implementation strategy will be performed, and in what way it will be assessed or monitored during and after its delivery to study participants (Box 22.10). This plan serves as a guide – by clearly prescribing *when*, and *who* should do *what, to whom*, and in *what manner* – for performing the process evaluation.

22.6 A Practical, Step-wise Approach to Process Evaluation

22.6.1 Step 1: Analysis of Implementation Strategy as Planned

After selecting one of the published frameworks for process evaluation, interviews with

---

Box 22.10   A Plan to Enhance and Monitor Fidelity in a Randomized Controlled Trial

In the SPHERE (Secondary Prevention of Heart DiseasE in GeneRal PracticE) study, a multifaceted implementation strategy was developed to improve secondary prevention of heart disease (Spillane et al. 2007). In line with the National Institutes of Health Behavior Change Consortium's fidelity recommendations (Bellg et al. 2004), the researchers outlined how they planned to enhance and monitor the performance of their implementation strategy. They developed clear procedures in five domains, as fidelity should be considered in relation to the study design, training providers, delivery of treatment/strategy, receipt of treatment/strategy, and enactment of treatment/strategy skills. More specifically:

- *Study design plan.* This specified for example:
  - The standardized strategy with clear guidelines.
  - The plan of how to include fidelity data in the analysis.
  - The planned observations of implementers (or providers) while delivering the strategies.
- *Provider training plan.* This specified for example:
  - The standardized training sessions.

- The role-plays and feedback to further standardize providers.
- *Strategy delivery plan.* This specified the measures to monitor the delivery of the strategy to patients (in this case, the participants to the strategy), for example:
  - Observation of randomly selected first consultations by a research member (quality assurance visit).
  - Observation of randomly selected follow-up intervention consultations by a research member (quality assurance visit).
- *Strategy receipt plan.* This specified the measures to monitor the receipt of the strategy, for example:
  - Follow-up telephone calls to patients after their first visit to review understanding.
  - Qualitative evaluation of patients' experiences.
- *Enactment of intended strategy outcomes plan.* This specified the measures to monitor the intended outcomes (i.e. the enactment of changed behavior in intended situations and at the appropriate time) of the strategy, for example:
  - Follow-up data collection – review of patient care plans, and patient questionnaires relating to self-reports of desired behavior.

Box 22.11   The WHO Strategy as Planned to Improve the Quality of Care for Respiratory Diseases

At a global level, the World Health Organization (WHO) develops generic guidelines that are not health system specific and need to be adapted to the particular local context. For example, to improve the quality of care for youths and adults with respiratory diseases, the WHO developed the generic PAL guideline, the Practical Approach to Lung health, in 1997. PAL was presented as a package that consists of the guideline and accompanying training materials (i.e. the implementation strategy). A context-specific PAL-Nepal adaptation was developed by a working group of Nepalese experts and potential stakeholders, and a pilot implementation was started in July 2002 (ten Asbroek et al. 2005). The authors ex ante assessed the feasibility of the successful implementation of PAL-Nepal by studying, among others, the implementation strategy as planned (i.e. the training) and its potential effectiveness. To assess this, they critically analyzed the planned strategy using the Hulscher et al. (2003) framework presented in Box 22.10. Input for this analysis was derived from the minutes of the working group meetings, training plans, and training manuals. This strategy as planned was, in the next step, compared with international literature on effective implementation of guidelines. In their critical analysis of the planned strategy and its comparison with the international literature, the authors identified potential areas for improvement. They suggested that there was a need to adapt (specifically to expand) the "mono-event" implementation strategy to increase the chances of successful implementation.

---

the program developers and other relevant individuals can provide information to describe the features of the implementation strategy. To supplement this process, it may be useful to use existing documentation such as a study plan, the program proposal, minutes of meetings, or existing records (Box 22.11). This analysis should elaborate the intervention components and the theory underlying the intervention effectiveness.

22.6.2   Step 2: Assessment of Intervention Fidelity

Next, the actual performance of these planned activities as part of the implementation strategy and the degree of participation in these activities need to be assessed to enable a comparison with the planned strategy. Both aspects can be measured retrospectively or prospectively (either continuously or periodically) among providers of the implementation strategy and/or participants in the

implementation strategy. After the project has been completed, interviews with or questionnaires among both groups can be used – while applying the selected framework – to retrospectively describe the features of the implementation strategy as delivered. Since the reliability of data reported in retrospect decreases as the complexity of the strategy and the interval since the start of the intervention increase, it is preferable to gather information during the process (i.e. prospectively) and to use these data to describe the strategy as delivered in its real-time form. Such data can be collected by using observation, interviews, questionnaires, and/or existing data sources (Box 22.12).

While carrying out the implementation strategy, it is sometimes permissible to vary the implementation activities across sites or time. The greater the variation permissible, the more attention must be paid to collecting process data for that specific feature or component of the strategy.

Box 22.12   A Decision Aid for Subfertile Couples

A multifaceted implementation strategy was developed to stimulate elective single embryo transfer (eSET) after in vitro fertilization (IVF; Kreuwel et al. 2013). The strategy consisted of four elements:

1) A decision aid containing information about chances and risks of singletons versus twin pregnancies.
2) A reimbursement offer for an extra IVF cycle for couples who did not achieve a pregnancy after eSET.
3) A counseling session with an IVF nurse to discuss the content of the decision aid and the financial offer.
4) A telephone conversation with the nurse to discuss any relevant questions that might have arisen during IVF treatment.

The strategy was tested in a randomized controlled trial; the control group received standard IVF care including a preparatory session in which the number of embryos transferred was discussed. The strategy significantly increased the eSET rate by 11% and reduced costs as well. To assess which elements of the strategy contributed most to its effectiveness, a process evaluation was performed using the Hulscher et al. 2003 framework (Box 22.10). On the one hand, couples' exposure (i.e. participation in the activities as part of the implementation strategy) to the different elements of the multifaceted strategy was evaluated. Data were collected using a checklist that not only provided the data for the evaluation; it was also useful for the IVF nurse, as it guided her activities and information provision. For each session and each telephone conversation the checklist provided, for example, information on the topics addressed and on the date and duration of the activity. On the other hand, couples' experiences with the various elements of the strategy were measured using a questionnaire. The questionnaire contained items (five-point Likert scales) asking about the couples' self-assessed influence of the specific elements on their final decision regarding the number of embryos transferred and about their assessment (e.g. comprehensibility, amount of necessary time investment) of each element.

Evaluation of exposure showed that almost 50% of all couples in the intervention group were exposed to all four elements of the strategy. Further analysis showed that these couples did not choose eSET more often than couples who only received the decision aid and the reimbursement offer. Regarding experiences, couples rated the reimbursement offer and the phone call as less important for their decision than the decision aid and the counseling session (p < 0.001). Combining these outcomes, the authors concluded that one element of the multifaceted strategy – the decision aid – was probably solely responsible for the increase in eSET rate. As IVF couples evaluated an additional counseling session with the IVF nurse as important and useful for their decision regarding the number of embryos transferred, the authors suggested it was important to consider – from a patient-centered point of view – the inclusion of a support session with an IVF nurse in a future implementation strategy for eSET.

22.6.3   Step 3: Assessment of Participant Experiences

Providers of the implementation strategy and participants in the implementation activities may be asked, during and/or after finishing the intervention, to provide information on how they experienced the activities. Their opinions on all the features of the implementation activities can be explored – while using the selected process evaluation framework –

Box 22.13 Active and Less Active Ingredients of a Multicomponent Complex Intervention to Reduce High-Risk Primary Care Prescribing

As described in Box 22.5, a strategy combining professional education with financial incentives and access to a web-based IT tool reduced high-risk prescribing from 3.7 to 2.2% (Grant et al. 2017). Reductions were sustained in the year after financial incentives stopped. In addition, there were reductions in emergency hospital admissions. The researchers performed a comprehensive mixed-methods process evaluation, alongside the pragmatic cluster-randomized controlled stepped-wedge trial in 33 Scottish general practices. They used a process evaluation framework they had previously developed (Grant et al. 2013; Box 22.3) to structure their process evaluation, mapping data collection to a logic model of how the implementation strategy was expected to work. The process evaluation was also informed by normalization process theory. The evaluation focused on practice participants' perceptions of the multifaceted implementation strategy delivered by the research team to participating practices, to examine whether and how the individual strategy components were effective from the perspective of the professionals using qualitative analysis of interview data.

All the components of the implementation strategy were perceived as active, but at different stages in the project: financial incentives primarily supported recruitment; education motivated the GPs to initiate implementation; the IT tool facilitated sustained implementation. Intervention sub-components also varied in whether and when they were active. For example, run charts providing feedback on change in prescribing over time were ignored in the IT tool, but were motivating in some practices in the regular emailed newsletter. Overall, GPs varied in terms of which components and sub-components they valued most or they perceived to be most active. There was no consistently identified set of inactive components, suggesting – as interpreted by the researchers – that all component parts should be delivered in a further roll-out.

---

including their opinion on the quality of delivery. They may also describe features they perceived as being most related to the success or failure of the strategy. In this way, information is gathered about experiences that are closely and directly linked to the implementation activities as part of the implementation strategy (Boxes 22.12 and 22.13). Participants may, for example after taking part in an "educational and feedback strategy," judge retrospectively that not all the professional specialisms involved in daily patient care were invited to the educational meetings; that the person who led the meeting (the provider) did not have the appropriate background and was not perceived as an opinion leader by the target group; that four educational meetings were too

much; that the meetings lasted too long; that the graphical feedback was difficult to interpret; that they lacked comparative information from colleagues; and that the second training meeting had contributed most to their changes in patient care. Researchers and evaluators can use this information to adjust the strategy to enhance its effectiveness.

22.6.4 Step 4: Exploration of Working Mechanisms

Working mechanisms can be explored quantitatively or qualitatively. In quantitative analyses, multivariate analysis can explore the mediating and moderating roles of (measured) factors. Under certain conditions, this may

---

Box 22.14   Improving Hand Hygiene with a State-of-the-Art Implementation Strategy

Researchers (Huis et al. 2013) compiled – based on a systematic literature review – an implementation strategy with proven effective components: education, reminders, feedback, and presence of adequate products and facilities for hand hygiene. This state-of-the-art strategy was applied in 47 nursing teams and resulted in an improvement in hand hygiene behavior from 22 to 44%. Improvement varied between the different teams. After the intervention, the researchers carried out a questionnaire study on 24 determinants of hand hygiene behavior. Analyses showed the importance of social influence (two questionnaire items: "My colleagues support each other in performing hand hygiene" and "Our team members address each other in case of undesirable hand hygiene behavior") and of leadership (five items: "My manager pays regular attention to the adherence of hand hygiene guidelines"; "Hand hygiene is not a priority at our ward"; "My ward manager addresses barriers to enable hand hygiene as recommended"; "My ward manager holds team members accountable for hand hygiene performance"; and "My ward manager encourages and motivates our team members to perform hand hygiene"). All seven items were significantly correlated with improvement of hand hygiene. The exploration of the relation between these determinants and hand hygiene compliance provided empirical evidence for social influence and leadership as important vehicles for changing hand hygiene behavior.

---

provide insight into potential causal mechanisms underlying the effectiveness of interventions. As previously stated, advanced knowledge of methodology and statistical methods is required for such analyses that take mediating and moderating factors into account.

In qualitative analyses (see Step 3), the perceptions of target groups and stakeholders of the mechanisms of change can be explored as well as the potential role of mechanisms, which emerge from the data in the context of chosen theories (e.g. May et al. 2018). In addition, analyzing barriers and facilitators – experienced while participating in the implementation activities and while introducing changes in daily patient care – can provide useful information on how the strategy brought about improvement, or not (see Box 22.4; Curran et al. 2013). This issue was discussed in Chapters 8 and 9. Ideally, a strategy that aims to change clinical practice is designed on the basis of an analysis of barriers and facilitators to change, linking the implementation activities to these influencing factors. In daily practice, however, this is not always the case; sometimes new barriers and facilitators present themselves during the course of the implementation project. For example, Jäger et al. found that about 30% of the determinants mentioned by professionals who had participated in the implementation activities had not been identified beforehand (Jäger et al. 2016). A complete analysis of "what works, for whom and under what circumstances" should therefore also include a post hoc analysis of barriers and facilitators, to collect information to, ultimately, increase the future effectiveness of the strategy tested (Box 22.14).

22.7 Conclusions

Process evaluation is an intensive task where attention to detail is indispensable and little standardization of methods and measures across studies is possible. A core component of any process evaluation is an assessment of the fidelity (and adaptation) of interventions and strategies in practice as compared to the plan. Process evaluation can also illuminate the factors, mechanisms, and processes responsible for the (lack of) improvement in the target group. In so doing, process evaluation makes a very relevant and important contribution to the development of successful implementation strategies, as well as to the body of scientific knowledge in the field.

References

ten Asbroek, A.H.A., Delnoij, D.M.J., Niessen, L. W. et al. (2005). Implementing global knowledge in local practice: a WHO lung health initiative in Nepal. *Health Policy Plan.* 20: 290–301.

Bellg, A.J., Borrelli, B., Resnick, B. et al. (2004). Enhancing treatment fidelity in health behaviour change studies: best practices and recommendations from the NIH behaviour change consortium. *Health Psychol.* 23: 443–451.

Bonell, C., Fletcher, A., Morton, M. et al. (2012). Realist randomized controlled trials: a new approach to evaluating complex public health interventions. *Soc. Sci. Med.* 75: 2299–2306.

Bryman, A. (1998). Barriers to integrating quantitative and qualitative research. *J. Mixed Methods Res.* 1: 8–22.

Carroll, C., Patterson, M., Wood, S. et al. (2007). A conceptual framework for implementation fidelity. *Implement. Sci.* 2: 40–48.

Craig, P., Dieppe, P., Macintyre, S. et al. (2008). Developing and evaluating complex interventions: the new Medical Research Council guidance. *BMJ* 337: 979–983.

Crocker-Buque, T., Edelstein, M., and Mounier-Jack, S. (2018). A process evaluation of how the routine vaccination programme is implemented at GP practices in England. *Implement. Sci.* 13: 132.

Curran, J.A., Brehaut, J., Patey, A.M. et al. (2013). Understanding the Canadian adult CT head rule trial: use of the theoretical domains framework for process evaluation. *Implement. Sci.* 8: 25.

Dixon-Woods, M., Leslie, M., Tarrant, C., and Bion, J. (2013). Explaining matching

Michigan: an ethnographic study of a patient safety program. *Implement. Sci.* 8: 70.

Dreischulte, T., Grant, A., Hapca, A., and Guthrie, B. (2018). Process evaluation of the Data-driven Quality Improvement in Primary Care (DQIP) trial: quantitative examination of variation between practices in recruitment, implementation and effectiveness. *BMJ Open* 8: e017133.

Dusenbury, L., Brannigan, R., Falco, M., and Hansen, W.B. (2003). A review of research on fidelity of implementation: implications for drug abuse prevention in school settings. *Health Educ. Res.* 18: 237–256.

Grant, A., Dreischulte, T., and Guthrie, B. (2017). Process evaluation of the data-driven quality improvement in primary care (DQIP) trial: active and less active ingredients of a multi-component complex intervention to reduce high-risk primary care prescribing. *Implement. Sci.* 12: 4.

Grant, E., Treweek, S., Dreischulte, T. et al. (2013). Process evaluations for cluster randomised trials of complex interventions: a proposed framework for design and reporting. *Trials* 14: 15.

Hermens, R.P.M.G., Hak, E., Hulscher, M.E.J.L. et al. (2001). Adherence to guidelines on cervical cancer screening in general practice: programme elements to successful implementation. *Br. J. Gen. Pract.* 51: 897–903.

Huis, A., Holleman, G., van Achterberg, T. et al. (2013). Explaining the effects of two different strategies for promoting hand hygiene in hospital nurses: a process evaluation alongside a cluster randomised controlled trial. *Implement. Sci.* 8: 41.

Hulscher, M.E., Laurant, M.G., and Grol, R.P. (2003). Process evaluation on quality improvement interventions. *Qual. Saf. Health Care* 12: 40–46.

Jäger, C., Steinhäuser, J., Freund, T. et al. (2016). Process evaluation of five tailored programs to improve the implementation of evidence-based recommendations for chronic conditions in primary care. *Implement Sci.* 11: 123.

Kreuwel, I.A., van Peperstraten, A.M., Hulscher, M.E. et al. (2013). Evaluation of an effective multifaceted implementation strategy for elective single-embryo transfer after in vitro fertilization. *Hum. Reprod.* 28: 336–342.

Masterson-Algar, P., Burton, C.R., and Rycroft-Malone, J. (2018). The generation of consensus guidelines for carrying out process evaluations in rehabilitation research. *BMC Med. Res. Methodol.* 18: 180.

May, C.R., Cummings, A., Girling, M. et al. (2018). Using normalization process theory in feasibility studies and process evaluations of complex healthcare interventions: a systematic review. *Implement. Sci.* 13: 80.

Michie, S., Johnston, M., Abraham, C. et al. (2005). Making psychological theory useful for implementing evidence based practice: a consensus approach. *Qual. Saf. Health Care* 14: 26–33.

Moore, G.F., Audrey, S., Barker, M. et al. (2015). Process evaluation of complex interventions: Medical Research Council guidance. *BMJ* 350: h1258.

Musuuza, J.S., Barker, A., Ngam, C. et al. (2016). Assessment of fidelity in interventions to improve hand hygiene of healthcare workers: a systematic review. *Infect. Control Hosp. Epidemiol.* 37: 567–575.

O'Cathain, A., Murphy, E., and Nicholl, J. (2008). The quality of mixed methods studies in health services research. *J. Health Serv. Res. Policy* 13: 92–98.

Odendaal, W., Atkins, S., and Lewin, S. (2016). Multiple and mixed methods in formative evaluation: is more better? Reflections from a South African study. *BMC Med. Res. Methodol.* 16: 173.

Pérez, D., Van der Stuyft, P., Zabala, M.C. et al. (2016). A modified theoretical framework to assess implementation fidelity of adaptive public health interventions. *Implement. Sci.* 11: 91.

Slaughter, S.E., Hill, J.N., and Snelgrove-Clarke, E. (2015). What is the extent and quality of documentation and reporting of fidelity to implementation strategies: a scoping review. *Implement. Sci.* 10: 129.

Spillane, V., Byrne, M.C., Byrne, M. et al. (2007). Monitoring treatment fidelity in a randomized controlled trial of a complex intervention. *J. Adv. Nurs.* 60: 343–352.

Spoorenberg, V., Hulscher, M.E., Geskus, R.B. et al. (2015). A cluster-randomized trial of two strategies to improve antibiotic use for patients with a complicated urinary tract infection. *PLoS One* 10: e0142672.

Swanborn, P.G. (1999). *Evalueren. Het ontwerpen, begeleiden en evalueren van interventies: een methodische basis voor evaluatie-onderzoek* [*The Design, Conduct and Evaluation of Interventions: A Methodological Foundation for Evaluation Research*]. Amsterdam: Uitgeverij Boom.

Tashakkori, A. and Creswell, J.W. (2007). The new era of mixed methods (editorial). *J. Mixed Methods Res.* 1: 3–7.

Vindrola-Padros, C., Pape, T., Utley, M., and Fulop, N.J. (2017). The role of embedded research in quality improvement: a narrative review. *Br. Med. J. Qual. Saf.* 26: 70–80.

Wiltsey Stirman, S., Baumann, A.A., and Miller, C.J. (2019). The FRAME: an expanded framework for reporting adaptations and modifications to evidence-based interventions. *Implement. Sci.* 14: 58.

Wiltsey Stirman, S., Miller, C.J., Toder, K., and Calloway, A. (2013). Development of a framework and coding system for modification and adaptations of evidence-based interventions. *Implement. Sci.* 8: 65.

Wolfenden, L., Yoong, S.L., Williams, C.M. et al. (2017). Embedding researchers in health service organizations improves research translation and health service performance: the Australian Hunter New England Population Health example. *J. Clin. Epidemiol.* 85: 3–11.

23

Economic Evaluation of Implementation Strategies

Johan L. Severens[1], Ties Hoomans[2], Eddy Adang[3], and Michel Wensing[4,5,6]

[1] *Erasmus School of Health Policy & Management and Institute of Medical Technology Assessment, Erasmus University Rotterdam, Rotterdam, The Netherlands*
[2] *Care Policy and Evaluation Centre, London School of Economics and Political Science, London, UK*
[3] *Department for Health Evidence, Radboud Institute for Health Sciences, Radboud University Medical Center, Nijmegen, The Netherlands*
[4] *Faculty of Medicine, University of Heidelberg, Heidelberg, Germany*
[5] *Department of General Practice and Health Services Research, Heidelberg University Hospital, Heidelberg, Germany*
[6] *Department IQ healthcare, Radboud Institute for Health Sciences, Radboud University Medical Center, Nijmegen, The Netherlands*

SUMMARY

- Economic evaluations of implementation strategies are explicit comparisons of alternative methods for introducing desirable changes in healthcare, relating the costs incurred to develop, execute, and participate in implementation activities to the (health) benefits obtained.

- Unlike economic evaluations of medical interventions, economic evaluations of implementation strategies incorporate measures of both care processes and patient outcomes.

- Economic evaluation of implementation strategies can be very informative, but they have been performed on only a limited scale so far.

- Economic research of implementation strategies is most efficiently conducted if the cost-effectiveness of the desired professional behavior or healthcare process in optimal conditions are known and subsequently can be used as a basis for comprehensive modeling.

23.1   Introduction

Previous chapters elaborated on outcome and process evaluation of implementation strategies. In this chapter, evaluation is extended to include the costs of implementation strategies, and to relate those costs to their effects on professional behavior and patient outcomes. Extension of implementation studies to include economic arguments may be considered the final component of evaluation before large-scale application of strategies is recommended and started. Box 23.1 provides an example of an economic evaluation of a complex intervention.

To date, there have been few examples of full economic evaluations of implementation strategies. In a review of 235 studies reporting 309 comparisons of strategies to implement clinical guidelines, only 29% of comparisons reported any economic data (Grimshaw et al. 2004; Vale et al. 2007). A few years later, the number of economic evaluations of implementation strategies had increased, although the

Improving Patient Care: The Implementation of Change in Health Care, Third Edition. Edited by Michel Wensing, Richard Grol, and Jeremy Grimshaw.
© 2020 John Wiley & Sons Ltd. Published 2020 by John Wiley & Sons Ltd.

Box 23.1   Randomized Controlled Economic Evaluation of Asthma Self-Management in Primary Healthcare

In this randomized controlled economic evaluation, implementation of guided asthma self-management was compared with usual asthma care according to guidelines for Dutch primary care (PC) physicians (Schermer et al. 2002). Nineteen family practices were randomized, and 193 adults with stable asthma (98 self-management, 95 usual care) were included and monitored for two years. Practices in the intervention group received training and support to implement the self-management program. Patient-specific cost data were collected, preference-based utilities were assessed, and incremental cost per quality-adjusted life year (QALY) and incremental

cost per successfully treated week gained were calculated. Self-management patients gained 0.039 QALY and experienced 81 successfully treated weeks in a period of two years; the corresponding figures for usual care were 0.024 and 75. Total costs were €1084 for self-management and €1097 for usual care. Self-management patients consumed 1680 puffs of budesonide, usual care patients 1897. When all costs were included, self-management was cost-effective for all outcomes. It was concluded that guided self-management is an efficient alternative approach compared with the asthma treatment usually provided.

---

methodological quality of these studies was low (Hoomans et al. 2007). Since then, the interest in economic evaluations of implementation strategies has remained limited (Lau et al. 2015), despite the fact that pressure on healthcare budgets seems to have increased. Most recently, a systematic review identified 30 economic evaluations of strategies to improve healthcare delivery and the uptake of evidence-based practices (Roberts et al. 2019).

Despite the lack of comprehensive economic evaluations, decision makers will often make an implicit estimate about the costs and consequences of a particular implementation strategy, or the competing costs of alternative strategies to introduce an innovation or change in practice. For instance, outreach visits to ambulatory practices require many more resources than sending written information. In an economic evaluation, the comparison of alternative implementation strategies in terms of both costs and effects is made explicit so that decisions about how to improve practice can be more evidence based. This chapter describes the principles and methods of economic evaluation of implementation strategies and illustrates these with examples.

23.2   The Basics of Economic Evaluation

As discussed earlier in this book, when a policy maker, healthcare manager, or clinician wants to change healthcare processes and promote particular behavior by healthcare professionals, there are numerous possible implementation strategies. These strategies can be effective, albeit the effects tend to be moderate and unpredictable (Grimshaw and Russell 1993; Grimshaw et al. 2012), but they all have costs. In many cases, these comprise time and other resources needed to develop, execute, and participate in activities (e.g. researcher time to develop feedback reports, and physician and nurse time to read these and plan actions).

Time and other resources tend to be scarce, so priorities have to be set. The costs of any implementation strategy, as with all interventions in healthcare, will come at the expense of other healthcare activities or other societal opportunity costs. It is possible that a clinical intervention that is cost-effective in the context of a clinical trial requires so many resources to implement in a routine care setting that its

Table 23.1 Criteria for a complete economic evaluation.

		Are both consequences and costs taken into consideration?		
		Consequences only	Costs only	Both consequences and costs
Are alternatives being compared?	No	Description of consequences	Description of costs	Description of cost and consequences
	Yes	Outcomes research	Cost analysis	Economic evaluation

Source: Based upon conclusions of Drummond et al. (2015).

cost-effectiveness deteriorates. Therefore, it is important to incorporate the cost-effectiveness of implementation in decisions about the uptake of clinical interventions (Hoomans et al. 2009c). The application of an implementation strategy can be considered part of the investment necessary to embed a new procedure or routine in the organization.

Economic evaluations are about efficiency in the allocation of scarce resources and so answering the "value for money" question, focusing on the relationship between the consequences achieved (e.g. better adherence to recommended practices) and the resources required to achieve those consequences. Economic evaluations aim to develop evidence that policy makers and healthcare managers can use to assess and make decisions about the allocation of resources.

As with economic evaluations of medical interventions, an economic evaluation of implementation strategies must meet two criteria (Table 23.1). First, there needs to be a choice between alternative mutually exclusive strategies. In implementation research, the choice consists of a comparison of two or more alternative implementation strategies, where one of the comparators usually involves "doing nothing" or "passive dissemination." Second, in economic evaluations, an explicit relationship has to be made between the inputs (use of people and resources) and the related consequences or actual results. The consequences and costs of an implementation strategy can then be considered in comparison with those of an alternative strategy, thus in fact presenting the incremental costs and consequences.

23.2.1 Definition of Cost-Effectiveness

Table 23.2 elaborates on economic evaluation research. If strategy A is associated with worse consequences and higher costs than strategy B, then strategy A is inferior and should not be pursued. The opposite occurs when an implementation strategy, here strategy B, has more

Table 23.2 Classification of the outcomes of economic evaluations that compares two alternative implementation strategies.

		Consequences of implementation strategy A compared to strategy B	
		A is worse than B	A is better than B
Costs of A Compared to B	Higher	A is inferior compared to B	Is a better outcome worth the higher costs?
	Lower	Is a worse outcome acceptable, considering the lower costs?	A is dominant compared to B

Source: Data from Sculpher (2000).

favorable consequences than its comparator and also incurs lower costs. This combination is known as dominance. The other two common situations (higher costs and better outcomes, or lower costs and worse outcomes) are known as consideration problems and there is then a need to decide on an acceptable ratio between costs and consequences.

23.3 Types of Economic Evaluation

There are four basic types of economic evaluation: (i) cost-minimization analysis; (ii) cost-effectiveness analysis; (iii) cost–utility analysis; and (iv) cost–benefit analysis. All of these can be relevant for the evaluation of implementation strategies. In addition, a cost–consequence analysis is considered to be a descriptive alternative to full economic evaluations. An overview of the methods of economic evaluation is shown in Table 23.3. Irrespective of the type of economic evaluation, it is important to realize that the effects on patient outcomes are determined not only by the implementation strategy evaluated, but also by the effectiveness of the clinical interventions that are implemented. Likewise, the costs are a function of both the implementation strategy and the clinical or preventive intervention.

A *cost-minimization analysis* is characterized by the assumption or evidence of equivalent consequences (outcomes, benefits) of the implementation strategies under comparison. In the face of such equivalence of effects, the economic evaluation of implementation strategies can be confined to analyzing all relevant costs, such as costs for development and execution of the implementation strategy, costs of healthcare provision and patients' use of healthcare, and non-medical costs. Of course, the least expensive alternative should be the preferred option to improve practice, under the assumption that outcomes are equal. Although this assumption is hardly ever met, Box 23.2 may provide an example.

Cost-effectiveness analysis expresses consequences in natural measurable consequences. Typically, implementation research focuses on behavioral or process measures, such as the number of physician practices reached by the implementation strategy (e.g. mailing of guidelines); the number of practices, departments, or professionals working in accordance with a specific guideline; or the number of patients receiving treatment in accordance with a protocol. These process measures can be considered intermediate outcomes that ideally have a (proven) relationship with patient outcomes. In using process measures, the analysis is focused on the performance of

Table 23.3 Types of economic evaluations.

Type	Level of measurement	Unit of measurement of consequences
Cost-minimization analysis	Not relevant, consequences of the implementation strategies are equivalent	Not applicable
Cost-effectiveness analysis	Multiple, including that of healthcare agencies, healthcare professional, or patient	Consequences in various measuring units
Cost–utility analysis	Patient	Health status, patient preferences, utilities
Cost–benefit analysis	Patient	Monetary units
Cost–consequence analysis	Multiple, including healthcare agencies, healthcare professional, or patient	Consequences in various measuring units

Box 23.2   Individual Feedback, Education on Guidelines, and Quality Improvement Sessions in Small Groups to Improve Test Ordering in Primary Care

This multicenter cluster-randomized study (randomization at local physicians group level) compared the costs and cost reductions of an innovative strategy aimed at improving test-ordering routines of PC physicians (14 groups) with those of a traditional strategy of individual feedback only (13 groups; Verstappen et al. 2004). In the experimental arm, physicians discussed each other's test-ordering behavior in regular quality meetings in local groups, related their behavior to clinical guidelines, and made individual and/or group plans for behavioral change. The cost analysis focused on the costs of developing the strategy, executing it ("running costs"), and the performed diagnostic tests (healthcare provision costs). This provided an estimate of costs per general practitioner (GP) using a six-month time horizon. The costs of the test-ordering behavior of GPs were retrospectively determined six months prior to the intervention.

The experimental strategy was found to incur higher costs related to development and execution than the conventional feedback system. These higher costs did not outweigh the lower costs related to test-ordering behavior, even in the case where the sunk costs of developing the implementation strategy were not taken into account. The overall conclusion was that individual feedback, education on guidelines, and quality improvement sessions in small groups as an innovative feedback system can be considered to be valuable, although further research into expected non-monetary benefits is warranted. The design may be defined as a cost-minimization analysis, as in this case equal patient outcomes are known or assumed. However, only healthcare provision costs related to diagnostic test ordering were analyzed, ignoring treatment cost and implicitly assuming that lower test ordering would not influence patient outcome.

healthcare providers (Wood and Freemantle 1999). Box 23.3 provides an example of cost-effectiveness analyses using process measures. Alternatively, cost-effectiveness analyses of implementation strategies may focus on patient outcomes, such as various morbidity and mortality measures (see Chapter 20 for a discussion of different types of outcomes in the evaluation of implementation strategies).

In *cost–utility analysis*, implementation strategies are compared with patients' eventual health being valued through the use of a utility measure (see Box 23.4 for an example). Utilities are usually based on the theory of choice (time trade-off utilities) under uncertainty (standard gamble utilities). This health-related utility is indicated by a number between 0 and 1, where 1 equals perfect health and 0 the worst imaginable health. Utilities can be combined with survival to provide a composite measure such

as QALYs, a measure that uses societal ratings of a patient's health condition and relates these to life span. Cost–utility analyses require patients to participate in a study and complete questionnaires. Within clinical evaluation studies this method of analysis is frequently used, but within implementation research it is used only sporadically, because changes in health professionals' behavior have usually only an indirect, long-term, and overall small impact on the survival and quality of life of patients.

Cost–benefit analysis measures both the costs (e.g. implementation activities, healthcare services) and the consequences (e.g. change in health processes, health status) in monetary terms (where for example the value of a life year gained is determined via contingent valuation techniques) and establishes a net monetary benefit of implementation strategies.

Box 23.3   Economic Analysis of Three Interventions for a Healthy Canteen Policy

This study compared three interventions of different intensity for improving implementation of a government health canteen policy in Australian schools (Reilly et al. 2018). Three different implementation interventions were compared to usual implementation. The outcome was a measure of adherence to policy by school canteens. The economic analysis was based on the cost of delivering the interventions by health service delivery staff to increase the proportion of schools that were adherent with the policy. The underlying assumption is that canteens promoting healthy food will lead to healthy behavior, reduction of overweight and obesity, and savings in healthcare utilization. The cost-effectiveness of the three interventions were AU$ 2982 (high intensity), $2627 (medium intensity), and $4730 (low intensity) per 1% increase in proportion of schools reporting adherence. The difference between "high" and "medium" was not significant. Student outcomes, such as aspects of healthy behavior, body mass, or disability-adjusted life years (DALYs), were not measured.

Box 23.4   A Cluster-Randomized Trial Examining Pay for Performance as a Cost-Effective Implementation Strategy

This study (Garner et al. 2018) found that pay for performance (P4P) may improve the implementation of high-quality care. Randomization was used to assign 29 organizations and their 105 therapists and 1173 patients to one of two conditions: IAU (implementation as usual, based on a multifaceted implementation strategy) being the control condition or IAU + P4P (experimental condition). IAU + P4P consisted of a bonus of US $50 for each month that care providers demonstrated competence in treatment delivery and $200 for each patient who received a specified number of treatment procedures and sessions found to be associated with significantly improved patient outcomes. The P4P strategy led to significantly higher average total costs compared to the IAU-only control condition, yet this average increase of 5% resulted in a 116% increase in the average number of months therapists demonstrated competency in treatment delivery (incremental cost-effectiveness ratio [ICER] $333), a 325% increase in the average number of patients who received the targeted dosage of treatment (ICER $453), and a 325% increase in the number of days of abstinence per patient in treatment (ICER $8.134). For P4P the cost per QALY was $8681 (95% confidence interval [CI] $1191–16 171), which makes it possible to compare the cost-effectiveness of this implementation strategy to other interventions in healthcare systems.

From the review of Hoomans et al. (2007), it became clear that none of the economic evaluation studies of implementation so far has attempted to express individual patient outcomes in monetary terms, as it is characterized in true cost–benefit analyses. The use of net monetary benefit calculations based on a threshold value for cost-effectiveness, instead of individual patient benefit, aims to facilitate the analysis of uncertainty associated with the costs and benefits of implementation strategies, and the consideration of the scale of implementation (Hoomans et al. 2011). Perhaps most importantly, it can be useful in establishing the upper bounds on the value that can be expected from implementation and thus in setting priorities among possible implementation projects (Fenwick et al. 2008; Hoomans et al. 2009b).

Cost–consequence analysis has been mentioned as a fifth, descriptive type of economic evaluation. This approach does not explicitly relate costs to a measure of effectiveness, one of the two prerequisites for a full economic evaluation. Instead, this method presents an overview of all the costs and consequences associated with an implementation strategy, without attempting to express the relationship between costs and effects in a single unit or indicating a value or preference for a specific strategy (Mauskopf et al. 1998). Such an approach may be useful when the effect sizes and cost differences of alternative implementation strategies are largely unknown or cannot be fully characterized or aggregated, or when decision makers prefer to consider the full range of economic and non-economic consequences when making implementation decisions. McIntosh et al. (1999) introduced the so-called *balance sheet approach*, which can be considered a specific type of cost–consequence analysis in which positive and negative consequences are simply stated in a table.

23.4 Policy Cost-Effectiveness

ICER can be calculated by dividing the differences in expected costs of various strategies by the corresponding differences in expected changes in aspects of professional behavior, healthcare processes, or patient outcomes. An example of such a process measure–based ratio is the implementation cost per guideline-treated patient. The ultimate goal in health economists' research is to express the efficiency of an implementation project in terms of patient outcomes, so as to help decision makers explore whether investing in change

is potentially worthwhile (see for example Box 23.1). To that end, Mason et al. (2001) developed an advanced approach to policy cost-effectiveness combining implementation cost-effectiveness with the cost-effectiveness of treatment or other clinical interventions.

Policy cost-effectiveness is calculated as follows:

$$\Delta CE_P = \frac{1}{d \cdot n_P \cdot p_d \cdot \Delta b_t} \cdot \Delta CE_i + \Delta CE_t = L_{CE} + \Delta CE_t$$

where Δb_t is the net health gain from improved treatment for a patient and ΔCE_t is the treatment cost-effectiveness per patient, with $\Delta CE_t = \Delta c_t / \Delta b_t$ and Δc_t the additional cost of better care. Δc_i, Δb_i, and ΔCE_i are the net cost, the proportion of patient care changed, and the implementation cost-effectiveness per practice ($\Delta c_i / \Delta b_i$); d is the duration of effect of the implementation method; n_p and p_d are the average practice size and population prevalence of the condition targeted; and L_{CE} is the loading factor on treatment cost-effectiveness (Mason et al. 2001).

This formula shows that multiple influences determine whether investing in activities to promote behavioral change is worthwhile. The preconditions are that there is a recommended clinical practice with proven cost-effectiveness and that gaps between current and recommended practice are substantial. Efficient improvement of healthcare from a policy viewpoint demands an implementation strategy that does not load treatment cost-effectiveness too much (Mason et al. 2001).

Decisions about recommended practices (e.g. clinical guidelines, standards of care) most commonly precede those about implementation strategies. This sequential approach to decision making does not necessarily lead to optimal patient care and resource use. Certain clinical guidelines and other recommended practices may be more expensive to implement than others. When decision makers consider two or more care alternatives for a particular health condition, and evidence suggests that these alternatives differ in both their efficiency and cost of implementation, the overall cost-effectiveness or net benefit of health policies should be considered such that clinical interventions are selected simultaneously with strategies for implementing them (Hoomans et al. 2009c).

23.5 Framing Economic Evaluations

When setting up an economic evaluation of interventions (e.g. implementation strategies), some key decisions are to be made so that the evaluation can produce results relevant for decision makers. These key decisions, called "framing" of an economic evaluation, relate to the choice of comparator, and the time horizon and perspective of the study. These decisions show overlaps with the decisions in the design of outcome evaluations generally (see Chapters 20 and 21).

23.5.1 Choice of Comparator

The choice of comparator(s) is a fundamental aspect of any evaluation. It is important to decide what the costs and effects of an implementation strategy are to be compared with. This could pertain to alternative implementation strategies, or perhaps a combination of interventions; a routinely used implementation strategy (such as the publication of guidelines); or no specific implementation strategy ("usual" care). Clearly, the implications of such differing comparisons could vary widely. Moreover, since healthcare decision makers in general strive to improve the healthcare system, "usual care" is a comparator that is almost always essential to inform decision makers most effectively.

23.5.2 Time Horizon of a Study

The time horizon of a study is the period of time over which a study aims to make a statement about the costs and consequences of implementation, for instance 1 year or 10 years. The time horizon should be sufficiently long to reflect all important differences in costs and consequences between the implementation strategies being compared. For example, if a study is to evaluate the impact of a strategy to modify the management of cardiovascular disease, and patient mortality is considered the most relevant clinical outcome, then the time horizon could be a period of several years up to a lifetime.

However, implementation research is frequently not primarily about the question of whether or not there have been effects on patients and at what cost, but rather about questions of how professional behavior or healthcare processes can be improved and at what cost. Ideally, the relationship between a clinical or prevention intervention and patient outcomes is known from clinical or public health research. The effect of an implementation strategy on patient outcomes could then be estimated using modeling studies, such as decision analytical models, Markov models, and Monte Carlo simulations (Buxton et al. 1997; Brennan and Akehurst 1999). In practice, there is nearly always uncertainty, so that the measurement of patient outcomes (e.g. as secondary outcomes) often adds value to the evaluation.

23.5.3 Study Perspective

Economic evaluations may be conducted from different perspectives, including financial, healthcare, or societal. The perspective of analysis determines the range and nature of both the costs and the consequences that are considered when comparing implementation strategies. Box 23.5 (Scheeres et al. 2008) illustrates this point. Of course, within one and the same study different perspectives may be presented; however, this often implies that a larger set of data need to be collected and various analyses need to be performed. When additional data collection is logistically feasible and not too costly, such evaluations may be conducted

---

Box 23.5   Implementation of Cognitive Behavior Therapy in Chronic Fatigue Syndrome

In a before–after comparison study (Scheeres et al. 2008), the costs and patient outcomes of implementing cognitive behavior therapy (CBT) for chronic fatigue syndrome (CFS) in a mental health center (MHC) were analyzed. The implementation interventions included informing physicians and CFS patients, training therapists, and instructing the MHC employees. Both the healthcare provision costs and the execution costs of implementing the treatment program were included in the analysis, as well as non-medical (productivity) costs during eight months of follow-up (time horizon). Patient outcomes were expressed as the percentage of patients recovered from CFS and the mean QALY gain. The researchers showed in this study that using a healthcare perspective, execution, and healthcare provision costs were related to the probability of recovering from CFS. In addition, since recovering from CFS implies lower productivity costs, using a societal perspective implementation of CBT was dominant (indication of a better outcome at lower costs) over not implementing CBT. This study clearly shows that the choice of the perspective of a study influences data collection on the conclusions drawn.

---

and reported from multiple perspectives so as to facilitate decision making.

From a *financial perspective*, for instance that of an insurer or third-party payer, the focus is on tariffs (or diagnosis-related groupings, DRGs) for efforts in healthcare. Such tariffs may include the cost of services, interventions, nursing days, and bed days. From a *healthcare perspective*, the costs will be rated in terms of actual costs incurred by the healthcare system. An example to demonstrate the difference between this perspective and a financial perspective is the payment of physician's services. In a system of contract payment, the medical specialist will get a standard compensation for consultations, regardless of the actual number of contacts with the patient during a full year; within a financial perspective, this standard cost would be an appropriate figure; while within a healthcare perspective, the number and cost of every consultation would be considered. A *societal perspective* includes the total costs as far as possible. This includes both costs within the healthcare sector as well as costs outside the healthcare sector that affect patients or third parties (such as costs related to sick leave). While the societal perspective is the most inclusive, the choice of perspective will be influenced by the relative contribution of health and non-health costs and pragmatic considerations around the logistics and costs of collecting data.

When interpreting the results of an economic evaluation, the reader should be aware of the perspective chosen for the analyses and from what perspective conclusions are drawn, since these may be contradictory. In a study of providing practice facilitation to a small PC practice, the authors transparently report positive variable costs from the perspective of an organization providing facilitation activities, but conclude that costs of practice facilitation have the potential to be cost neutral from a societal perspective (Culler et al. 2013).

A study perspective that is not part of the common perspectives of economic evaluations of clinical interventions, yet is very important for users of implementation research, is the *perspective of the healthcare provider and healthcare institution*. This perspective is relevant because it considers the costs and consequences that are directly experienced by healthcare providers or healthcare institutions trying to implement an innovation and participating in an implementation strategy. In contrast to the above-mentioned healthcare perspective, this approach also indicates which party is bearing the costs or experiencing the

Table 23.4 Hypothetical example of a cost–consequence analysis of implementing reduced waiting lists for treatment from a healthcare provider's perspective.

Costs	Responsible party	Consequences	Responsible party
Appointment of consultant	Institution	Reduced waiting list	Patient
Investment of 20-hour preparation and administration by physician	Physician	One polyclinic visit less per patient	Physician/ patient
Patient saving time and traveling expenses	Patient	Time for other activities, such as paid work	Patient
Reduction of emergency operations	Institution/ physician	Extra free rooms in polyclinic	Institution/ physician

Source: Data from McIntosh et al. (1999).

consequences. In this approach, the costs are usually described but not aggregated (similar to cost–consequence analysis). Table 23.4 itemizes the costs and consequences of a hypothetical analysis of an implementation strategy intended to reduce the waiting lists for treatment (McIntosh et al. 1999).

23.6 Cost Analysis

Cost analysis is a major part of the economic evaluation of implementation strategies. Within implementation research a clear distinction can be made between on the one hand healthcare costs related to patientcare itself, and on the other hand costs related to activities to develop and execute an implementation strategy. Within these categories, four types of costs are relevant: directly attributable, indirectly attributable, fixed, and variable costs.

23.6.1 Directly Attributable, Indirectly Attributable, Fixed, and Variable Costs

When considering healthcare provision for an individual patient, a distinction is made between those costs directly attributable to the healthcare process and other, indirectly attributable costs. *Directly attributable costs* include the time a physician spends with a patient and the materials used during that time. *Indirectly attributable costs* (also known as overhead costs) include the time a physician spends on extra education, any activities of staff that cannot be attributed to a specific patient, the time a consultant spends providing individual feedback to healthcare providers, and the costs of developing a change proposal or new procedure.

Within a cost analysis, further distinctions are made between fixed and variable costs. *Fixed costs* are supposed not to vary with the level of output and are fixed given a certain observation period (in principle, in the long run, all costs are variable and an economic evaluation based on a long time horizon should take this into account); they have no link to the scale of use of the specific (healthcare) provision. For example, if consensus meetings are used to develop a clinical pathway, the costs will remain the same whether 1 or 100 physicians later use it. Attribution of the fixed costs to patients or healthcare providers might occur on the basis of a simple division. A fixed cost of €10 000 for consensus meetings and 10 physicians subsequently using the pathway with 10 patients each gives fixed costs for that pathway of €1000 per physician and €100 per patient. If 20 physicians and nurses follow a protocol with 10 patients each, these costs become €500 per professional and €50 per patient.

The *variable costs* of an implementation strategy are dependent on both intensity and the degree to which a protocol, guideline, or procedure is followed. For example, education that lasts two days is more expensive than education that lasts two hours. The variable costs are illustrated with a recommendation that advises that patients at increased risk of cardiovascular disease be called on a regular basis for check-ups to measure blood pressure. Here, the number of patients affected by the recommendation determines the amount of the costs. If the number of patients is zero, then the number of consultations based on the recommendation is zero, incurring zero (variable) costs; equally, 130 patients invited and consulting incur 130 unit costs. In case variable costs are considered to be equal distributed over the unit of measurement (patients, healthcare providers), such costs can be attributed simply through a division of total costs by number of measuring units (practice, physician, or patient). This means these particular variable costs do not add variability to the total cost measure. In case such costs vary between units of measurement, these have to be measured empirically for each unit of measure. For the latter, prospective measurement of activities is essential, as is shown in the previously mentioned study of providing practice facilitation to small PC practices (Culler et al. 2013). In this study, detailed prospective registration took the place of such variable costs as recorded time, mileage, and materials associated with all activities.

An economic evaluation assumes a steady-state or stable long-run situation. This steady state is only achieved when all of the shadows of the previous technology or organizational state have disappeared, in other words when (i) the new technology is fully functional; (ii) staff have mastered the new technology; (iii) a more or less constant occupancy rate for the new technology has been achieved; (iv) all costs for the old technology have dissipated; and (v) there is no spill-over of effects from the old technology into the new situation any longer. In the short run, these conditions are seldom met. During this time period, costs may be induced for both technologies, and clinical effectiveness for the new technology is likely not to be optimal yet. This may very well result in a negative deviation from the long-run cost-effectiveness outcome during the short run. A successful implementation strategy should also aim at optimizing the short run (Adang and Wensing 2008; van de Wetering et al. 2012). Box 23.6 illustrates the importance of the time frame of a study (O'Brien et al. 2000).

23.6.2 Categories of Costs

Within economic evaluations in the healthcare sector, a distinction is made between several categories of costs whose inclusion are

---

Box 23.6   Implementation of Clinical Guidelines for Treating Colon Injuries

Based on retrospective discharge database analyses, in one study a cost-minimization analysis was performed (O'Brien et al. 2000). A comparison between different ways of treating penetrating intra-peritoneal colon injuries by different surgical approaches (primary repair versus diverting colostomy) exemplified how implementation of a clinical guideline can affect the cost of care. Cost data contained stay in hospital, diagnostic tests, and treatment procedures. Implementing a guideline for primary repair turned out to be more costly in the short term; however, in the longer term fixed costs per patient decreased because of a higher number of patients being subjected to the guideline. The development and execution costs were in the long run expected to be compensated by lower healthcare provision costs. This study clearly shows that the time frame of a study can influence the number of patients that benefit and that an implementation program might become efficient.

dependent on the choice of study perspective and time horizon: healthcare costs, implementation costs, and non-medical costs. Medical, nursing, or paramedical costs are costs that are linked directly to a patient's healthcare process, such as the costs for diagnostics or therapy. The directly attributable costs of implementation strategies are also part of this cost category. The costs of implementation strategies that are focused on improving healthcare delivery can be subdivided into different phases of the implementation process (Severens 2003). First, there are costs related to the *research and development of the innovation* itself. Ideally, these (fixed) developmental costs should be part of a cost analysis. In reality, however, the availability of an innovation (a new procedure, a protocol, a guideline) is usually taken as a given and not included in an economic evaluation. Next, there are costs associated with the *research and development of a specific implementation strategy*. For example, if implementing a new care pathway for a chronic disease includes using outreach visitors who need to visit practices, teams, or physicians, training of the visitors is needed. Such costs are usually one-off costs and therefore can also be considered fixed costs. In contrast, the costs of the *execution of the implementation strategy* (e.g. implementation team spending time visiting physicians, practices, or hospitals) are usually considered variable costs. Also variable are those costs associated with a *change in*

healthcare provision as a result of the application of an implementation strategy, for instance a decrease of test ordering. Change in care provision might be observed in the immediate target of the implementation strategy; however, relevant spill-over consequences might occur in non-targeted providers, patients, practices, and behaviors.

Non-medical costs are costs that are incurred outside the healthcare sector. These include the patient's costs, such as costs for time and traveling (direct non-medical costs), and other societal costs, also known as indirect non-medical costs, such as costs resulting from absence from work due to health problems, costs of special education, and legal costs. Table 23.5 summarizes the relevance of the costs in the different stages of implementation strategies.

23.6.3 Volumes and Cost Prices

A cost analysis starts with the determination of volumes, such as the number of outreach visits, educational hours, consultations, tests, or treatments. Volumes are all the units of "expenditure" or resource use that are measured one way or another and that form the basis for the cost analysis. When looking at professional performance, for instance if physicians work in line with a care pathway, the number and duration of contacts between PC physicians and medical specialists can be used as a volume parameter. If, however, the health

Table 23.5 Costs in the different stages of implementation strategies.

Stages	Relevance
Research and development of a guideline, protocol, or new procedure	Ideally, these fixed costs are passed on to the cost-effectiveness measure through a division calculation
Research and development of the implementation strategy	Ideally, these fixed costs are passed on to the cost-effectiveness measure through a division calculation
Execution of the implementation strategy	These costs are always taken into consideration
Change in healthcare provision and patients' use of healthcare	These costs are taken into consideration when measurement at a patient level is conducted
Non-medical costs	These costs are taken into consideration when measurement at a patient level is conducted

condition of the individual patient is used as a cost-effectiveness measure, the number of contacts between physician and patient is relevant as well. Box 23.7 (Frijling et al. 2001) provides an example of a cost analysis of an implementation program.

Once volumes have been measured, the next step is to attribute prices to each unit of volume. The volume parameter is usually stochastic by nature (thus associated with random fluctuation), whereas the price parameter is usually deterministic (fixed cost price). In a system of managed competition prices may vary between providers. However, these prices concern strategic information and are not publicly available. In reality, it is almost impossible to empirically collect specific cost price data for all volumes. Therefore, it is customary to use pre-existing data on cost prices, for which several sources can be used. First, cost prices may have been reported in the *scientific literature*. When using these data, researchers need to ask themselves whether or not the definition of the unit price agrees with the one in their own study, and whether or not the situation on which the cost price is based is comparable. All cost prices must relate to the same year or, if not, be indexed to one specific year. Alternatively, *guideline prices* may be used if available. These are (usually) national data on the costs and production volume of healthcare institutions, giving estimates of average integral cost prices. Using such national guideline prices are therefore only recommended if the general approach suffices. Third, *current tariffs* can be used. As mentioned before, current tariffs are

---

Box 23.7   Cost Analysis of an Implementation Strategy

The explanation of cost analyses of implementation strategies can be illustrated using the Dutch CARPE (Common Assessments for Repeated Paramedic service Encounters) study. This randomized trial (Frijling et al. 2001) evaluated the use of trained outreach visitors or facilitators to encourage the use of the recommendations of seven national PC guidelines (hypertension, cholesterol, diabetes mellitus II, peripheral arteriosclerosis, angina pectoris, heart failure, and cerebrovascular accident or transient ischemic attack) with patients with cardiovascular risk indicators or diseases. The cost analysis addressed the question: "What are the costs of the intervention compared to no active implementation strategy?" (zero implementation costs). The analysis used a healthcare perspective and the time horizon was limited to the 18 months during which the visitors were active. The cost analysis of the several stages of implementation was limited to execution of the implementation strategy. During the study the facilitators prospectively recorded cost volumes for each visit to the practices. This involved the number of visits by the visitor to each practice as well as the preparation, travel, and consultation time per visit, the preparation and execution time that physician(s) and practice assistant(s) spent during each visit, and the number of miles the visitor had to travel. The recorded volumes were rated against the actual cost prices in accordance with Dutch guidelines (Oostenbrink et al. 2002). Data were collected on 934 consultation visits in 62 practices. Results are shown in Table 23.6. The number of visits to each practice ranged from 3 to 17 visits (mean 14.8 visits). Partly because of this, the costs per practice varied. It was also the case that the number of physicians and assistants who actively participated in the implementation strategy (by preparing and attending consultation visits) varied for each practice: one to four physicians and zero to five assistants per practice, respectively. In particular, it turned out that the costs of the time investment of the physicians largely determined the variation in costs of the implementation strategy.

Table 23.6 Costs of the outreach visitor intervention (in euros) per practice.

	Mean	Minimum	Maximum
Traveling expenses outreach visitor	339	0	1522
Time costs outreach visitor			
Costs for preparation time/traveling	935	184	1609
Costs for presence at practice visit	276	53	419
Time costs practice assistant			
Costs for preparation time	271	0	1395
Costs for presence at visit	296	0	728
Time costs physician			
Costs for preparation time	1245	53	4493
Costs for presence at visit	955	239	3084
Total time costs	3978	574	8673

used for evaluations from a financial perspective. Tariffs can also be used in situations in which it can be assumed that the tariff will not deviate much from the actual cost price. However, for those volumes for which it is decided that an exact cost price needs to be determined, a *cost price study* will have to be performed. Obviously, this is also required for those volumes for which no approximate cost price is available at all, for new methods of treatment, for example, or for a new implementation strategy. A cost price study is also recommended for those volumes that make a large contribution to the cost differences between several implementation alternatives. Cost price research can be a time-consuming job.

23.7 Sensitivity Analysis, Quantitative Modeling, and Budget Impact

23.7.1 Sensitivity Analysis

As with all scientific data, cost and cost-effectiveness estimates are based on available data and as such there is always uncertainty surrounding values of variables in any calculation. Cost and cost-effectiveness calculations are based on both stochastic and deterministic variables. Stochastic variables are variables that have been measured per unit of measurement (patient, physician, hospital, practice) of the study and thus show some random variation. Therefore, it is possible to calculate a mean value with a corresponding standard deviation and the uncertainty can be expressed as a confidence interval. Deterministic variables are variables that have been determined once in a fixed "point estimate." For example, when measured empirically the *number* of physician/patient consultations per patient is a stochastic variable, and the *cost price* for a consultation (which can be an estimate, a derivation, or a measurement) is a deterministic variable. Even if the cost price is based on cost price research with more than one workplace measurement, only a single (deterministic) average cost price for the volume unit can be used. Alternatively, the number of physician/patient consultations per patient is considered a deterministic variable in cases where the value is equally defined for all patients by expert opinion.

In order to determine how changes in uncertain variables influence the results of a study, sensitivity analysis can be performed (Briggs et al. 1994). In such an analysis, the effect of changes in the most important factors on overall cost and cost-effectiveness is examined. There are several techniques for sensitivity analysis. For example, the estimate of a deterministic variable (e.g. €20 for a consultation with a PC physician) is either decreased (e.g. to €15) or increased (e.g. to €25) in order to judge the influence of these changes on the results of the analysis. This is called a one-way deterministic sensitivity analysis. When several deterministic variables are varied at the same time, it is called a multiway deterministic sensitivity analysis.

Stochastic variables can also be subject to deterministic sensitivity analyses. As each variable has a confidence interval, it is possible to examine the impact of using the value of the upper or lower confidence interval instead of the mean. It can also be used to compensate for research design problems. For example, patients in a clinical trial may visit their physicians more frequently, not only for their routine healthcare but also for pre-specified contacts for trial-related measurements. The latter contacts and their associated costs are driven by research protocol (Drummond et al. 2015), and should not be part of a cost analysis. However, if these two types of contact cannot be reliably distinguished, the stochastic parameters of the total number of contacts with PC physicians can be arbitrarily decreased in a sensitivity analysis.

An additional method to assess the sensitivity of cost-effectiveness results to uncertainty of empirical data is a so-called non-parametric bootstrap analysis. In such an analysis the original patient data are resampled with replacement into a second, third, up to for example 1000 iterations to obtain a large number of estimates of the ICER. In a cluster-randomized trial comparing a distant learning program for GPs compared to written guidelines in the management of lower urinary tract symptoms in older men, the authors showed that the ICERs could vary from −€423 to €239 per point on the urinary symptom scale. Authors are aware of the difficulty of the interpretation of

negative ICERs and, in this specific case, indicate that while the effects on urinary symptoms remained neutral, the costs were lower in the intervention group (Wolters et al. 2006). To overcome the problem of interpreting negative ICERs, the net monetary benefit approach can be used.

23.7.2 Quantitative Modeling

Empirical evaluation of comprehensive cost-effectiveness is not always possible. When this is the case, or policy makers need information before empirical data can be available, quantitative modeling can be used. Modeling synthesizes available evidence supplemented, where necessary, with assumptions to estimate the costs and consequences of interventions to improve healthcare.

Health economic models are used to generalize from the data observed in one situation to others, such as from trials to routine healthcare practice (Gold et al. 1996; Buxton et al. 1997). Health economic models are used in three situations. First, decision analytical models are used to adjust or extrapolate data, where the relevant effectiveness studies have not been conducted or did not include economic data. Second, statistical models like extrapolation models, epidemiological models and Markov models, can be used where intermediate outcomes need to be connected with final outcomes or to extrapolate beyond short-term follow-up. Third, modeling is often performed to explore the uncertainty of the effect of healthcare interventions on patient outcomes and costs, and to establish the value of doing further research on these interventions.

Especially in implementation research, modeling is an evident tool to make sure that economic evaluation is performed efficiently. For instance, resource-consuming empirical data collection may be avoided if estimates of incremental cost per QALY ratios can be linked to behavior change and to health-related outcomes in quantitative models. Moreover, instead of carrying out economic evaluations after inefficiency has been identified as a problem of implementation, Hoomans and Severens (2014) propose a three-step ex ante process of evaluation and decision making, by explicit cost-effectiveness modeling.

It is an important responsibility of model developers to conduct modeling studies to the highest standards and to complement the model results with faithful disclosure of the underlying assumptions, with the caution that conclusions are conditional upon the assumptions and data on which the model is build (Weinstein et al. 2003). A common concern about the use of decision analytical modeling is that pieces of information from different studies and populations are combined into the same model; this has been termed a "Frankenstein's monster" form of economic evaluation, because the analyst brings different parts together to form a model (or monster) that hopefully will behave in a predictable way (O'Brien 1996).

Criteria for assessing the quality of models and the usefulness of modeling results for decision making generally fall into three areas: model structure, data used as inputs, and model validation. Model assumptions about causal structure and parameter estimates should be continually assessed against data, and models should be revised accordingly. Structural assumptions and parameter estimates should be reported clearly and explicitly, and opportunities for users to appreciate the conditional relationship between inputs and outputs should be provided through sensitivity analyses. As in empirical studies, the influence of uncertainty of the values of variables in models need to be assessed for both deterministic and stochastic parameters. The distribution of stochastic parameters is used as a basis for a so-called probabilistic sensitivity analysis, where simultaneously for each stochastic parameter in the model a value is drawn from each specific distribution, and the calculations are performed based on the alternative parameter values. In a probabilistic sensitivity analysis, in this way the cost-effectiveness is recalculated a large number of times (>1000),

leading to an estimation of the (un)certainty of the ICER.

Economic modeling has also been used in implementation research (Richardson 2004; Harmsen et al. 2009; Hoomans et al. 2009a). An example is presented in Box 23.8 (Harmsen et al. 2009). A good example of the advantages of economic modeling is presented by Basu et al. (2017). In the latter example, the authors show, based on sensitivity analyses in their model for assessing the financial impact for PC practices of integrating behavioral health services (a collaborative care model), that their outcomes were sensitive to rates of patient referral acceptance, presentation, and therapy completion. However, the collaborative care model remained consistently financially viable compared to the PC behaviorist model, so despite uncertainty of inputs, uncertainty of outputs was within an acceptable range.

23.7.3 Budget Impact Analysis

An economic evaluation leads to insights into the additional costs per unit of analysis (e.g. patient, physician, hospital, or practice) and the incremental cost-effectiveness of the implementation strategy compared with an alternative strategy. However, this does not provide information about the influence of a large-scale application of an implementation strategy in the healthcare sector. So information about cost-effectiveness does not indicate whether an intervention is affordable, for which budget impact analysis is relevant (Bilinski et al. 2017).

A budget impact analysis shows the effects of such a broad introduction of an implementation strategy within a healthcare system, or on a national scale, on the total costs and savings generated. For this analysis, it is necessary to know – in addition to investments and possible savings at the level of individual patient or healthcare provider – how many patients, professionals, hospitals, and practices are eligible for the implementation strategy.

In a budget impact analysis, who bears the costs is not taken into account, since in

---

Box 23.8 Modeling the Cost-Effectiveness of a Maximum Care Model for Urinary Tract Infections in Children

A study (Harmsen et al. 2009) aimed to assess the cost-effectiveness of a maximum care model for urinary tract infection (UTI) in children, implying more testing and antibiotic treatment, compared with current practice. Childhood UTI can lead to renal scarring and ultimately to terminal renal failure, which has a high impact on quality of life, survival, and healthcare costs. This indicates that in the short term healthcare provision costs might increase due to the maximum care model, but in the longer term costs of treating renal failure might be saved. Therefore, the researchers decided to use a time horizon of 30 years, which made it necessary to model longer-term costs and outcomes mathematically. For this purpose, a so-called Markov model was developed in which a theoretical (cohort of) patient(s) will be situated in a specific health state (in this case no UTI, UTI, renal scarring, chronic kidney disease,

renal failure including dialysis, and death). Each of these states is defined by a health state value and a cost value. Progress of disease and treatment effect are reflected by transition probabilities over time between states, and these were defined based upon the literature. Of course, transition probabilities differed for analyzing current care versus the maximum care model. Based on the modeling calculations performed, the authors concluded that maximum care for childhood UTI was dominant in the long run over current care, meaning that it delivered more quality of life at lower costs. They indicated that their findings should be interpreted cautiously given the lack of data and the results of extensive sensitivity analyses. Furthermore, because the differences in QALYs and costs were relatively small, implementation strategies for the maximum care model for UTI should not incur high investment.

---

cost-effectiveness from a healthcare or societal perspective all costs are summed. In effect, it is assumed that budgets can easily be shifted, for instance between healthcare sectors or from one caregiver to another. In practice, however, this assumption is seldom met: budgets are often fixed and shifting from one alternative to another or from one sector to another is difficult. To assess the inflexibility of budgets of stakeholders involved in the process of implementation, Adang et al. (2005) developed a checklist.

23.8 Ex Post Evaluation of the Efficiency of Implementation

Till now an ex ante economic evaluation was presented and explained. Such an ex ante evaluation addresses the question of which

implementation strategy, from a set of mutually exclusive alternatives, can be expected to be most efficient. An ex post economic evaluation of the implementation strategy addresses the question of which factors determine optimal implementation in terms of efficiency. A study aimed at determining the (technical) efficiency of practices delivering recommended cardiovascular risk management provides a methodological framework for how to deal with ex post evaluation of implementation. For that purpose, a data envelopment analysis (DEA) complemented with a truncated regression analysis, a so-called two-stage approach, was used (see Box 23.9).

23.9 Conclusions

Strategies for implementing changes in healthcare use resources, such as the time of health professionals. To inform decisions

---

Box 23.9   Efficiency of the Implementation of Cardiovascular Risk Management in Primary Care Practices

A study aimed at determining the technical efficiency of PC practices delivering recommended cardiovascular risk management (CVRM) for patients with established cardiovascular disease and also aimed to identify factors associated with the variation in efficiency (Adang et al. 2016). Here, technical efficiency is associated with the use of optimal procedures (i.e. optimal implementation of procedures) and was defined as the extent to which a PC practice delivers evidence-based CVRM in relation to its inputs in terms of medical labor. The researchers used a two-stage DEA approach. The first step was to calculate the efficiency scores by using a DEA, while the second step used an econometric approach (truncated regression) to analyze the impact of explanatory variables on the level of efficiency by which PC practices deliver CVRM (dependent variable). DEA is a benchmarking method that finds its origins in management science, mathematical programming, and operations research. The econometric counterpart of DEA is stochastic frontier analysis. Both approaches deliver efficiency scores that can be used as input for the second stage, regressing explanatory factors on the efficiency score. Based on the two-stage DEA approach, the authors found that not all PC practices delivered recommended CVRM and consequently were positioned on the efficient frontier. This variation in technical efficiency between PC practices delivering CVRM was associated with training practice status. Whether CVRM clinical tasks were performed by a practice nurse or a GP did not influence technical efficiency in a statistically significant way, and neither did practice size. From this the authors conclude that "being a training practice" was the most important factor for the efficient implementation of CVRM.

---

about actively implementing clinical interventions in settings in which the resources are limited, economic evaluations can be used to compare the cost-effectiveness of alternative implementation strategies. The cost-effectiveness of an implementation strategy is essentially a product of four elements: the cost-effectiveness of the recommended clinical or prevention practices; the degree to which health professionals, and/or patients, automatically or immediately adopt these practices; the costs of an implementation strategy; and the effectiveness of an implementation strategy (Sculpher 2000). Economic evaluations of implementation have not been widely conducted, even in countries that conduct many economic evaluations of clinical and prevention interventions. Unlike economic evaluations of clinical interventions, economic evaluations of implementation strategies can use both healthcare processes and patient outcomes as outcomes of interest. Nevertheless, economic evaluation is most informative if the cost-effectiveness ratio of the recommended clinical or prevention practice is also measured or known and found to be acceptable, or if it can at least be assumed to be favorable.

References

Adang, E.M., Gerritsma, A., Nouwens, E. et al. (2016). Efficiency of the implementation of cardiovascular risk management in primary care practices: an observational study. *Implement. Sci.* 11: 67.

Adang, E., Voordijk, L., van der Wilt, G.J., and Ament, A. (2005). Cost-effectiveness analysis in relation to budgetary constraints and reallocative restrictions. *Health Policy* 74: 146–156.

Adang, E.M.M. and Wensing, M. (2008). Economic barriers to implementation of innovations in healthcare: is the long run–short run efficiency discrepancy a paradox? *Health Policy* 88: 256–262.

Basu, S., Landon, B.E., Williams, J.W. et al. (2017). Behavioral health integration into primary care: a microsimulation of financial implications for practices. *J. Gen. Intern. Med.* 32: 1330–1341.

Bilinski, A., Neumann, P., Cohen, J. et al. (2017). When cost-effective interventions are unaffordable: integrating cost-effectiveness and budget impact in priority setting for global health programs. *PLoS Med.* 14: 10.

Brennan, A. and Akehurst, R. (1999). Modelling in economic evaluation: what is its place? What is its value? *Pharmacoeconomics* 17: 445–459.

Briggs, A.H., Sculpher, M., and Buxton, M.J. (1994). Uncertainty in the economic evaluation of healthcare technologies: the role of sensitivity analysis. *Health Econ.* 3: 95–104.

Buxton, M.J., Drummond, M.F., van Hout, B.A. et al. (1997). Modelling in economic evaluation: an unavoidable fact of life. *Health Econ.* 6: 217–227.

Culler, S.D., Parchman, M.L., Lozano-Romero, R. et al. (2013). Cost estimates for operating a primary care facilitation program. *Ann. Fam. Med.* 11: 207–211.

Drummond, M.F., Sculpher, M.J., Claxton, K. et al. (2015). *Methods for the Economic Evaluation of Healthcare Programmes*, 4e. Oxford: Oxford Medical Publications.

Fenwick, E., Claxton, K., and Sculpher, M. (2008). The value of implementation and the value of information: combined and uneven development. *Med. Decis. Making* 28: 21–32.

Frijling, B.D., Spies, T.H., Lobo, C.M. et al. (2001). Blood pressure control in treated hypertensive patients: clinical performance of general practitioners. *Br. J. Gen. Pract.* 51: 9–14.

Garner, B.R., Lwin, A.K., Strickler, G.K. et al. (2018 Jul 4). Pay-for-performance as a cost-effective implementation strategy: results from a cluster randomized trial. *Implement Sci.* 13: 92.

Gold, M.R., Siegel, J.E., Russell, L.B., and Weinstein, M.C. (1996). *Cost-Effectiveness in Health and Medicine*. New York: Oxford University Press.

Grimshaw, G.M. and Russell, I.T. (1993). Effect of clinical guidelines on medical practice: a systematic review of rigorous evaluations. *Lancet* 342: 1317–1322.

Grimshaw, G.M., Thomas, R.E., MacLennan, G. et al. (2004). Effectiveness and efficiency of guideline dissemination and implementation strategies. *Health Technol. Assess.* 8 (iii–iv): 1–72.

Grimshaw, J.M., Eccles, M.P., Lavis, J.N. et al. (2012). Knowledge translation of research findings. *Implement. Sci.* 7: 50.

Harmsen, M., Adang, E.M., Wolters, R.J. et al. (2009). Management of childhood urinary tract infections: an economic modeling study. *Value Health* 12: 466–472.

Hoomans, T., Abrams, K.R., Ament, A.J.H.A. et al. (2009a). Modelling the value for money of changing clinical practice change: a stochastic application in diabetes care. *Med. Care* 47: 1053–1061.

Hoomans, T., Ament, A.J., Evers, S.M., and Severens, J.L. (2011). Implementing guidelines into clinical practice: what is the value? *J. Eval. Clin. Pract.* 17: 606–614.

Hoomans, T., Evers, S.M.A.A., Ament, A.J.H.A. et al. (2007). The methodological quality of economic evaluations of guideline implementation into clinical practice: a systematic review of empiric studies. *Value Health* 10: 305–316.

Hoomans, T., Fenwick, E.A., Palmer, S., and Claxton, K. (2009b). Value of information and value of implementation: application of an analytic framework to inform resource allocation decisions in metastatic hormone-refractory prostate cancer. *Value Health* 12: 315–324.

Hoomans, T. and Severens, J.L. (2014). Economic evaluation of implementation strategies in healthcare. *Implement. Sci.* 9: 168.

Hoomans, T., Severens, J.L., Evers, S.M., and Ament, A.J. (2009c). Value for money in changing clinical practice: should decisions about guidelines and implementation strategies be made sequentially or simultaneously? *Med. Decis. Making* 29: 207–216.

Lau, R., Stevenson, F., Ong, B.N. et al. (2015). Achieving change in primary care – effectiveness of strategies for improving implementation of complex interventions: systematic review of reviews. *BMJ Open* 5: e009993.

Mason, J., Freemantle, N., Nazareth, I. et al. (2001). When is it cost-effective to change the behaviour of health professionals? *JAMA* 286: 2988–2992.

Mauskopf, J.A., Paul, J.E., Grant, D.M., and Stergachis, A. (1998). The role of cost-consequence analysis in healthcare decision making. *Pharmacoeconomics* 13: 277–288.

McIntosh, E., Donaldson, C., and Ryan, M. (1999). Recent advances in the methods of cost-benefit analysis in healthcare. Matching the art to the science. *Pharmacoeconomics* 15: 357–367.

O'Brien, B.J. (1996). Economic evaluation of pharmaceuticals: Frankenstein's monster or vampire of trails? *Med. Care* 34(Suppl.): DS99–DS108.

O'Brien, J.A., Jacobs, L.M., and Pierce, D. (2000). Clinical practice guidelines and the costs of care; a growing alliance. *Int. J. Technol. Assess. Healthcare* 16: 1077–1091.

Oostenbrink, J.B., Koopmanschap, M.A., and Rutten, F.F.H. (2002). Standardisation of costs; the Dutch manual for costing in economic evaluations. *Pharmacoeconomics* 20: 443–454.

Reilly, K.L., Reeves, P., Deeming, S. et al. (2018). Economic analysis of three interventions of different intensity in improving school implementation of a government health canteen policy: costs, incremental and relative cost-effectiveness. *BMC Public Health* 18: 378.

Richardson, G. (2004). Cost-effectiveness of implementing new guidelines for treatment of hypertension in general practice. *Br. J. Gen. Pract.* 54: 765–771.

Roberts, S.L.E., Healey, A., and Sevdalis, N. (2019). Use of health economic evaluation in the implementation and improvement science

fields – a systematic review. *Implement. Sci.* 14: 72.

Scheeres, K., Wensing, M., Bleijenberg, G., and Severens, J. (2008). Implementing cognitive behaviour therapy for chronic fatigue syndrome in mental healthcare: a costs and outcomes analysis. *BMC Health Serv. Res.* 8: 175.

Schermer, T.R., Thoonen, B.P., van den Boom, G. et al. (2002). Randomized controlled economic evaluation of asthma self-management in primary healthcare. *Am. J. Respir. Crit. Care Med.* 166: 1062–1072.

Sculpher, M. (2000). Evaluating the cost-effectiveness of interventions designed to increase the utilization of evidence-based guidelines. *Fam. Pract.* 17: S26–S31.

Severens, J.L. (2003). Value for money of changing healthcare services? Economic evaluation of quality improvement. *Qual. Saf. Healthcare* 12: 366–371.

Vale, L., Thomas, R., MacLennan, G., and Grimshaw, J. (2007). Systematic review of economic evaluations and cost analyses of guideline implementation strategies. *Eur. J. Health Econ.* 8: 111–121.

Verstappen, W.H., van Merode, F., Grimshaw, J. et al. (2004). Comparing cost effects of two quality strategies to improve test ordering in primary care: a randomized trial. *Int. J. Qual. Healthare* 16: 391–398.

Weinstein, M.C., O'Brien, B.J., Hornberger, J. et al. (2003). Principles of good practice of decision analytic modelling in healthcare evaluation: report of the ISPOR Task Force in Good Research Practices. Modelling studies. *Value Health* 6: 9–17.

van de Wetering, G., Woertman, W.H., and EMM, A. (2012). A model to correct for short-run inefficiencies in economic evaluations in healthcare. *Health Econ.* 21: 270–281.

Wolters, R., Grol, R., Schermer, T. et al. (2006). Improving initial management of lower urinary tract symptoms in primary care: costs and patient outcomes. *Scand. J. Urol. Nephrol.* 40: 300–306.

Wood, J. and Freemantle, N. (1999). Choosing an appropriate unit of analysis in trials of interventions that attempt to influence practice. *J. Health Serv. Res. Policy* 4: 44–48.

Index

Page numbers in *italic* indicate figures; page numbers in **bold** indicate tables; page numbers suffixed with 'b' indicate boxes. US spelling is used in this index.

Improving Patient Care: The Implementation of Change in Health Care, Third Edition. Edited by Michel Wensing, Richard Grol, and Jeremy Grimshaw.
© 2020 John Wiley & Sons Ltd. Published 2020 by John Wiley & Sons Ltd.

Printed and bound by CPI Group (UK) Ltd, Croydon, CR0 4YY

27/10/2024

14580358-0002